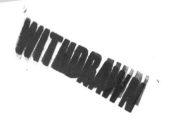

# Handbook on
# Dementia Caregiving

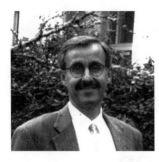
**Richard Schulz, PhD,** is Professor of Psychiatry, Director of Gerontology and Director of the University Center for Social and Urban Research at the University of Pittsburgh. He has spent most of his career doing research and writing on adult development and aging. His work has focused on the social-psychological aspects of aging, including the role of control as a construct for characterizing life-course development, adult age-related changes in the experience, perception, and expression of affect, and the impact of disabling late life disease on patients and their families. Dr. Schulz has more than two decades of experience carrying out research on caregiving. This body of work is reflected in numerous publications that have appeared in major medical and aging journals, including *Journal of the American Medical Association, Annals of Behavioral Medicine,* the *Journals of Gerontology,* and *Psychology and Aging.*

# Handbook on Dementia Caregiving

## Evidence-Based Interventions for Family Caregivers

# Richard Schulz, PhD
Editor

 Springer Publishing Company

Copyright © 2000 by Springer Publishing Company, Inc.

Springer Publishing Company, Inc.
536 Broadway
New York, NY 10012-3955

*Acquisitions Editor:* Bill Tucker
*Production Editor:* Jean Hurkin-Torres
*Cover design by* James Scotto-Lavino

00 01 02 03 04 / 5 4 3 2 1

**Library of Congress Cataloging-in-Publication Data**

Handbook on dementia caregiving : evidence-based interventions in family caregiving / Richard Schulz, editor.
    p.   cm.
    Includes bibliographical references and index.
    ISBN 0-8261-1312-5 (Hardcover)
    1. Dementia—Patients—Care—Handbooks, manuals, etc.
    2. Dementia—Patients—Care—Cross-cultural studies—Handbooks, manuals, etc.   3. Dementia—Patients—Family relationships—Handbooks, manuals, etc.   4. Caregivers—Mental health services—Handbooks, manuals, etc.   I. Schulz, Richard, 1947-
    RC521.H355   2000
    362.1'9683—dc21                                              99-053867
                                                                      CIP

Printed in the United States of America

# Contents

# Contributors

**Patricia Arean, Ph.D.**
University of California, San
  Francisco
Department of Psychiatry
2330 Post St. Suite 300
San Francisco, CA 94115

**Trinidad Arguelles, M.S.**
Center on Adult Development
  and Aging
University of Miami
1425 N.W. 10th Avenue, Suite
  210
Miami, FL 33136

**Steven Belle, Ph.D.**
Epidemiology Data Center—
  Department of Epidemiology
Graduate School of Public
  Health
127 Parran Hall
University of Pittsburgh
Pittsburgh, PA 15261

**Louis Burgio, Ph.D.**
The University of Alabama
Applied Gerontology Program
210 Osband Hall
Tuscaloosa, AL 35487-0315

**Robert Burns, M.D.**
VA Medical Center (11H)
1030 Jefferson Avenue
Memphis, TN 38104

**David Coon, Ph.D.**
Veterans Affairs Medical Center
795 Willow Road
Menlo Park, CA 94025

**Mary Corcoran, Ph.D., OTR/L**
George Washington University
Department of Health Care Ser-
  vices, Room 2B409
2150 Pennsylvania Avenue, NW
Washington, DC 20037

**Sara Czaja, Ph.D.**
Center on Adult Development
  and Aging
University of Miami
1425 N.W. 10th Avenue
Miami, FL 33136

**Carl Eisdorfer, Ph.D., M.D.**
Center on Adult Development
  and Aging
University of Miami
1425 N.W. 10th Avenue
Miami, FL 33136

**Dolores Gallagher-Thompson, Ph.D.**
Veterans Affairs Medical Center
795 Willow Road
Menlo Park, CA 94025

**Laura Gitlin, Ph.D.**
Center for Collaborative Research
Thomas Jefferson University
130 South 9th Street, Suite 2200
Philadelphia, PA 19107-5233

**William Haley, Ph.D.**
Department of Gerontology—
College of Arts and Sciences
University of South Florida
4202 East Fowler Avenue, SOC 107
Tampa, FL 33620-8100

**Brooke Harrow, Ph.D.**
HRCA Research and Training Institute
Hebrew Rehabilitation Center for Aged
1200 Centre Street
Boston, MA 02131-1097

**Joel Kennet, Ph.D.**
Department of Human Development and Family Studies
College of Health and Human Development
The Pennsylvania State University
110 Henderson Bldg. South
University Park, PA 16802

**David Loewenstein, Ph.D.**
4300 Alton Road
Miami Beach, FL 33140

**Diane Feeney Mahoney, Ph.D.**
HRCA Research and Training Institute
Hebrew Rehabilitation Center for Aged
1200 Centre Street
Boston, MA 02131-1097

**Charlotte Malone, M.A.**
VA Medical Center (11H)
1030 Jefferson Avenue
Memphis, TN 38104

**Jennifer Martindale-Adams, Ph.D.**
VA Medical Center (11-H)
1030 Jefferson Avenue
Memphis, TN 38104

**Ana Menéndez**
Veterans Affairs Medical Center
795 Willow Road
Menlo Park, CA 94025

**Linda Nichols, Ph.D.**
VA Medical Center (11H)
1030 Jefferson Avenue
Memphis, TN 38104

**Marcia Ory, Ph.D.**
National Institute on Aging
Behavioral and Social Science Program
Gateway Building, Suite 533
7201 Wisconsin Avenue MSC 9205
Bethesda, MD 20892-9205

**Mark Rubert, Ph.D.**
Center on Adult Development
and Aging
University of Miami
1425 N.W. 10th Avenue
Miami, FL 33136

**Richard Schulz, Ph.D.**
University of Pittsburgh
University Center for Social
and Urban Research
121 University Place
Pittsburgh, PA 15260

**Galen E. Switzer, Ph.D.**
University of Pittsburgh
502 Iroquois Building
Forbes Avenue
Pittsburgh, PA 15260

**Jose Szapocznik, Ph.D.**
Center on Adult Development
and Aging
University of Miami
1425 N.W. 10th Avenue
Miami, FL 33136

**Kellie Takagi, Ph.D.**
Veterans Affairs Medical Center
795 Willow Road
Menlo Park, CA 94025

**Barbara Tarlow, Ph.D.**
HRCA Research and Training
Institute
Hebrew Rehabilitation Center
for Aged
1200 Centre Street
Boston, MA 02131-1097

**Sharon L. Tennstedt, Ph.D.**
New England Research
Institutes (NERI)
9 Galen Street
Watertown, MA 02172

**Larry Thompson, Ph.D.**
Veterans Affairs Palo Alto
Health Care System
Mail Code: 182C/MP
795 Willow Road
Menlo Park, CA 94025

**Laraine Winter, Ph.D.**
Center for Collaborative Research
Thomas Jefferson University
130 South 9th Street, Suite 2200
Philadelphia, PA 19107-5233

**Stephen R. Wisniewski, Ph.D.**
Epidemiology Data Center—
Department of Epidemiology
Graduate School of Public
Health
127 Parran Hall
University of Pittsburgh
Pittsburgh, PA 15261

**Jennifer L. Yee, Ph.D.**
University of Pittsburgh
University Center for Social
and Urban Research
121 University Place
Pittsburgh, PA 15260

# Introduction and Overview

Alzheimer's disease and other dementing illnesses are some of the most prevalent and costly conditions of late life. Current estimates indicate that as many as two million individuals suffer from Alzheimer's disease alone and this number is expected to increase dramatically over the next half century. The costs and burdens of providing care for dementia patients rests primarily on the shoulders of one critical resource—the family members of the patient. Caring for a relative with dementia involves significant expenditure of instrumental and emotional resources over potentially long periods of time. It often involves unpleasant and uncomfortable tasks, nonsymmetrical (i.e., one-sided) interactions, and the assumption of unanticipated roles. Providing care to a relative suffering from dementia has been likened to being exposed to a severe, long-term, chronic stressor. As a result, high levels of burden and distress are reported in virtually all Alzheimer's disease and related dementia caregiving studies published in the last 20 years.

Over the past decade, the needs of caregivers have become a prominent focus of professionals in a variety of academic disciplines and applied settings. In recent years, there has been an explosion of papers on this subject presented at professional meetings and published in professional journals. There has also been a concomitant increase in funding of caregiver research by the National Institutes of Health, as well as support of caregiver research and demonstration programs by numerous private foundations.

Research on caregiving has evolved through a predictable pattern common to new research domains in the social sciences. Early caregiver studies were action- and advocacy-oriented. They attempted to describe the roles, needs, and burdens of family caregivers, often in the words of caregivers themselves, and typically without a guiding theoretical framework. These studies served an important role in focusing attention on the nature of the problem—the needs of family caregivers. This was followed by attempts to develop better conceptualizations and quantitative measures of the concept of burden itself. Numerous burden scales were developed. Researchers sought to link a variety of caregiver and care recipient demographics, personalities, health and functional status, and contextual variables (e.g., social support) to the experience of burden. These studies also introduced a variety of theoretical frameworks to guide data collection, analysis, and interpretation of the data. More recently the focus of research has shifted to "harder" caregiver outcomes such as psychiatric and physical morbidity, and formal service utilization. This shift was also accompanied by a search for behavioral and biological mediating mechanisms that might causally account for observed health effects. Paralleling the research stream exploring causes of caregiver burden and morbidity have been interventions studies designed to decrease caregiver burden and improve caregiver health and functioning. This book represents a convergence of these two research streams.

The purpose of this book is to provide a thorough treatment of intervention approaches to dementia caregiving. This book includes a) a review and critique of existing knowledge about dementia caregiving, b) a conceptual framework for organizing caregiver interventions of all types, c) a discussion of the pragmatics of implementing an intervention study in the community, d) the challenges of designing and carrying out intervention research with culturally diverse populations, e) a strong emphasis on issues related to assessing mechanisms of action in intervention studies, f) a review and evaluation of appropriate measurement strategies for assessing caregiver intervention studies, g) a discussion of the challenges of translating/ intervention research into public policy, and h) an assessment of the future of caregiving and caregiving intervention research.

This is the ideal time for this book to be released because of a number of converging factors. First, almost two decades of descriptive research have established that family caregiving is a burdensome role with potentially high costs to the caregiver. Second, there exists a rich theoretical literature that helps us understand under what circumstances caregiving is most burdensome and provides a theoretical rationale for designing and targeting interventions aimed at diminishing caregiver burden. Third, the intervention literature has matured to a point where a systematic and organized statement of intervention approaches to caregiving is warranted and is likely to benefit both the academic and practitioner communities. A broad range of interventions has been described in the literature—from educational programs to therapeutic interventions, technology-based approaches, as well as interventions targeting the physical environment. Unfortunately, the literature describing these methods is widely dispersed, fragmented, and generally not easily accessible. We are at a pivotal stage in the development of caregiver interventions both from a scientific and public policy perspective. A major goal of this book is to bring order to what we know and provide direction for the future development of this critical area.

Despite the relatively large number of contributors to this book, it should be noted that it is not a traditional edited volume, but rather an integrated and focused book written by a team of experts with extensive knowledge of the proposed topic and with a history of working closely together as a research team and as a writing group.

Richard Schulz
University of Pittsburgh

# 1

# The Extent and Impact of Dementia Care: Unique Challenges Experienced by Family Caregivers

*Marcia G. Ory, Jennifer L. Yee,*
*Sharon L. Tennstedt, and Richard Schulz*

Caregiving is a family issue, as evidenced by the much cited fact that the bulk of care for chronically ill or disabled older people is provided by family and friends (e.g., Schulz & O'Brien, 1994). This is especially true when considering care for persons with dementia. With the aging of the population, the number of people with Alzheimer's disease and related disorders is expected to increase from nearly two million Americans age 65 and over afflicted with the disease in 1995 to nearly three million Americans by the year 2015 (General Accounting Office, 1998). The personal, social, and financial impacts of dementia caregiving have been well documented (Schulz, O'Brien, Bookwala, & Fleissner, 1995), with a recent study providing more precise estimates on the costs of both family and institutional care at different stages of illness (Leon, Cheng, & Neumann, in press).

Given the characteristic cognitive, behavioral, and affective losses associated with the progression of the disease, caring for someone with dementia is assumed to be more difficult and burdensome than caring for loved ones with other chronic conditions and disabilities (Light, Niederehe, & Lebowitz, 1994). However, this assertion has never really been adequately examined in a large representative population of both dementia and nondementia caregivers.

Recent innovations—such as the development of new cognitive-enhancing drugs or the emergence of new residential care facilities—are likely to affect the course and care of people with dementia. Similarly with a rapidly expanding population of older adults, smaller family sizes, and more women in the paid labor force, there are concerns regarding the availability and willingness of future generations of family caregivers (Hooyman & Gonyea, 1995; Kaye & Applegate, 1990; Marks, 1996). However, functional deficits are still likely to occur, particularly at the later stages of the disease, and there is no reason to believe that, for the foreseeable future, families will not remain primary caregivers throughout most of the course of illness.

The purpose of this introductory chapter is to provide an overview on the prevalence of caregiving in general, with specific attention to dementia caregiving. Discussing the implications of different definitions of caregiving, we will review national data describing who is providing what kinds of and how much care. Also summarized will be the various impacts associated with caregiving tasks and responsibilities. Using data from the 1997 National Survey on Family Caregiving (National Alliance for Caregiving, 1997), differences between dementia and nondementia care will be highlighted. The chapter will introduce major research and policy themes which will receive further elaboration in this volume.

## HEALTH EFFECTS OF DEMENTIA CAREGIVING

The extent to which caregiving affects the physical and mental health of the caregiver is an important policy question and has been addressed by numerous studies carried out in the past decade. Research on caregiving remains a priority because of the need to strengthen family members' abilities to provide care without jeopardizing caregivers' own health or well-being or relinquishing their caregiver responsibilities prematurely (Schulz & Quittner, 1998).

Researchers have assessed psychiatric morbidity attributable to caregiving by using standardized self-report measures such as the CES-D (Radloff, 1977) or Beck Depression Inventory (Beck, Ward, Mendelson, Mock, & Erbaugh, 1961), structured diagnostic interviews, such as the Diagnostic Interview Schedule (DIS) or the Hamilton Depression Rating Scale (Hamilton, 1967), as well as indicators of psychotropic drug use (see Schulz et al., 1995). On the whole, studies using self-report inventories show a consistent pattern of increased depression and anxiety symptomatology among dementia caregivers when compared to age and gender based norms (e.g., Collins & Jones, 1997; Haley et al., 1995; Irwin et al., 1997; King & Brassington, 1997; Majerovitz, 1995; MaloneBeach & Zarit, 1995; Rose-Rego, Strauss, & Smyth, 1998; Schulz et al., 1997). Studies that include clinical diagnoses as an outcome report elevated rates of major depression among dementia caregivers when compared to age-matched controls, and in some studies, elevated rates of generalized anxiety (Irwin et al., 1997; Redinbaugh, MacCullum, & Kiecolt-Glaser, 1995; Vitaliano, Russo, Scanlan, & Greeno, 1996; Vitaliano, Scanlan, Krenz, Schwartz, & Marcovina, 1996; Schulz et al., 1995). The use of psychotropic drugs as an indicator of psychiatric morbidity has been examined in only a few studies and the results have varied widely, making it difficult to reach conclusions about the effects of caregiving on the use of these medications (Schulz et al., 1995).

Studies of physical health outcomes among caregivers have used a broad range of measurements, which can be classified into four major types of outcomes: self-rated global health; the presence of chronic conditions, illnesses, physical symptoms, and disabilities; health-related behaviors, medication use, and health service utilization; and physiological indices (Bookwala, Yee, & Schulz, 1998). In contrast to the consistent findings for psychiatric health effects among Alzheimer's disease related disorders (ADRD) caregivers, findings based on physical health outcomes are less conclusive.

A common assessment of physical health status that has been employed in caregiving studies is a single question that asks respondents to rate their current overall health on a scale from poor to excellent. In general, most studies have found that caregivers perceive their health to be somewhat poorer than noncaregivers or community samples (Beach, Schulz, Yee, & Jackson, 1998; Mui, 1995;

Pruchno, Peters, & Burant, 1995; Rose-Rego et al., 1998; Schulz et al., 1997).

Contrary to the findings for self-rated global health, findings concerning the other types of physical health measures are more equivocal. With respect to self-reported physical illness and disability, common measures employed by researchers include symptoms checklists such as the Cornell Medical Health Index or the Physical Health Section of the OARS (Duke University, 1978), and asking respondents to report if they have experienced various illnesses or diseases. A few recently published studies suggest that caregiving may be related to the presence of illness, physical symptoms, and disabilities (Bass, Noelker, & Rechlin, 1996; Canning, Dew, & Davidson, 1996; Cochrane, Goering, & Rogers, 1997; Fuller-Jonap & Haley, 1995; Jutras & Lovoie, 1995). For example, Fuller-Jonap and Haley (1995) reported that caregiving husbands reported more respiratory problems than a comparison group. Jutras and Lovoie (1995) noted that more caregivers than noncaregivers reported having diabetes and back problems than those that did not reside with a disabled elder. In addition, Cochrane et al. (1997) reported that caregivers mentioned having more physical health problems in the previous year, and more "limited activity days" and "days that required extreme effort" compared to noncaregiving controls. However, in contrast to these studies, other studies have failed to find an association between caregiving and self-reported illness or disability (Brodaty & Hadzi-Pavlovic, 1990; Irwin et al., 1997; Pruchno et al., 1995; Shaw et al., 1997).

With regard to health-related behaviors, some studies have found that caregivers report less physical activity, sleep, and rest than noncaregivers (Burton, Newsom, Schulz, Hirsch, & German, 1997; Fuller-Jonap & Haley, 1995; Glaser & Kiecolt-Glaser, 1997; Kiecolt-Glaser, Glaser, Gravenstein, Malarkey, & Sheridan, 1996; Schulz et al., 1997). However, inconsistent evidence was found with regard to differences in other health-related behaviors, such as alcohol consumption, smoking, weight change, finding time to see the doctor, and missing doctor's appointments. In terms of medication use, Schulz et al. found increased medication use among caregivers and Burton et al. reported that caregivers were more likely to forget to take their medications. A few studies examined utilization of health services, such as hospitalizations and physician visits as physical health indicators. However, a consistent association has not been found between caregiving and health care utilization (Schulz et al., 1995).

An important emerging area of caregiving health outcomes research focuses on changes in subclinical disease such as immune functioning, hypertension, pulmonary function, blood chemistries, and cardiac arrhythmias as indicators of health status. However, evidence supporting the association between caregiving and such physiological indices is mixed. In two recent studies, Kiecolt-Glaser and her colleagues reported that compared to matched controls, caregivers showed poorer immune response after exposure to an influenza virus vaccine and to infection by a latent herpes simplex virus (Glaser & Kiecolt-Glaser, 1997; Kiecolt-Glaser et al., 1996). Similarly, Pariante and associates (1997) found that caregivers had lower levels of T cells, a higher percentage of T suppressor/cytotoxic cells, and a lower T helper: suppressor ratio compared to matched controls. With regard to cardiovascular risk factors and functioning, Vitaliano, Russo, Scanlan, and Greeno (1996) found that men caregivers had higher lipids than age- and sex-matched controls and women caregivers reported less aerobic activity than their noncaregiving counterparts. In addition, Moritz, Kasl, and Ostfeld (1992) showed increased systolic blood pressure among male ADRD caregivers. Although some studies found caregiving to be related to physiological indices of health, others found no association (e.g., Irwin et al., 1997; Schulz et al., 1997).

If we ask the question, what factors predict negative health effects among caregivers, two distinct patterns emerge. One pattern of findings indicates that predictors generally known to be risk factors for negative health outcomes in all populations emerge in these studies as well. Thus, physical and psychiatric morbidity is associated with being female, low financial adequacy, high levels of stress, and personality variables, such as high levels of neuroticism, and low levels of mastery (e.g., Bookwala & Schulz, 1998; Burton et al., 1997; Draper, Poulos, Poulos, & Ehrlich, 1995; Dura, Stukenberg, & Kiecolt-Glaser, 1991; Hooker, Monahan, Frazier, & Shifren, 1998; Morrissey, Becker, & Rupert, 1990; Mui, 1995). Similarly, the relation between depression, anxiety, social support, and physical health morbidity have been frequently reported in the literature and are characteristic of the caregiving literature as well (e.g., Li, Seltzer, & Greenberg, 1997; Redinbaugh et al., 1995). The second pattern concerns those associations that are unique to the caregiving context. For dementia caregivers, two factors are important in predicting negative health effects in addition to those already listed above. Patient problem behaviors are consistently linked to both psychiatric and physical morbidity of the caregiver and patient cognitive impairment is consistently related to physical morbidity of the caregiver (Li et al., 1997; Majerovitz, 1995; Moritz et al., 1992; Schulz et al., 1995).

Evaluating links between caregiving stress and health outcomes will ultimately require us to specify complex, multivariate models that are tested prospectively. Minimally, such models will include objective measures of stressors, assessments of how those stressors are perceived by caregivers, and a repertoire of health outcomes that includes categorical clinical disease, subclinical disease markers, health care utilization data, and self-reported health. In developing and testing such models, it is important to keep in mind that we must identify not only patterns of relations among variables but also that the observed morbidity effects exceed some absolute standard for classifying an individual as ill or at risk of illness. This can be achieved by selecting health measures with well-established age and gender norms.

In articulating such stress-health models, it may be fruitful to focus on outcomes that reflect the exacerbation of existing health conditions. The demands of caregiving may not precipitate an illness event per se, but rather may aggravate existing vulnerabilities. Thus, attempts should be made to assess whether illness results from existing conditions being exacerbated or represents new conditions unrelated to prior medical history or risk factors. Illness effects will most likely be found among individuals with elevated risk factors who are exposed to higher levels of stress (Vitaliano, Schulz, Kiecolt-Glaser, & Grant, 1997).

Finally, to the extent that illness effects are observed in future studies of caregiving, it will be important to determine the mechanisms that account for those effects. It must be remembered that mechanisms accounting for symptom reporting, health care utilization, and disease processes may differ from each other.

## DEFINITION OF CAREGIVING

As a dynamic process that unfolds and changes over time, the family caregiving role evolves from preexisting social expectations and obligations (e.g., Kosloski & Montogomery, 1993; Stoller, Forster, & Duniho, 1992). Caregiving and care receiving can occur at any point in the life course, and is typically associated with chronic illnesses or disabilities which result in losses of independence and functioning. This chapter will draw on studies examining caregiving for older adults, although it is not restricted to caregiving by older adults.

There is no standard definition of family caregiving, which has been used consistently from one study to another (National Alliance for Caregiving and the American Association of Retired Persons, 1997 report). What is meant by the term caregiving is not always clear and frequently varies with the purpose for which such definitions are used (Schulz et al., 1997).

The provision of support or assistance by one family member to another is a normative and pervasive aspect of human interactions. Giving help to a family member with a chronic illness or disability is sometimes not very different from the tasks and activities that characterize interactions among families without the presence of illness or disability (Schulz & Quittner, 1998). For example, when a wife provides care to her husband with Alzheimer's disease by preparing his meals or keeping the house clean, she is engaging in an activity she might normally do for her husband. However, assistance with personal care activities, such as bathing or dressing, is more clearly seen as caregiving. The defining difference is that providing help with bathing or dressing or assisting with complex medical routines reflects "extraordinary" care and exceeds the bounds of what is "normative" or "usual" for spousal responsibilities (Schulz & Quittner, 1998). This may help explain why adult children sometimes report more caregiving burdens than do spouses, despite providing fewer hours of actual care.

Whether episodic or chronic, extraordinary care often involves a significant expenditure of time and energy. This may require the performance of tasks that may be physically demanding or unpleasant and disruptive of other social and family roles.

Family caregivers may perform tasks similar to those carried out by paid health or social service providers. Another defining feature of informal caregiving is that family members perform these services for no compensation and do so either voluntarily or because they feel they have no other alternative (Schulz & Quittner, 1998).

While there may be a growing consensus that family caregiving is characterized by some degree of extraordinary care, in reality, different studies have used widely variant definitions of caregiving. Estimates of the prevalence of caregiving and the characteristics of caregivers may vary depending on whether a restrictive or inclusive definition of caregiving is employed (Bookwala et al., 1998). We will illustrate the variability in caregiving definitions by presenting two examples: 1) a collaborative intervention study designed to enhance family caregiving, and 2) a national survey designed to document the extent and impact of family caregiving.

## REACH

Established in 1995, the Resources for Enhancing Alzheimer's Caregiver Health (REACH) Project was funded by the National Institute on Aging and The National Institute of Nursing Research, NIH to characterize and test the most promising behavioral, social, technological, or environmental interventions for enhancing family dementia care (Coon, Schulz, & Ory, in press). Interventions are carried out at six sites (Birmingham, Boston, Memphis, Miami, Palo Alto, Philadelphia) that have all adopted a common measurement battery.

The modest results of previous caregiver intervention studies are attributed, in part, to the fact that the studies were designed to reduce stress and caregivers who agree to be in studies may not be overly stressed at baseline, or may not be performing substantial caregiving tasks (Bourgeois, Schulz, & Burgio, 1996).

Thus, several selection criteria were established to ensure that caregivers were involved in caregiving tasks and experienced caregiving responsibilities that could be taxing. This included requiring that the caregiver be a family member living with the person with dementia; that they had been in the caregiver role for at least six months; and that they provided at least four hours of supervision or direct assistance per day for the care recipient. REACH targeted adult caregivers since it was felt that younger caregivers would be relatively rare and have very different needs. Both genders were solicited except in one site where only women were recruited.

Logistical requirements were also specified with caregivers competent in languages specified by the individual studies, having a telephone, and planning to remain in the geographic area for at least six months. Caregivers were included if they did not have conditions associated with severe disability or death. Additionally, to avoid possible confounding effects, caregivers were not recruited if they were participating in any other caregiver intervention study. It was assumed that some care recipients might be put in new drug studies over the course of the study, and this was to be monitored for its effects on behaviors that might affect caregiver outcomes. While a formal cognitive screen was not conducted on caregivers, if the interviewer reported problems in administering the caregiver screen or interview, a standard protocol was developed for administering a short cognitive assessment.

An underlying theme in establishing these criteria was to minimize the exclusion criteria so that a broad net could be cast for persons with dementia and their primary caregiver. This is important for ensuring generalizability of treatment effects and for easing the recruitment process. Each inclusion and exclusion criterion was presented and defended as absolutely necessary for examining longterm intervention effects.

## A National Survey on Family Caregiving in the U.S.

In 1996, the National Alliance for Caregiving, in conjunction with the American Association of Retired Persons, sponsored a national telephone survey of over 1,500 family caregivers (National Alliance for Caregiving and the American Association of Retired Persons, 1997). The purpose was to document the magnitude, intensity, and types of informal caregiving along with a profile of caregiving impacts in four racial/ethnic groups across the country (Whites, Blacks, Hispanics, and Asians). Given the study purposes, a broad definition of caregiving was utilized to assess the type of informal care provided to older persons. This survey documented the use of a variety of caregiving activities ranging from long-distance care, occasional hands-on care to round-the clock personal care.

The following definitions were used in this study:

"By caregiving, I mean providing unpaid care to a relative or friend who is aged 50 or older to help take care of themselves."

"Caregiving may include help with personal needs or household chores. It might be taking care of a person's finances, arranging for outside services, or visiting regularly to see how they are doing. This person need not live with you" (National Alliance for Caregiving and the American Association of Retired Persons, 1997 report, p. 6).

In contrast to the REACH study, this national survey took a very broad view of caregiving and caregivers. The target was an adult caregiver that had provided informal care to a relative or friend at some point during the past 12 months. There were no restrictions on the amount, frequency, duration, or place of care.

The caregivers were asked about the health status of the care-recipients. Those who said they provided care to someone with Alzheimer's disease, confusion, dementia, or forgetfulness were classified as "dementia" caregivers. A hallmark of dementia care versus care for physical illnesses is the need to provide supervision and cueing to enable the care recipient to carry out activities of daily living.

## PREVALENCE OF FAMILY CAREGIVING IN THE U.S.

Estimates of the magnitude and nature of family caregiving will be influenced by the definition utilized. Data from the National Alliance for Caregiving Survey on Family Caregiving will be utilized since this is among one of the largest, most representative family caregiving studies conducted to date.

Another major advantage is that this survey is large enough to include both dementia and nondementia caregivers, permitting a comparison of these two types of caregivers on several different domains. To date, few studies have been conducted that examined differences between dementia and nondementia caregivers. The results of these prior studies have been inconsistent with respect to the impact of caregiving on dementia versus nondementia caregivers. Some studies have reported few differences between dementia and nondementia caregivers in terms of burden or depression (Cattanach & Tebes, 1991; Draper, Poulos, Cole, Poulos, & Ehrlich, 1992). In contrast, some investigators have noted that dementia caregivers suffer more negative effects, such as increased depression and anxiety levels, than nondementia caregivers (Hooker et al., 1998; Moritz, Kasl, & Berkman, 1989). However, most of these studies suffered from small sample sizes. In addition, these studies have primarily investigated differences in caregiver's mental health and have not included detailed descriptions concerning characteristics of dementia and nondementia caregivers. Thus, the National Alliance survey provides us with the opportunity to develop a detailed profile of the differences between dementia and nondementia caregivers.

## NUMBERS OF CAREGIVERS

Using the entry criteria described above, this study estimated that nearly one in four U.S. households with a telephone contained at least one caregiver. This translates into over 22 million caregiving households nationwide that met these criteria in the past 12 months. The majority of households (approximately 18 million) were White, non-Hispanic. A dementia-related condition was reported in more than 20 percent of the households. Nationwide, this translates into over five million households providing care for someone with dementia or related symptoms.

### Caregiver Characteristics

This study of caregiving over the life course found that the typical caregiver was a middle-aged, married woman who was working either full- or part-time (National Alliance for Caregiving and American Association of Retired Persons, 1997). As seen in Table 1.1, several notable differences were observed in terms of demographics between caregivers providing care for persons with dementia as compared to those providing care for persons without this condition. Such differences in caregiving roles (e.g., spousal relationships) have been shown to be important predictors of perceived stress and burden. Dementia caregivers were more likely than nondementia caregivers to be spouses versus adult children (7.2% v. 3.1% spouses; 48.9% v. 52.8% adult children). There were significant differences between dementia and nondementia caregivers in terms of employment sta-

**TABLE 1.1 Demographic Characteristics of Dementia and Nondementia Caregivers**

| Demographic variable | Dementia | Nondementia | Statistic |
|---|---|---|---|
| | Dementia status | | |
| Mean age | 46.26 (14.85) | 42.99 (14.05) | $t(1496) = 3.65^*$ |
| Mean age of care recipient | 78.39 (10.10) | 75.65 (10.67) | $t(1496) = 4.11^*$ |
| Percent female | 72.5 | 68.1 | $X^2(1, N = 1498) = 2.30$ |
| Race (percent) | | | |
| White | 42.8 | 41.0 | $X^2(3, N = 1498) = 21.25^*$ |
| Black | 26.9 | 18.4 | |
| Asian | 10.3 | 19.4 | |
| Hispanic | 19.4 | 20.5 | |
| Relationship to recipient (percent) | | | |
| Spouse/partner | 7.2 | 3.1 | Test of dementia vs. |
| Parent/parent-in-law | 48.9 | 52.8 | nondementia for spouse, |
| Sibling/sibling-in-law | 3.1 | 2.9 | parent, or other relationship: |
| Child | 0.0 | 0.2 | $X^2(2, N = 1494) = 11.65^{**}$ |
| Grandparent/grand-parent-in-law | 16.9 | 18.0 | |
| Aunt/uncle | 8.8 | 6.2 | |
| Other relative | 0.6 | 0.9 | |
| Nonrelative/friend | 14.4 | 16.0 | |
| Median income category | $30,000 but less than $40,000 | $30,000 but less than $40,000 | |
| Median highest education level | Some college | Some college | |
| Marital status (percent) | | | |
| Married/living with partner | 62.3 | 63.8 | $X^2(3, N = 1488) = 4.73$ |
| Single, never married | 14.2 | 17.4 | |
| Divorced/separated | 16.5 | 12.5 | |
| Widowed | 7.0 | 6.3 | |
| Children present (percent) | 43.5 | 49.0 | $X^2(1, N = 1488) = 5.21$ |

**TABLE 1.1** *(continued)*

| Demographic variable | Dementia status | | Statistic |
| | Dementia | Nondementia | |
| --- | --- | --- | --- |
| Employment status | | | |
| Full- or part-time | 61.6 | 68.3 | $X^2(2, N = 1495) =$ |
| (percent) | | | 8.77*** |
| Retired | 16.6 | 10.8 | |
| Not employed | 20.9 | 21.9 | |

*p < .001; **p < .01; ***p < .05
*Note:* Values in parentheses are standard deviations.

tus. For example, compared to nondementia caregivers, dementia caregivers were less likely to report being employed full- or part-time and more likely to be retired (61.6% v. 68.3% employed; 16.6% v. 10.8% retired). In addition, differences were observed between dementia caregivers and nondementia caregivers with regard to the age of the caregiver and care recipient. Dementia caregivers were significantly older than nondementia caregivers ($M = 46.26$ v. M = 42.99) and dementia caregivers were caring for recipients that were significantly older than nondementia caregivers ($M = 78.39$ v. $M = 75.65$). In terms of race, dementia caregivers were overrepresented in the Black sample (26.9% v. 18.4%) and underrepresented in the Asian sample (10.3% v. 19.4%). No differences between dementia and nondementia caregivers were found with regard to gender, marital status, income, education, and the presence of children in the household.

## Amount of Care Provided

The typical caregiver in this study had been in a caregiving relationship for about five years. When comparing duration of care and estimated hours of care provided per week between dementia and nondementia caregivers, we see that there is no difference in duration of care, but that there is a substantial difference in amount of care provided. As indicated in Table 1.2, the average duration of care is about five years for both types of caregivers. However, caregivers

**TABLE 1.2 Means of Caregiving Involvement Characteristics
for Dementia and Nondementia Caregivers**

| Caregiver involvement characteristic | Dementia | Nondementia | t-test |
|---|---|---|---|
| Duration of care | 5.10 | 5.07 | $t(1429) = .056$, n.s. |
| (years) | (1.28) | (1.28) | |
| | ($N = 309$) | ($N = 1122$) | |
| Hours of care | 17.06 | 12.45 | $t(1243) = 4.61^*$ |
| | (17.37) | (14.54) | |
| | ($N = 251$) | ($N = 994$) | |

$^*p < .001$.
*Note:* Values in parentheses are standard deviations.

providing care for someone with dementia provide over 17 hours of care a week, compared to slightly over 12 hours of care provided by nondementia caregivers.

These averages mask the widespread variability in intensity of care reported. At one extreme, there are many caregivers that only provide 8 hours or less of care a week (36.8% of the dementia caregivers and 51.8% of the nondementia caregivers). At the other extreme, there are a significant minority of caregivers who are providing constant care. In this study, dementia caregivers were more likely than nondementia caregivers to be providing such care (16.1% of the dementia caregivers reported providing constant care versus 10.9% of the nondementia caregivers).

## Caregiving Tasks

This study provided detailed information on what types of activities caregivers provided assistance with. For example, help may be needed on managing everyday living (e.g., transportation, grocery shopping, housework, preparing meals, managing finances, arranging/supervising outside services, and giving medicine). Assistance may also be needed with basic activities of daily living, defined as getting out of bed or a chair, dressing, bathing, toileting, feeding, and help with continence or diapers.

As indicated in Table 1.3, dementia caregivers provided assistance with more tasks overall as compared to nondementia caregivers (an average of 7.07 v. 5.73 tasks performed by each group respectively). Dementia caregivers were particularly more likely to be helping with basic activities of daily living (an average of 2.29 ADL tasks performed by dementia caregivers versus 1.36 tasks performed by nondementia caregivers).

## Caregiving Impacts

The duration, amount, and intensity of caregiving tasks have been related to reported stresses and burdens, although studies repeatedly show variability based on caregiver role and other mediating factors. Table 1.4 summarizes data on reported physical, emotional, and financial strain as well as interference with other activities.

We see that in general, many caregivers report some negative effects, but that those caring for people with dementia are more likely to report negative effects. The impact on social and personal time is especially notable, with a greater proportion of dementia caregivers reporting having to give up pleasurable personal activities

**TABLE 1.3  Means of ADL and IADL and Total Task Performance for Dementia and Nondementia Caregivers**

| Types of tasks performed | Dementia ($N = 320$) | Nondementia ($N = 1178$) | $t$-test |
|---|---|---|---|
| IADLs | 4.78 | 4.37 | $t(1496) = 3.47^*$ |
|  | (1.97) | (1.83) |  |
| ADLs | 2.29 | 1.36 | $t(1496) = 7.86^*$ |
|  | (2.12) | (1.82) |  |
| Total | 7.07 | 5.73 | $t(1490) = 7.04^*$ |
|  | (3.22) | (7.07) |  |

$^*p \leq .001$.

*Note.* Values in parentheses are standard deviations.

Activities of daily living (ADLs) include: getting in or out of beds or chairs; getting dressed; getting to and from the toilet; bathing and showering; continence or dealing with diapers; feeding.

Instrumental activities of daily living (IADLs) include: giving medicines, pills, injections; managing finances; grocery shopping; housework; preparing meals; transportation; arranging services.

**TABLE 1.4  The Effects of Physical, Emotional, Financial and Role Stress on Dementia and Nondementia Caregivers**

| Item | Dementia status | | Statistic |
|------|------------------------|------------------------|-----------|
|      | Dementia ($N = 320$) | Nondementia ($N = 1176$) | |
| Give up vacations, hobbies or your own activities (percent) | 55.0 | 40.9 | $X^2$ (1, $N = 1496$) = 20.30[*] |
| Less time for other family members (percent) | 52.0 | 38.1 | $X^2$ (1, $N = 1494$) = 20.05[*] |
| Other relatives doing their fair share of caregiving (percent) | 59.4 | 74.1 | $X^2$ (1, $N = 1072$) = 19.03[*] |
| Extent of family conflict over caregiving (mean out of a one to three range) | 1.55 (0.96) | 1.34 (0.76) | $t(1134) = 3.67$[*] |
| Emotional strain of caregiving (mean out of a one to five range) | 2.99 (1.48) | 2.22 (1.36) | $t(1490) = 8.74$[*] |
| Physical strain of caregiving (mean out of a one to five range) | 2.40 (1.42) | 1.80 (1.16) | $t(1490) = 7.72$[*] |
| Did you suffer mental or physical problems as a result of caregiving (percent) | 22.3 | 12.6 | $X^2$ (1, $N = 1494$) = 18.66[*] |
| Financial hardship of caregiving (mean out of a one to five range) | 1.87 (1.34) | 1.50 (0.99) | $t(1488) = 5.48$[*] |
| Own money spent a month (mean) | 104.00 . | 106.22 | $t(1283) = 0.12$ |

[*]$p < .001$

*Note:* Values in parentheses are standard deviations.

(55% v. 40.9%) or having less time for other family members (52% v. 38.1%). In addition to having less time for other family, dementia caregivers were more inclined than nondementia caregivers to perceive that other family members were not doing their fair share (59.4% v. 74.1%) of caregiving and to report a greater degree of family conflict ($M = 1.55$ v. $M = 1.34$).

In terms of emotional and physical strain overall, caregivers reported a moderate degree of strain (means are approximately 2 to 3 on a 5-point scale). However, dementia caregivers reported a higher level of emotional ($M = 2.99$ v. $M = 2.22$) and physical strain ($M = 2.40$ v. $M = 1.80$) than nondementia caregivers. Furthermore, dementia caregivers were more likely than nondementia caregivers to mention that they had suffered mental or physical problems as a result of caregiving (22.3% v. 12.6%), although such caregivers were in the minority.

Overall, caregivers reported a low degree of financial hardship (means were between 1 and 2 on a 5-point scale), although dementia caregivers reported higher levels of financial hardship ($M = 1.87$ v. $M = 1.50$) than nondementia caregivers. However, dementia caregivers and nondementia caregivers reported spending about the same amount of money per month on caregiving (approximately $105 per month).

## Overall Feeling

In addition to reporting the amount of strain, family conflict, and interference with other activities resulting from caregiving, respondents were asked to state the one feeling that best describes their caregiving experience. Caregiving was seen in both positive and negative terms, with some differences reported by dementia caregiving status. As indicated in Table 1.5, more than half of caregivers in this study (both dementia and nondementia) reported positive feelings with regard to caregiving. However, there were significant differences between caregivers and noncaregivers in terms of negative feelings about caregiving. Although anger is not a predominant response, dementia caregivers were more likely to express this feeling (5.1% v. 1.5%) than nondementia caregivers. In addition, related

**TABLE 1.5  Percentages of Dementia and Nondementia Caregivers
Reporting the Feeling That Best Describes Caregiving**

| Feeling category | Dementia status | | Chi-square |
|---|---|---|---|
| | Dementia ($N = 237$) | Nondementia ($N = 923$) | |
| Anger | 5.1 | 1.5 | $X^2(1, N = 1169) = 11.01^*$ |
| Sadness/fear | 2.5 | 1.5 | $X^2(1, N = 1169) = 1.19$ |
| Burden | 15.2 | 10.6 | $X^2(1, N = 1169) = 4.07^{**}$ |
| Obligation | 11.0 | 12.9 | $X^2(1, N = 1169) = 0.56$ |
| Love | 17.3 | 18.4 | $X^2(1, N = 1169) = 0.13$ |
| Happiness | 48.9 | 54.5 | $X^2(1, N = 1169) = 2.35$ |

$^*p < .001;$ $^{**}p < .05$

to the results on caregiving strain, a slightly greater proportion of dementia caregivers reported feeling burdened (15.2% v. 10.6%).

To summarize, caregiving had a greater impact on dementia caregivers in terms of time for other activities, family conflict, caregiving strain, the experience of mental and physical problems, financial hardship, and negative feelings. In general, however, most caregivers did not report extremely negative effects as a result of caregiving and many reported feeling positively about their caregiving responsibilities.

## VARIATIONS IN CAREGIVING EXPERIENCES

While the direct relationship between the care recipient's needs for care and the care provided by informal caregivers has been firmly established, the types and amounts of help also have been related to several sociodemographic characteristics of the caregiver. The characteristics frequently investigated include caregiver gender and race, relationship to the care recipient, and coresidence with the care recipient. These factors are related not only to the pattern of care but also to the size and composition of the caregiving network.

Consistently across all studies of caregiving and as has been reported in the National Alliance for Caregiving (NAC) study, spouses are the first source of caregiving assistance. Perhaps related to the nature of the marital relationship, spouses are often the sole caregiver (Stone, Cafferata, & Sangl, 1987; Tennstedt, McKinlay, & Sullivan, 1989) and provide the most extensive and comprehensive care (Cantor, 1983; Horowitz, 1985a; Johnson, 1983; McKinlay & Tennstedt, 1986; Shanas, 1979; Soldo & Myllyuoma, 1983; Stephens & Christianson, 1986; Stone et al., 1987). This holds true for caregivers of elders with dementia or with functional disabilities only. Offspring are usually the next source of informal care, also for both groups. However, caregiving for elders with dementia is less frequent among extended kin or nonkin, likely because of the greater commitment and involvement required.

The type and amount of help provided has also been related to the caregiver's gender, again with no difference between caregivers of elders with dementia and those with noncognitive functional disabilities only. Female caregivers provide more help and assist with a wider range of tasks (e.g., Horowitz, 1985b). With gender-specific division of labor, some studies show that male caregivers are more likely to assist with home repairs, financial management, and transportation (Collins & Jones, 1997; Fredriksen, 1996; Young & Kahana, 1989), whereas females provide personal care, meal preparation, and other household management tasks (e.g., Dwyer & Coward, 1991; Horowitz, 1985b). However, there is more support in the literature for a gendered division of labor for female-oriented than male-oriented caregiving tasks. Perhaps one exception to this division of labor is the role of spousal caregivers. More likely to be the only source of help, husbands and wives may provide more similar amounts and types of care to their spousal care recipients than adult children provide to parent recipients (Tennstedt, Crawford, & McKinlay, 1993a).

The proximity of the caregiver to the care recipient is a critical factor in determining the pattern of care. In particular, if the caregiver and care recipient co-reside, there will be greater caregiving involvement and less use of formal services (Chappell, 1991; Diwan, Berger, & Manns, 1997; Tennstedt et al., 1993a), regardless of caregiver relationship (Tennstedt et al., 1993a). Coresidence is more likely for dementia caregivers, especially at later stages of disease, which likely accounts for the greater caregiving involvement when compared to all nondementia caregivers. However, the relationship between co-residence and lower use of selected dementia services has also been reported (Gill, Hinrichsen, & DiGiuseppe, 1998). Proximity to the care recipient is less of an issue in the provision of short-term or "crisis" care. Himes, Jordan, and Farkas (1996) have reported no difference in amount of care by those living with or very near the care recipient and by those caregivers more distant when the care was for a time-limited period. This is less relevant for primary caregivers in the care of elders with dementia, underscoring the importance of proximity or coresidence in the provision of care.

The relationship between race or ethnicity and patterns of care have been studied only more recently. Most of the research on care of minority elders has been conducted with African Americans and Hispanics. Comparative studies are limited, usually comparing a single minority group with Whites. Connell and Gibson (1997) reviewed 12 studies since 1985 that examined the impact of race, culture, and/or ethnicity on the dementia caregiving experience. Compared to White caregivers, non-White caregivers were less likely to be a spouse and more likely to be offspring, another relative, or friend. Some of the studies included in this review reported that non-White caregivers received more instrumental support from others than did White caregivers.

Most of these studies did not report amount of care by White and non-White caregivers. In a study of functionally disabled African-American, Puerto-Rican and White caregivers, Tennstedt and Chang (1998) reported that, controlling for level of disability, non-White caregivers provided more care than White caregivers. Given reports of more strongly held attitudes of filial support among minority caregivers than among White caregivers (Lawton, Rajagopal, Brody, & Kleban, 1992; Cox, 1993; Cox & Monk, 1990), it is reasonable to assume that non-White dementia caregivers also provide more care than do White caregivers, who indicate a greater willingness to institutionalize a care recipient with a dementing illness (Hinrichsen & Ramirez, 1992).

It is commonly thought that the size and composition of the caregiving network influences the organization and provision of care.

Larger networks of caregivers, closely related and/or very committed to providing care, are thought to result in sharing of caregiving responsibilities. This would seem particularly relevant in care for elders with dementing illness for whom needs for care are frequently great. The composition of the caregiving network evolves over time, influenced by the age, gender, and race of the care recipient, but is generally stable (Peek, Zsembik, & Coward, 1997). Burton and colleagues (1995) have reported that the number of caregivers does not differ by race although others have reported that minority elders have more caregivers due to the involvement of modified extended families (Chatters, Taylor, & Jackson, 1985, 1986; Miller, McFall, & Campbell, 1994; Hatch, 1991; Cox & Monk, 1990).

Yet in light of these data, it has been reported consistently that the primary caregiver provides most of the care. In a study by Stommel and colleagues (1995), which included both dementia and non-dementia caregivers, the primary caregiver provided assistance with instrumental activities of daily living (IADLs) almost exclusively, but help with ADLs was shared with others. Data from this study revealed no threshold at which secondary caregivers are involved, but involvement was more likely when a high frequency of care was needed. The primary pattern of division of labor was one of supplementation, i.e., that secondary caregivers shared the responsibility for specific tasks with the primary caregiver rather than a splitting up of tasks (or specialization) among the caregivers. Other data reported by these investigators (Stommel, Given, & Given, 1998) indicate that division of labor is influenced by race. Consistent with the larger caregiving networks of African Americans, these caregivers are more likely than White caregivers to share care with secondary helpers but again remain involved in most activities

## INTERFACE OF INFORMAL AND FORMAL CARE

Division of labor also extends to the involvement of formal service providers. This interface between the informal and formal sources of care has been of public policy interest in response to the concern that changing social trends—smaller family size, increased geographic mobility, greater participation of women in the workforce, and rising rates of marital disruption—will decrease the availability or willingness of family members to provide care to a disabled elder. Division of formal and informal labor is of concern from a clinical perspective in terms of timely and appropriate use of formal services to ensure the well-being of both care recipient and caregiver.

The involvement of a coresiding caregiver consistently has been related to lower use of formal services by elders with (Gill et al., 1998) and without dementing illness (Tennstedt et al., 1993a; Tennstedt, Harrow, & Crawford, 1996). Initial use, or increased use, of formal services usually occurs in the presence of informal care but when care needs increase or when there is a change in the primary caregiver (Tennstedt, Crawford, & McKinlay, 1993b; Tennstedt et al., 1996). The use of formal services is more likely when the elder has ADL deficits (Diwan et al., 1997). There are no longitudinal data about these transitions in dementia care. Similar to findings for elders with physical disabilities, cross-sectional data indicate that use of formal services is greater by elders with dementia who have greater functional impairment, live alone, and have higher incomes (Bass, Looman, & Ehrlich, 1992; Caserta, Lund, Wright, & Redburn, 1987; Gill et al., 1998; Mullan, 1993, Penning, 1995). Caregiver burden has not been unequivocally established as a correlate or predictor of service use (Bass et al., 1992; Caserta et al., 1987; Gill et al., 1998; Penning, 1995). However, Hamilton (1996) has reported that the primary caregiver's sense of personal competence or caregiving mastery was related to nonuse of services to which they had been referred.

## RESEARCH NEEDS

Despite the increase in the magnitude and quality of dementia care research over the past decade, there are still substantial gaps in our knowledge. As discussed throughout this volume, what is known about dementia and dementia caregiving is heavily influenced by who ends up in our studies. Basic variations in the definition of family caregiver can influence our estimates of the magnitude and impact of dementia care. We are just beginning to address the complexities in untangling the differential effects associated with particular caregiver situations and characteristics across different domains of impact (e.g., personal, social, or health impacts).

Too often caregiver research is static. The dynamic aspects of care needs, caregiving roles, and care outcomes need to be examined more fully. We need more attention to how changing disease processes interact with caregiving needs, responsibilities, and available treatments and services. Those who have come to the attention of clinicians and researchers are often providing care for persons at later stages in the disease. Less is known about factors influencing early detection in the community and the process that family members go through in detecting and labeling dementia related symptoms. Although there has been a recent push to include minority and ethnic populations in dementia research, with few exceptions, most studies are still conducted in primarily White, middle-class populations. Even when minority differences are highlighted for attention, comparisons are typically made across groups, and the more subtle within group differences ignored.

There has been progress in the conceptualization of caregiving impacts, with the development of carefully specified conceptual models linking caregiver stressors to health outcomes. Still needed in most research studies is a clearer delineation of terms such as caregiver roles, responsibilities, stresses, burdens, and impacts. Additional conceptualization and measurement of caregiver outcomes is essential to understand better the natural consequences of caregiving responsibilities as well as to evaluate the impact of interventions designed to ameliorate caregiving burdens. For example, outcome measures should be more sensitive to detecting small changes over time, and assess both positive as well as negative caregiver outcomes. The other chapters in this volume will describe in greater depth research advances and challenges involved in designing and evaluating the effectiveness of caregiver interventions.

## IMPLICATIONS FOR POLICY AND PRACTICE

The care of disabled older adults can be burdensome. However, empirical evidence does not support the universality of caregiving stress. For many caregivers of elders with dementia, caregiving is emotionally and physically stressful. Yet, data from some studies of caregivers of elders with functional disabilities indicate that, other than the shared restrictions on personal and leisure time, caregiving is not always perceived as stressful by caregivers (Tennstedt, Cafferata, & Sullivan, 1992; McKinlay, Crawford, & Tennstedt, 1995). From a policy perspective, it is important not to generalize the findings from studies of dementia caregivers to nondementia caregivers and vice versa. Doing so would likely result in over- or under-estimates respectively of the need for support and services. The strains and needs of both groups of caregivers should be acknowledged yet clearly distinguished for at least two reasons: 1) to accurately identify how best to assist caregivers in each group since their stressors, perceived stress, and resulting needs may differ; and 2) to more accurately estimate the demand for long-term care and caregiver support services, both types and amount.

Contrary to the continued concerns of public policy makers, families do not relinquish their caregiving role unnecessarily. Data from a longitudinal study by Tennstedt and colleagues (1993b) support the conclusion that services are used as intended—to support and sustain the informal caregiving arrangement or to fill gaps in needed care. While home and community-based services are used by many, informal care typically predominates in these mixed care arrangements (Tennstedt, Sullivan, McKinlay, & D'Agostino, 1990; Tennstedt et al., 1993b, 1996).

In the case of dementia care, use of formal services is not only appropriate but also clinically indicated as severity increases. From a practice perspective, it is important to determine the optimal mix of formal services and informal care in order to ensure the well-being of both care recipient and caregiver. Transition to a special care environment is another important juncture in this regard. Assistance with appropriate timing and with negotiating a role for continued involvement of the caregiver(s) will facilitate what might be interpreted as another in a series of losses by a caregiver who sees this transition as loss of an important role.

From a policy perspective, the issue of eligibility criteria for services is important. For both publicly and privately (i.e., third party payer) funded services, eligibility typically is based on functional disability in the performance of specified ADLs. The Advisory Panel on Alzheimer's Disease (1989) has advocated for the expansion of eligibility criteria to provide services in situations where the degree of cognitive impairment interferes with the person's ability to complete either IADLs or ADLs without substantial supervision. The cost analyses performed by Paveza and associates (1998) "suggest that changes in cognitive impairment are independent factors affecting cost regardless of the magnitude of ADL/IADL impairment" (p. 79). Similar findings from the National Long-Term Care Channeling Demonstration Project were reported by Liu, McBride, and Coughlin (1990). These findings support the notion of applying a cognitive weighting factor to the degree of ADL/IADL impairment in establishing eligibility for services.

Finally, we should not lose sight of the fact that caregiving is imbedded in the family experience, history, and values. How caregivers respond to the presenting needs for care, how they perceive the personal impact of that care, and how they interface with the formal service system will by shaped by their personal situation. As we have argued for recognition of the heterogeneity of older adults, as researchers, practitioners, and policy makers we must recognize the heterogeneity of their caregivers.

## ACKNOWLEDGMENTS

We would like to thank the National Alliance for Caregiving and American Association of Retired Persons for the use of their data obtained in the *Family Caregiving in the U.S.: Findings from a National Survey*, National Alliance for Caregiving and American Association for Retired Persons, 1997.

## REFERENCES

Advisory Panel on Alzheimer's Disease. (1989). *Report of the Advisory Panel on Alzheimer's Disease*. DHHS. Pub. No. (ADM) 89–1644. Washington, DC: Supt. of Docs., U.S. Government Printing Office.

Bass, D.M., Looman, W., & Ehrlich, P. (1992). Predicting the volume of health and social services: Integrating cognitive impairment into the modified Andersen Framework. *The Gerontologist, 32*, 33–43.

Bass, D.M., Noelker, L.S., & Rechlin, L.R. (1996). The moderating influence of service use on negative caregiving consequences. *Journal of Gerontology: Social Sciences, 51B*, S121–S131.

Beach, S.R., Schulz, R., Yee, J.L., & Jackson, S. (1998). Negative (and positive) health effects of caring for a disabled spouse: Longitudinal findings from the Caregiver Health Effects Study. Manuscript submitted for publication to *Psychology and Aging*.

Beck, A.T., Ward, C.H., Mendelson, M., Mock, J., & Erbaugh, J. (1961). An inventory for measuring depression. *Archives of General Psychiatry, 4*, 561–571.

Bookwala, J., & Schulz, R. (1998). The role of neuroticism and mastery in spouse caregivers' assessment and response to a contextual stressor. *Journal of Gerontology: Psychological Sciences, 53B*, P155–P164.

Bookwala, J., Yee, J.L., & Schulz, R. (1998). Caregiving and Detrimental Mental and Physical Health Outcomes. Manuscript in preparation.

Bourgeois, M.S., Schulz, R., & Burgio, L. (1996). Interventions for caregivers of patients with Alzheimer's Disease: A review and analysis of content, process, and outcomes. *The International Journal of Aging and Human Development*.

Brodaty, H., & Hadzi-Pavlovic, D. (1990). Psychosocial effects on carers of living with persons with dementia. *Australian and New Zealand Journal of Psychiatry, 24*, 351–361.

Burton, L., Kasper, J., Shore, A., Cagney, K., LaVeist, T., Cubbin, C., & German, P. (1995). The structure of informal care: Are there differences by race? *The Gerontologist, 35*, 744–752.

Burton, L.C., Newsom, J.T., Schulz, R., Hirsch, C.H., & German, P.S. (1997). Preventative health behaviors among spousal caregivers. *Preventative Medicine, 26*, 162–169.

Canning, R.D., Dew, M.A., & Davidson, S. (1996). Psychological distress among caregivers to heart transplant recipients. *Social Science and Medicine, 42*, 599–608.

Cantor, M. (1983). Strain among caregivers: A study of experience in the United States. *The Gerontologist, 23*, 597–604.

Caserta, M.S., Lund, D.A., Wright, S.D., & Redburn, D.E. (1987). Caregivers to dementia patients: The utilization of community services. *The Gerontologist, 27*, 209–214.

Cattanach, L., & Tebes, J.K. (1991). The nature of elder impairment and its impact on family caregivers' health and psychosocial functioning. *The Gerontologist, 31*, 246–255.

Chappell, N. (1991). Living arrangement and sources of caregiving. *Journal of Gerontology: Social Sciences, 46*, S1–S8.

Chatters, L.M., Taylor, R.J., & Jackson, J.S. (1985). Size and composition of the informal helper networks of elderly Blacks. *Journal of Gerontology, 40*, 605–614.

Chatters, L.M., Taylor, R.J., & Jackson, J.S. (1986). Aged Blacks' choice for an informal helper network. *Journal of Gerontology, 41*, 94–100.

Cochrane, J.J., Goering, P.N., & Rogers, J.M. (1997). The mental health of informal caregivers in Ontario: An epidemiological survey. *American Journal of Public Health, 87,* 2002–2007.

Collins, C., & Jones, R. (1997). Emotional distress and morbidity in dementia carers: A matched comparison of husbands and wives. *International Journal of Geriatric Psychiatry, 12,* 1168–1173.

Connell, C.M., & Gibson, G.D. (1997). Racial, ethnic, and cultural differences in dementia caregiving: Review and analysis. *The Gerontologist, 37,* 355–364.

Coon, D.W., Schulz, R., & Ory, M.G. (in press). Innovative intervention approaches with Alzheimer's Caregivers. In D. Biegel & A. Blum (Eds.), *Innovations in Practice Service and Delivery Across the Lifespan.* New York: Oxford.

Cox, C. (1993). Services needs and interests: A comparison of African American and White caregivers seeking Alzheimer assistance. *American Journal of Alzheimer's Disease,* May/June, pp. 33–40.

Cox, C., & Monk, A. (1990). Minority caregivers of dementia victims: A comparison of Black and Hispanic families. *Journal of Applied Gerontology, 9,* 340–354.

Diwan, S., Berger, C., & Manns, E.K. (1997). Composition of the home care service package: Predictors of type, volume, and mix of services provided to poor and frail older people. *The Gerontologist, 37,* 169–181.

Draper, B.M., Poulos, C.J., Cole, A.D., Poulos, R.G., & Ehrlick, F. (1992). A comparison of caregivers for elderly stroke and dementia victims. *Journal of the American Geriatrics Society, 40,* 896–901.

Draper, B.M., Poulos, R.G., Poulos, C.J., & Ehrlich, F. (1995). Risk factors for stress in elderly caregivers. *International Journal of Geriatric Psychiatry, 11,* 227–231.

Duke University, Center for the Study on Aging. (1978). *Multidimensional functional assessment: The OARS methodology* (2nd ed.). Durham, NC: Duke University.

Dura, J.R., Stukenberg, K.W., & Kiecolt-Glaser, J.K. (1991). Anxiety and depressive disorders in adult children caring for demented parents. *Psychology and Aging, 6,* 467–473.

Dwyer, J.W., & Coward, R.T. (1991). A multivariate comparison of the involvement of adult sons versus daughters in the care of impaired parents. *Journal of Gerontology: Social Sciences, 46,* S259–S269.

Fredriksen, K.I. (1996). Gender differences in employment and the informal care of adults. *Journal of Women and Aging, 8,* 35–53.

Fuller-Jonap, F., & Haley, W.E. (1995). Mental and physical health of male caregivers of a spouse with Alzheimer's disease. *Journal of Aging and Health, 7,* 99–118.

General Accounting Office. (1998). Alzheimer's disease: Estimates of prevalence in the United States (GAO/HEHS—98–16). Washington, DC: United States General Accounting Office, Health, Education, and Human Services Division.

Gill, C.E., Hinrichsen, G.A., & DiGiuseppe, R. (1998). Factors associated with formal service use by family members of patients with dementia. *The Journal of Applied Gerontology, 17*, 38–52.

Glaser, R., & Kiecolt-Glaser, J.K. (1997). Chronic stress modulates the virus-specific immune response to latent herpes simplex type 1. *Annals of Behavioral Medicine, 19*, 78–82.

Haley, W.E., West, C.A.C., Wadley, V.G., Ford, G.R., White, F.A., Barrett, J.J., Harrell, L.E., & Roth, D.L. (1995). Psychological, social, and health impact of caregiving: A comparison of Black and White dementia family caregivers and noncaregivers. *Psychology and Aging, 10*, 540–552.

Hamilton, E.M. (1996). Factors associated with family caregivers' choice not to use services. *American Journal of Alzheimer's Disease, 11*, 29–38.

Hamilton, M. (1967). Development of a rating scale for primary depressive illness. *British Journal of Social and Clinical Psychology, 6*, 278–296.

Hatch, L. (1991). Informed support patterns of older African-American and White women. *Research on Aging, 13*, 144–170.

Himes, C.L., Jordan, A.K., & Farkas, J.I. (1996). Factors influencing parental caregiving by adult women. *Research on Aging, 18*, 349–370.

Hinrichsen, G.A., & Ramirez, M. (1992). Black and White dementia caregivers: A comparison of their adaptation, adjustment, and service utilization. *The Gerontologist, 32*, 375–381.

Hooker, K., Monahan, D.J., Frazier, L.D., & Shifren, K. (1998). Personality counts for a lot: Predictors of mental and physical health of spouse caregivers in two disease groups. *Journal of Gerontology: Psychological Sciences, 53B*, P73–P85.

Hooyman, N.R., & Gonyea, J. (1995). *Feminist perspectives on family care: Policies for gender justice.* Thousand Oaks, CA: Sage.

Horowitz, A. (1985a). Family caregiving to the frail elderly. In M.P. Lawton & G. Maddox (Eds.), *Annual review of geriatrics and gerontology* (pp. 194–246). New York: Springer.

Horowitz, A. (1985b). Sons and daughters as caregivers to older parents: Differences in role performance and consequences. *The Gerontologist, 25*, 612–617.

Irwin, M., Hauger, R., Patterson, T., Semple, S., Ziegler, M., & Grant, I. (1997). Alzheimer caregiver stress: Basal natural killer cell activity, pituitary-adrenal cortical function, and sympathetic tone. *Annals of Behavioral Medicine, 19*, 83–90.

Johnson, C. (1983). Dyadic family relations and social support. *Gerontologist, 23*, 377–383.

Jutras, S., & Lavoie, J.P. (1995). Living with an impaired elderly person: The informal caregiver's physical and mental health. *Journal of Aging and Health, 7*, 46–73.

Kaye, L.W., & Applegate, J.S. (1990). *Men as caregivers to the elderly: Understanding and aiding unrecognized family support.* Lexington, MA: Lexington Books/DC Heath.

Kiecolt-Glaser, J.K., Glaser, R., Gravenstein, S., Malarkey, W.B., & Sheridan, J. (1996). Chronic stress alters the immune response to influenza virus vaccine in older adults. *Proceedings of the National Academy of Sciences, USA, 93*, 3043–3047.

King, A.C., & Brassington, G. (1997). Enhancing physical and psychological functioning in older family caregivers: The role of regular physical activity. *Annals of Behavioral Medicine, 19*, 91–100.

Kosloski, K.D., & Montogomery, R.J. (1993). Caregiver career lines: Markers and determinants, 30th meeting of the International Institute of Sociology, Paris, France.

Lawton, M.P., Rajagopal, D., Brody, E., & Kleban, M.H. (1992). The dynamics of caregiving for a demented elder among Black and White families. *Journal of Gerontology: Social Sciences, 47*, S156–S164.

Leon, J., Cheng, C.K., & Neumann, P.J. (in press). Health service utilization costs and potential savings for mild, moderate, and severely impaired Alzheimer's disease patients, *Health Affairs.*

Li, L.W., Seltzer, M.M., & Greenberg, J.S. (1997). Social support and depressive symptoms: Differential patterns in wife and daughter caregivers. *Journal of Gerontology: Social Sciences, 52B*, S200–S211.

Light, E., Niederehe, G., & Lebowitz, B.D. (1994). *Stress effects on family caregivers of Alzheimer's patients: Research and interventions.* New York: Springer.

Liu, K., McBride, T.D., & Coughlin, T.A. (1990). Costs of community care for disabled elderly persons. *The policy Implications Inquiry, 27*, 61–72.

Majerovitz, S.D. (1995). Role of family adaptability in the psychological adjustment of spouse caregivers to patients with dementia. *Psychology of Aging, 10*, 447–457.

MaloneBeach, E.E., & Zarit, S.H. (1995). Dimensions of social support and social conflict as predictors of caregiver depression. *International Psychogeriatrics, 7*, 25–38.

Marks, N.F. (1996). Caregiving across the lifespan: National prevalence and predictors. *Family Relations, 45*, 27–36.

McKinlay, J.B., Crawford, S.L., & Tennstedt, S.L. (1995). The everyday impacts of providing informal care to dependent elders and their consequences for the care recipients. *Journal of Aging and Health, 7*, 497–528.

McKinlay, J.B., & Tennstedt, S.L. (1986). "Social Networks and the Care of Frail Elders." Final Report to the National Institute on Aging, Grant No. AG03869. Boston: Boston University.

Miller, B., McFall, S., & Campbell, R.T. (1994). Changes in sources of community long-term care among African-American and White frail older persons. *Journal of Gerontology: Social Sciences, 49,* S14–S24.

Moritz, D.J., Kasl, S.V., & Berkman, L.F. (1989). The impact of living with a cognitively impaired elderly spouse: Depressive symptoms and social functioning. *Journal of Gerontology: Social Sciences, 44,* S17–S27.

Moritz, D.J., Kasl, S.V., & Ostfeld, A.M. (1992). The health impact of living with a cognitively impaired elderly spouse. *Journal of Aging and Health, 4,* 244–267.

Morrissey, E., Becker, J., & Rupert, M.P. (1990). Coping resources and depression in the caregiving spouses of Alzheimer patients. *British Journal of Medical Psychology, 63,* 161–171.

Mui, A. (1995). Perceived health and functional status among spouse caregivers of frail older persons. *Journal of Aging and Health, 7,* 283–300.

Mullan, J.T. (1993). Barriers to the use of formal services among Alzheimer's caregivers. In S.H. Zarit, L.I. Pearlin, & K.W. Schaie (Eds.), *Caregiving systems: Informal and formal helpers* (pp. 241–259). Hillsdale, NJ: Lawrence Erlbaum.

National Alliance for Caregiving and the American Association of Retired Persons. (1997). *Family caregiving in the US: Findings from a national survey. Final Report.* Bethesda, MD: National Alliance for Caregiving.

Pariante, C.M., Carpiniello, B., Orru., M.G., Sitzia, R., Piras, A., Farci, A.M.G., Del Giacco, G.S., Piludu, G., & Miller, A.H. (1997). Chronic caregiving stress alters peripheral blood immune parameters: The role of age and severity of stress. *Psychotherapy and Psychosomatics, 66,* 199–207.

Paveza, G.J., Mensah, E., Cohen, D., Williams, S., & Jankowski, L. (1998). Costs of community-based long-term care services to the cognitively impaired aged. *Journal of Mental Health and Aging, 4,* 69–82.

Peek, C.W., Zsembik, B.A., & Coward, R.T. (1997). The changing caregiving networks of older adults. *Research on Aging, 19,* 333–361.

Penning, M.J. (1995). Cognitive impairment, caregiver burden, and the utilization of home health services. *Journal of Aging and Health, 7,* 233–253.

Pruchno, R.A., Peters, N.D., & Burant, C.J. (1995). Mental health of coresident family caregivers: Examination of a two-factor model. *Journal of Gerontology: Psychological Sciences, 50B,* P247–P256.

Radloff, L.S. (1977). The CES-D scale: A self-report depression scale for research in the general population. *Applied Psychological Measurement, 1,* 385–401.

Redinbaugh, E.M., MacCullum, R.C., & Kiecolt-Glaser, J.K. (1995). Recurrent syndromal depression in caregivers. *Psychology in Aging, 10*, 358–368.

Rose-Rego, S.K., Strauss, M.E., & Smyth, K.A. (1998). Differences in the perceived well-being of wives and husbands caring for persons with Alzheimer's disease. *The Gerontologist, 38*, 224–230.

Schulz, R., Newsom, J., Mittelmark, M., Burton, L., Hirsch, C., & Jackson, S. (1997). Health effects of caregiving: The caregiver health effects study, an ancillary study of the cardiovascular health study. *Annals of Behavioral Medicine, 19*, 110–116.

Schulz, R., & O'Brien, A.T. (1994). Alzheimer's disease caregiving: An overview. *Seminars in Speech and Language, 15*, 185–193.

Schulz, R., O'Brien, A.T., Bookwala, J., & Fleissner, K. (1995). Psychiatric and physical morbidity effects of dementia caregiving: Prevalence, correlates, and causes. *The Gerontologist, 35*, 771–791.

Schulz, R., & Quittner, A.L. (1998). Caregiving through the life span: An overview and future directions. *Health Psychology, 17*, 107–111.

Shanas, E. (1979). The family as a social support system in old age. *Gerontologist, 19*, 169–174.

Shaw, W.S., Patterson, T.L., Semple, S.J., Ho, S., Irwin, M.R., Hauger, R.L., & Grant, I. (1997). Longitudinal analysis of multiple indicators of health decline among spousal caregivers. *Annals of Behavioral Medicine, 19*, 101–109.

Soldo, B., & Myllyluoma, J. (1983). Caregivers who live with dependent elderly. *Gerontologist, 23*, 605–611.

Stephens, S., & Christianson, J. (1986). *Informal care of the elderly.* Lexington, MA: Lexington Books.

Stoller, E.P., Forster, L.E., & Duniho, T.S. (1992). Systems of parent care within sibling networks. *Research on Aging, 14*, 313–330.

Stommel, M., Given, B.A., Given, C.W., & Collins, C. (1995). The impact of the frequency of care activities on the division of labor between primary caregivers and other care providers. *Research on Aging, 17*, 412–433.

Stommel, M., Given, C.W., & Given, B.A. (1998). Racial differences in the division of labor between primary and secondary caregivers. *Research on Aging, 20*, 199–217.

Stone, R., Cafferata, G.L., & Sangl, J. (1987). Caregivers of the frail and elderly: A national profile. *The Gerontologist, 27*, 616–626.

Tennstedt, S.L., Cafferata, G.L., & Sullivan, L. (1992). Depression among caregivers of impaired elders. *Journal of Aging and Health, 4*, 58–76.

Tennstedt, S.L., & Chang, B. (1998). The relative contribution of ethnicity versus socioeconomic status in explaining differences in disability and receipt of informal care. *Journal of Gerontology: Social Sciences, 53*, S1–S10.

Tennstedt, S.L., Crawford, S.L., & McKinlay, J.B. (1993a). Determining the pattern of community care: Is coresidence more important than caregiver relationship? *Journal of Gerontology: Social Sciences, 48,* S74–S83.

Tennstedt, S.L., Crawford, S.L., & McKinlay, J.B. (1993b). Is family care on the decline? A longitudinal investigation of the substitution of formal long-term care services for informal care. *The Milbank Quarterly, 71,* 601–624.

Tennstedt, S.L., Harrow, B., & Crawford, S. (1996). Informal vs. formal services: Changes in patterns of care over time. *Journal of Aging and Social Policy, 7,* 71–92.

Tennstedt, S.L., McKinlay, J.B., & Sullivan, L. (1989). Informal care for frail elders: The role of secondary caregivers. *The Gerontologist, 29,* 677–683.

Tennstedt, S.L., Sullivan, L., McKinlay, J.B., & D'Agostino, R. (1990). How important is functional status as a predictor of service use by older people? *Journal of Aging and Health, 2,* 439–461.

Vitaliano, P.P., Russo, J., Scanlan, J.M., & Greeno, K. (1996). Weight changes in caregivers of Alzheimer's care recipients: Psychobehavioral predictors. *Psychology and Aging, 11,* 155–163.

Vitaliano, P.P., Scanlan, J.M., Krenz, C., Schwartz, R.S., & Marcovina, S.M. (1996). Psychological distress, caregiving, and metabolic variables. *Journal of Gerontology: Psychological Sciences, 51B,* P290–P299.

Vitaliano, P.P., Schulz, R., Kiecolt-Glaser, J.K., & Grant, I. (1997). Research on physiological and physical concomitants of caregiving: Where do we go from here? *Annals of Behavioral Medicine, 19,* 117–123.

Young, R.F., & Kahana, E. (1989). Specifying caregiver outcomes: Gender and relationship aspects of caregiving strain. *The Gerontologist, 29,* 660–666.

# 2

## Understanding the Interventions Process: A Theoretical/Conceptual Framework for Intervention Approaches to Caregiving

*Richard Schulz, Dolores Gallagher-Thompson,
William Haley, and Sara Czaja*

### THEORETICAL PERSPECTIVES ON CAREGIVING

The goal of this chapter is to introduce a number of relevant theoretical perspectives useful in understanding caregiving. While our attention primarily will be focused on theories concerning the impact of caregiving on the caregiver, we also present a conceptual framework for characterizing interventions for dementia caregivers. We will begin by asking a question that has not been addressed directly by researchers in this area, namely: Why do people help? Next, we present Family Systems Theory as a perspective for understanding the impact of dementia on the family. This is followed by a discussion of both generic and caregiver specific models of stress-coping that attempt to predict the impact of caregiving at the individual level. Finally, we present a conceptual framework for characterizing caregiver interventions in order to stimulate comparisons across studies and to better identify which features of interventions and which delivery methods are most effective in achieving desired outcomes for the patient and caregiver.

## WHY DO PEOPLE HELP?

Human beings throughout the world provide care to relatives and friends each year, often at great cost to the quality of their own lives as well as their health (see chapter 1). Why do people provide such large quantities of help, particularly in view of the apparent personal costs often associated with providing care? To some, the answer to this question may be self-evident. There exist strong normative expectations in most cultures that we help our kin. Although cultural norms provide at a least a partial answer to this question, it is clearly not the complete answer. The purpose of this section is to address this question from multiple perspectives.

### Motives for Helping

Attempts to identify specific motives for helping have yielded two types of explanations. One assumes that helping serves an egoistic or self-serving motive while the other centers on empathy and altruism (Batson & Coke, 1983). The egoistic explanation argues that helping is motivated by the anticipation of rewards for helping and punishment for not helping. These rewards and punishments may be either external (such as praise) or intrapsychic (such as avoiding guilt). Individuals may help for obvious reasons, such as the expectation of payment, gaining social approval (Baumann, Cialdini, & Kendrick, 1981), avoiding censure (Reis & Gruzen, 1976), receiving esteem in exchange for helping (Hatfield, Walster, & Piliavin, 1978), complying with social norms (Berkowitz, 1972), seeing oneself as a good person (Bandura, 1977), or avoiding guilt (Hoffman, 1982). For example, caring for a relative in order to prevent institutionalization can be interpreted in terms of avoiding censure, complying with social norms, and/or seeing oneself as a good person (Brody, Poulshock, & Masciocchi, 1978).

Guilt and indebtedness are the motives alluded to by the often heard comment made by caregivers, "I know I'm doing everything

I can for my mother, but somehow I still feel guilty" (Brody, 1985, p. 26), or in the idea that providing care is a repayment in kind for care provided by the parent at an earlier age. Feelings of guilt may also be the motivating force for individuals who feel they must atone for past sins (e.g., neglect, bad treatment) against their spouse or parent.

A theoretical basis for indebtedness as a motive is provided by Greenberg (1980) who states that feeling indebted has motivational properties, such that the greater its magnitude, the greater the resultant arousal and discomfort, and hence, the stronger the ensuing attempts to deal with or reduce it. Feelings of indebtedness should be higher to the extent that individuals feel the help provided them was based on altruistic motives on the part of the helper, help was given in response to requests or pleas for help from the recipients, and the helper incurred costs in providing the help. All of these factors apply to spousal and parent-child relationships and may be factors worthy of attention in our efforts to understand who becomes the caregiver, the magnitude of the costs the caregiver is willing to incur in providing help to a relative, and the amount of residual guilt experienced by the caregiver.

A substantially different perspective on human nature is provided by a theory of helping that is based on purely altruistic motivation. According to this view, individuals help others because they are able to adopt the perspective of the other, experience an emotional response—empathy—congruent with the other's welfare, and empathic emotion evokes a motivation aimed at reducing the other's needs. The magnitude of the altruistic motivation is assumed to be a direct function of the magnitude of the empathic emotion. Unlike the egoistic perspective described earlier, the primary goal of empathically evoked altruism is to benefit the other and not the self, even though benefits to oneself may be a consequence of helping (see Batson & Coke, 1983, for a review of the relevant literature). It seems reasonable to assume, although it has not been demonstrated empirically, that the ability to empathize may be based on such variables as kinship, similarity, prior interaction, attachment, or some combination of these, all of which are relevant to the intrafamilial caregiving situation. This suggests that higher levels of similarity, attachment, and prior positive interaction should result in greater levels of caregiving, although they may also lead to higher levels of distress among caregivers (Cantor, 1983; Horowitz, 1985).

Although helping an elderly relative is likely to be based on both altruistic and egoistic motivations, it would be interesting to know whether the two motives differentially affect caregiver well-being. Since emotions are a central feature of altruistically motivated helping, one might hypothesize that the emotional status of the patient plays an important role in determining the amount of help provided and the affect of the helper. Moreover, the nature of the cognitive declines associated with a disease such as Alzheimer's suggests that altruistic motivation may be more relevant to the early stages of the disease when cognitive function is still more or less intact and the caregiver can readily empathize with the patient, and that egoistically motivated helping is the driving force in later stages of the disease when cognitive function is debilitated.

## Social Norms and Helping

Sociological explanations for why people help frequently emphasize the role of social norms, such as reciprocity, equity, or social responsibility. The reciprocity norm enjoins us to pay back what others give to us, and the equity norm underscores the importance of costs and rewards in a relationship. Simply stated, a relationship is equitable if those involved receive a return from it proportional to what they have invested in it. According to the social responsibility norm, helping others in need—the sick, infirm, or very young—is a duty that should not be shirked, although the manner in which and how much we help another may depend on our beliefs about who or what is responsible for the cause and solution of the recipient's problem (see Brickman et al., 1982: Thompson & Pitts, 1992).

These norms may differ substantially due to cultural and contextual variables. For example, in Cuban-American families there is often an extremely strong culturally based expectation that daughters should provide care for an impaired relative (Haley, Han, & Henderson, 1998). In some Asian cultures, the wives of the oldest son are deemed to have a similarly high expectation of providing care (Haley et al., 1998). African-American family caregivers are far less likely to place their relatives in nursing homes than White families (Skinner, 1995), and in White families nursing home placement is lower when the family caregiver is a daughter than in other caregiving relationships (Moen, Robison, & Fields, 1994).

Social norms are obviously relevant to understanding caregiver behavior. For example, they may be useful in predicting caregiving behavior among successive cohorts of caregivers, but the existence of norms does not in itself explain why people adhere to them. We still need to answer the questions: Why do these norms exist? Where do they come from? To address these questions we need to examine some underlying characteristics about the nature of human beings.

## Sociobiology of Helping

The social-psychological theories of helping described above are based on the notion that social behavior in humans is developed through experience and learning, rather than through instinct. A new theoretical approach that can have direct relevance for understanding the helping process—sociobiology—challenges this orthodoxy. Sociobiology suggests that the fundamental goal of the organism is not mere survival or survival of its offspring, but "inclusive fitness," to pass on the maximum number of genes to the next generation (Hamilton, 1964). Sociobiology believes that human helping can only be understood in terms of the human evolutionary past—close relatives help each other, even at risk of their lives, in order to increase the chance that their genes will survive in their relatives (Forsyth, 1987). Sociobiology thus takes a positive view of human nature, believing that human beings are innately helpful to each other albeit for a "selfish" purpose, the preservation of the gene pool. Beyond the clear benefit of helping one's own family members, evolutionary psychology and sociobiology suggest that personality characteristics or patterns of adaptive behavior such as empathy to the distress of others may be generally adaptive (Wilson, 1998). Similarly, cooperation may be generally adaptive in ensuring survival or strength of the individual, family, and community (Axelrod, 1984).

To date, tests of this theory, which have relied primarily on research with nonhumans, indicate that helping is much more common among close relatives than among strangers and in dense rather than dispersed communities (Barash, 1982). Applying this theory to family caregiving, it can be argued that, in general, intrafamily helping behaviors enhance the survival of the familial gene pool. Thus intrafamilial helping of all types is desirable—the old helping the young as well as the young helping the old. This general rule, however, has at least one qualification: When resource constraints demand that priorities be set among those who can be helped, this perspective would predict that resources would be allocated to the young rather than the old. It should also be noted that sociobiological explanations of family caregiving have one very important limitation: family caregiving for older adults enhances the survival of individuals who are generally no longer able to reproduce. In addition, human evolution occurred for the most part during a historical period in which survival to old age was extremely uncommon. Thus cultural explanations remain important in explaining late life caregiving.

There are clearly substantial cultural differences in norms for the provision of care to older adults. One extreme example is the Niue culture from an independent Polynesian island. According to an ethnographic analysis (Barker, 1997), the Niue place an extreme value on reciprocity. Frail elders, particularly cognitively impaired elders, are viewed as unable to contribute to the well-being of the society. Families and neighbors will not summon freely available medical care, even for treatable conditions, for frail older adults. This culture apparently views neglect as appropriately hastening the death of older adults who are no longer productive.

Our discussion of why people help raises a number of important questions regarding the instigation and perpetuation of intrafamilial helping, but it does not directly address questions concerning patient and family outcomes associated with caregiving. In order to address this issue, we will describe family *systems theory*, which attempts to understand chronic illness in the context of the entire family. This will be followed by discussion of how humans cope with stressors like caregiving at the individual level.

## THEORETICAL PERSPECTIVES ON THE COSTS AND BENEFITS OF PROVIDING CARE

### Impact on the Family

An overarching perspective on family caregiving may be found in theories that view the family unit itself as the object of analysis. These theories are explicitly discipline-spanning, since they stem from the premises of general systems theory (von Bertalanffy, 1968). *General systems theory* sees units at all levels of analysis as containing interacting components that function in a coordinated way to deal with the environment. The pattern of interactions among components is established as the system attempts to adapt to the demands of the external environment. When an effective and efficient adaptation is achieved, the system is in balance, or equilibrium. Systems seek such homeostasis because they demand the least effort from each component. These basic assumptions of systems theory lead to the premise that one can understand the actions of any system element only by examining the relationships that exist within all components of a system.

The family has been analyzed extensively from a systems perspective. Family members are viewed as interacting elements in a *family system* that attempts to synchronize its efforts to deal with its social environment. Each family, over time, develops a stable pattern of interaction that permits it to meet environmental demands in an effective and efficient manner. From a systems perspective, the behaviors of one family member can be understood only by examining his or her interrelationships with other family members. This framework emphasizes such system variables as role relationships and communication patterns that emerge and stabilize in the family's efforts to best fulfill its needs (Parsons & Bales, 1955). Once the family system of defined role patterns attains a functional equilibrium, it tends to be perpetuated until an external change serves as a stimulus for a new adaptation (Bowan, 1966).

Another related theoretical framework is found in *crisis theory*. Because systems tend to freeze into stable patterns of interaction, any situational change may represent a potential crisis, requiring restructuring of all family interaction patterns. Such crises create severe stress on family members as they react to the disequilibrium created by the life event. Because stress is a threat to the ongoing functioning of the system, members mobilize energy to establish a new equilibrium as quickly as possible.

We can distinguish between two types of family crises, maturational and situational (Gray-Price & Szczesny, 1985). Maturational family crises are associated with normal developmental stages, occurring at such major life transitions as childbirth, school entry, children leaving home, and retirement (Haley & Ranson, 1976; Minuchin, 1974). Because these predictable life-stage events inevitably require major restructuring of family interactions, adaptation is facilitated by the prior awareness that most people have of these transition points. Thus, such transitions can be anticipated and prepared for, thereby softening their impact.

In contrast, unpredictable crises, such as the illness of a family member, may be viewed as sudden major disruptions to the entire family system. Its ability to maintain itself in achieving its goals is undermined (Cassileth & Hamilton, 1979). The inevitable immediate consequence of such a crisis is anxiety and disequilibrium, not only to the patient but to all other members of the family system. Family systems theory focuses on how the entire family copes with the crisis of illness of one family member. It analyzes the ways the family adapts to the task demands of different stages of this crisis (Giacquinta, 1977; Kaplan, 1982; Leventhal, Leventhal, & Nguyen, 1985; Mailick, 1979). For example, family members must quickly learn to negotiate with the medical system in order to gain needed information and mediate for the patient. These demands occur while family members are also confronting their own initial fears regarding the overall impact of the patient's illness on their lives, as well as the possibility of losing their loved one. Another task demand involves the need to figure out a mode of dealing with the patient as he or she reacts to the illness, which may involve withdrawal from normal family patterns of interaction (Singer, 1983).

Giacquinta (1977), for example, has developed a model that identifies ten phases of family functioning during four different stages of cancer and its aftermath. Her model begins with the initial disorganizing impact that a cancer diagnosis has on family functioning, and proceeds through the patient's decline and death to the family's post-bereavement efforts to establish a new equilibrium. Giacquinta also identifies specific hurdles that the family must overcome at each phase, from despair over the initial diagnosis to alienation for families who cannot expand their social networks again after bereavement.

Since chronic illnesses such as dementia involve long-term changes in the family members' abilities to perform expected family roles, new role patterns need to be established within the family system (Bruhn, 1977; Mailick, 1979). Wellisch (1985) suggests that an illness impacts marital processes relating to the independence of each spouse, their intimacy and communication patterns, and their sexual relationship. Such role realignments are often accompanied by resentment, in part because of the need to take on additional and unfamiliar role behaviors (Singer, 1983; Vettese, 1981). And because family roles vary at different stages of the family life cycle, adaptation problems and resolutions will also differ (Gray-Price & Szczesny, 1985; Herz & McGoldrick, 1980: Leventhal et al., 1985).

Because of the extensive demands on families dealing with serious illness, it is not surprising that some families of the chronically ill fail to adapt, experiencing severe disruption and breakdown (Bruhn, 1977; Giacquinta, 1977; Kaplan, 1982; Vettese, 1981). The level of family functioning prior to the crisis appears to be a factor central to its ability to cope with the crisis of illness. Families with better communication, better problem-solving skills, and flexible role relationships are viewed as having better ability to cope realistically with the crisis. In contrast, families that have more rigid interaction styles may experience more difficulty (Quinn & Herndon, 1986). Even highly functional families may need help in dealing with the crisis of serious illness (Gray-Price & Szczesny, 1985; Kaplan, 1982; Mailick, 1979; Singer, 1983; Vettese, 1981).

The family systems perspective summarized here has provided a central theoretical framework for many therapeutic interventions of family reactions to illness. Family-based intervention research focused on AD caregivers is designed to assist family members manage and live with the dementing illness at the highest level of effectiveness. The underlying assumption is that with rare exceptions, primary caregivers have resources within themselves as well as their families and communities that can be harnessed to reduce or solve problems associated with caring for a demented patient. The challenge for family-based intervention research is to identify the specific problems caregivers are experiencing, the efficacy of family problem-solving styles and solutions, the range of useable family resources available to the caregiver and their formal support systems, the range of useable community resources available and accessible to the family, and the capacity of caregivers and their families to collaborate in the caregiving effort (Szapocznik & Kurtines, 1989). In the case of caregiving, the target problem is defined by the caregiver's burden and the goal is to identify those patterns of family interactions that may be linked to the symptom of caregiver burden. Such patterns may include, for example, sequences of behaviors in which family members offer help to a complaining caregiver, and the caregiver— angry for not having received help before—vents her anger at the offering family member, thereby bringing about an interruption of the offered help in an already ambivalent family member. The intervention in such an instance may involve helping the family member to understand the caregiver's feelings and respond to the feelings of frustration with understanding rather than with a sense of rejection.

## Impact on the Individual

Clinical observations about family caregiving have highlighted the fact that caregivers react with marked individual differences to seemingly similar circumstances. Some family caregivers react with guilt, depression, and poor health, while other families provide care with either no ill effects or even experience positive consequences. Thus, theorists have developed models explaining individual differences in caregiving. Much of the literature on caregiving can be characterized as an attempt to link some antecedent variables to outcomes assessing the well-being of individuals who provide support to ill relatives. Common independent variables in this conceptualization might be the functional or behavioral status of the patient, and a representative dependent variable any one of a number of measures assessing the psychosocial status or physical and mental health of the caregiver, such as morale, life satisfaction, depression, or perceived strain or burden. A large number of individual and situational conditioning variables characteristic of all stress-coping models may moderate or mediate the relation between stressors and caregiver well-being. Examples include age, gender, socioeconomic status, type and quality of relationship between caregiver and patient, social support, as well as personality attributes of the caregiver such as self-esteem and locus of control. The need for conditioning or intervening variables is justified by data demonstrating only moderate relationships between independent variables such as patient impairment (e.g., ability to perform activities of daily living (ADL) tasks) and caregiver outcomes, such as mental health (Coppel, Burton,

Becker, & Fiore, 1985; Pagel, Becker, & Coppel, 1985; Schulz, O'Brien, Bookwala, & Fleissner, 1995).

A number of theorists have proposed stress process models that share common features (e.g., Cohler, Groves, Borden, & Lazarus, 1989; Haley, Levine, Brown, & Bartolucci, 1987; Montgomery, Stull, & Borgatta, 1985; Schulz, Tompkins, Wood, & Decker, 1987; Schulz, Tompkins, & Rau, 1988). On the whole, these models provide a convenient framework for organizing the large number of variables relevant to understanding the caregiving process.

*The Basic Stress-Coping Model.* Probably the most basic way of conceptualizing the caregiving experience is in terms of a framework for interactions between the individual and the environment (Eliott & Eisdorfer, 1982). This model, illustrated in Figure 2.1, has three primary elements: a potential activator (x), an individual's reaction (y) to the activator, and the consequences (z) or sequaele to the reactions. Mediators are thought to be the filters and modifiers that act on each stage of the x-y-z sequence to produce individual variations. In the laboratory, specifying the x-y-z sequence can be relatively straightforward. For example, injecting an antigenic sub-

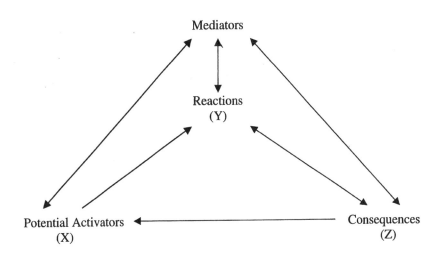

**FIGURE 2.1   The basic x-y-z stress model (from Elliot & Eisdorfer, 1982).**

stance (x) under the skin of a healthy individual results in an immunologic response (y) that produces local swelling, redness, and tenderness (z) (Elliott & Eisdorfer, 1982). Few nonlaboratory situations, however, are as easy to characterize or understand. A given activator may elicit a strong reaction in one person and none at all in another, or it may result in a response at one point in time but not another. Moreover, distinctions between reactions and consequences are often difficult to make.

The basic x-y-z model has been elaborated and applied to many caregiving situations and has been very useful in identifying and organizing variables thought to affect caregiving outcomes (see Biegel, Sales, & Schulz, 1991, for a review of stress models applied to caregiving). One of the most recent iterations of a stress process model may be particularly applicable to the dementia caregiving in as much as it attempts to link environmental stressors to health outcomes (Cohen, Kessler, & Gordon, 1995). An adaptation of this model is presented in Figure 2.2.

The sequential relations between components of this model can be described as follows. The primary stressors or environmental demands include the functional limitations and problem behaviors of the dementia patient and related social and environmental stressors. When confronted with these stressors, people evaluate whether the demands pose a potential threat and whether sufficient adaptive capacities are available to cope with them. If they perceive the environmental demands as threatening and at the same time view their coping resources as inadequate, they perceive themselves as under stress. The appraisal of stress is presumed to result in negative affect, which under extreme conditions may directly contribute to the onset of affective psychiatric disorders. Negative emotional responses may also trigger behavioral or physiological responses that place the individual at increased risk for psychiatric or physical illness.

It is also conceivable, although less likely when applied to dementia caregiving, that stressors are appraised as benign and/or that individuals feel that they have the capacity to deal with the stressors. This in turn leads to positive emotional responses that may lead to salutary physiological and behavioral responses. Although this pathway is theoretically possible and has been demonstrated empirically in some instances, it is important to note that this pathway is both less common and, on the whole, has less empirical support.

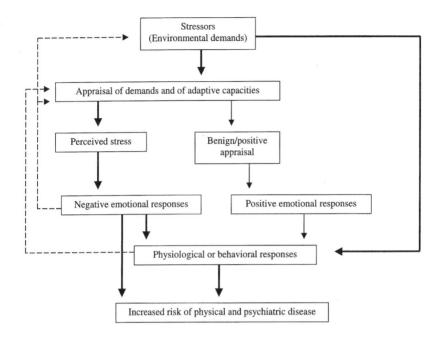

**FIGURE 2.2 A unified model of the stress-health process applied to dementia caregiving (adapted from Cohen, Kessler, and Gordon, 1995).**

Two other features of this model are important to point out. One critical feature is that environmental stressors can place the individual at risk for negative health outcomes even when the appraisal of the stressor does not result in perceptions of stress or negative emotional responses. This is illustrated by the arrow linking stressors to physiological and behavioral responses. For example, a caregiver may take pride in doing an excellent job of caring for a demented relative without realizing that they are neglecting their own needs such as eating regularly or seeing a doctor to attend to their own health problems. The second feature of this model concerns the existence of many possible feedback loops, a few of which are illustrated with dashed lines. Although the model is primarily unidirectional, it should be noted that dealing with stressors is a complex, dynamic process in which responses at one stage of the model may subsequently feed back to earlier stages. One example of this process is represented by the dashed line linking emotional responses to the stressor and the appraisal process. A negative emotional response to a stressor might subsequently increase the stressor itself or impact negatively on the appraisal of the stressor. This might happen, for example, when a caregiver becomes distressed in response to the disruptive behavior of a care recipient, who then becomes more disruptive because of the caregivers response, and so on.

*Enduring Outcomes—Caregiving Endpoints.* Caregiving endpoints are the prolonged or cumulative consequences of being exposed to the demands of caregiving. The stress-health model presented here focuses on health as the primary outcome of the stress health process because there exists strong consensus that health is an important outcome at both the individual and societal level and because stress and health have been consistently linked in the empirical literature. In addition, one of the goals of most interventions for caregivers is to improve or maintain the psychological and physical well-being of the caregiver. Nevertheless, our focus on health should be viewed as illustrative rather than as definitive. Other important outcomes examined in the caregiving literature include institutionalization of the care recipient, and a variety of role strains such as family conflict and economic problems which may further exacerbate the distress experienced by the caregiver and compromise the health of the caregiver (Pearlin, Mullan, Semple, & Skaff, 1990). Specific examples of the latter category include the multiple role conflicts caused by the demands of caregiving. Daughters caring for a disabled parent must often juggle multiple roles including care provision to parents and children, meeting the needs of their spouse, and fulfilling the demands of working full time.

*Contextual Variables/Mediators and Moderators.* All models of caregiving recognize that contextual or situational and individual difference variables contribute to caregiving outcomes. This category of variables is broadly defined to include the social networks and support systems of caregivers; characteristics of caregivers including socioeconomic status, health, gender, and relationship to patients, the quality of the relationship between caregiver and care recipient, number of competing roles such as mother, wife and worker; as well as personality attributes such as orientation toward control and neuroticism. It also includes factors characterizing the environment, such as the availability and utilization of professional services.

The large number of studies focused on these variables has paid off in a significant body of reliable findings (e.g., see chapter 1; Horowitz, 1985; U.S. House of Representatives, 1987, Schulz et al., 1995). At the descriptive level, investigators have characterized the caregiving population in terms of gender, age, race, ethnicity, marital status, employment, economic status, health status, and living arrangements. For example, we know that (a) most caregivers are female; (b) their average age is about 57 years; (c) about 70% of all caregivers are married; (d) one third of informal caregivers are employed, although as a group both men and women caregivers are less likely to be employed than similarly aged counterparts; (e) compared to their age peers in the general population, male and female caregivers are more likely to report adjusted family incomes below the poverty line; (f) their self-assessed health is lower than their age peers; and (g) approximately three quarters of caregivers live with the disabled family member or friend (see chapter 1 for descriptive data on dementia and nondementia caregivers).

A second body of research examines these variables in terms of their direct relationship to caregiving impact. As one would expect, living arrangements between caregivers and care recipients are major predictors of caregiver involvement, behavior, and burden. Caregivers who live with the impaired elderly are more involved with the daily care of patients and experience greater limitations on their personal lives. Employed caregivers frequently experience conflict between the demands of work and the needs of patients. Caregivers with a great deal of social support cope better with the demands of caregiving than those with little support.

A third body of research treats these variables as interactive conditioning factors that moderate the relationships between stressors and their impact on caregivers. One example of this approach is the stress-buffering hypothesis applied to social support. According to this view, individuals exposed to high levels of caregiving stress benefit from support received from others, but individuals who are not stressed or who experience low levels of stress as a result of caregiving exhibit no beneficial effects attributable to social support.

One of the important contributions of research on social support is its emphasis on the search for mechanisms through which caregiving stressors exert their impact on caregiver outcomes. For example, support may play a role at two different points in the causal chain linking stress to illness. It may intervene between the stressor and a stress reaction by attenuating or preventing a stress appraisal response, or it may intervene after the stress is experienced and prevent the onset of pathological outcomes by reducing the emotional reaction, dampening physiologic processes, or altering maladaptive behavior responses (Cohen, 1988). Thus knowing that others will be available to help care for patients when necessary may prevent caregivers from feeling burdened or stressed. Alternatively, the availability of social support may dampen the impact of a perceived stressor by providing helpful information or assistance or by facilitating healthful behaviors.

Clearly, a comprehensive model of the caregiving experience would be much more complex than Figure 2.2 illustrating the stress-health process. This complexity represents both a challenge and an opportunity. On the one hand, we are never likely to fully understand the caregiving experience and its many individual variations. On the other hand, the rich and interactive nature of the caregiving experience presents many opportunities for the creative interventionist interested in enhancing the life of the caregiver.

## DEVELOPING A CONCEPTUAL MODEL
## FOR DEMENTIA INTERVENTIONS

As indicated in our review of the intervention literature (see chapter 3), formal interventions for dementia caregivers have existed for almost two decades. Attempts to characterize interventions used in dementia caregiving studies have typically focused on the broad goals of the intervention (e.g., Knight, Lutzky, & Macofsky-Urban, 1993; Bourgeois & Schulz, 1996; Dunkin & Anderson-Hanley, 1998). For example, interventions have been classified in terms of key functions they provide such as education, support, or respite, but they have not been explicitly linked to a general stress process framework described above. The goal of this section of this chapter is to describe a comprehensive classification system for dementia interventions that captures the content, process, and goals of an intervention in a theoretically relevant manner.

The first question we address is, how does our characterization of the caregiver stress process relate to the intervention strategies used with dementia caregivers? Given the complex, multifaceted nature of most interventions for dementia caregivers, one could characterize them along many different dimensions. Based on the stress process model presented above, we focus on four relatively orthogonal dimensions: 1) the primary entity being targeted by the intervention (i.e., the caregiver, the care recipient, or the social/ physical environment); 2) the primary domain being targeted (i.e., cognitive skills, knowledge, behavior, or affect); 3) the intensity of the intervention (i.e., amount of time or frequency of interventionist contact with caregiver/care recipient); and 4) personalization (i.e., extent to which intervention is tailored to the individual needs of the participant). The first two dimensions were derived from the general stress-health model while the latter two dimensions capture pragmatics of the delivery system that may attenuate the impact of a specific intervention. Each of these dimensions is further defined below and in the accompanying tables.

*Primary Entity Being Targeted (See Table 2.1).* We recognize that the caregiver serves as the vehicle through which all interventions are delivered, but the interventions vary with respect to the locus of their primary intended effect. With some interventions the primary goal is to change the physical or social environment, while with others it is to induce change (e.g., behavior, affect) within the caregiver or the care recipient.

*Primary Domain Being Targeted (See Table 2.1).* Interventions also vary with respect to the primary domain being targeted. For example, some interventions are designed to be primarily informational and increase the knowledge of the caregiver about themselves, the care recipient, or the social environment. Other interventions emphasize more generalizable cognitive skills that could be applied to many different situations. Alternatively, an intervention might focus on changing the behavior of the caregiver or caregiver affect.

*Delivery System Characteristics—Intensity and Personalization (See Table 2.2).* This category includes a broad array of factors that character-

**TABLE 2.1  Definitions Used to Characterize Interventions in Terms of Entity and Domain Targeted**

| | Primary Entity Targeted | | |
|---|---|---|---|
| Primary domain targeted | Caregiver | Care recipient | Family/social and physical environment |
| **Cognition—Knowledge** | **Problem:** Lack of information/insight about the caregiving process and the role of caregivers. | **Problem:** Lack of information about the disease affecting patient, prognosis of illness, and factors affecting care recipient behavior. | **Problem:** Lack of information about the potential role of other family members in caregiving, the secondary impacts of caregiving, and factors in the physical environment that might impede caregiving. |
| | **Goal:** Acquire information and knowledge about caregivers and their role in the caregiving process. | **Goal:** Increased information and knowledge about care recipients and their role in the caregiving process. | **Goal:** Provide knowledge and information about the social and physical environment and how they might influence caregiver transactions. |
| | **Examples:** This category includes information and knowledge related to caregiving that concerns primarily the caregiver. For example, it might include information about how caregiving affects the caregiver, how others respond to caregiving, as well as information that might be useful in accessing resources and support directly relevant to the caregiver. | **Examples:** This category includes information and knowledge about the care recipient that might be useful to the caregiver. This might include information about services available for care recipients, knowledge about the disease and its progression, as well as information about patient behavior and the reasons for that behavior. | **Examples:** This might include information on how family members other than the caregiver respond to caregiving; characteristics of the physical environment that might impede or facilitate caregiving, as well as information about available resources for altering the physical environment. |

**TABLE 2.1** *(continued)*

Primary Entity Targeted

| Primary domain targeted | Caregiver | Care recipient | Family/social and physical environment |
|---|---|---|---|
| **Cognition— Skills** | **Problem:** Lack of skills enabling caregiver to analyze and understand their own situation impairs caregiver's ability to function effectively.<br><br>**Goal:** Acquire basic skills of self-monitoring, appraisal, discrimination, and modification of one's own cognitions.<br><br>**Examples:** Cognitive behavior therapy (CBT) and problem solving skills training applied to oneself typify this cell. Includes generalizable cognitive skills training applicable to varied settings and goals. Cognitive skills training aimed at caregiver depression would be partially allocated to this cell to the extent that the skills training goes beyond dealing with affect. | **Problem:** Lack of skills enabling analysis of care recipient memory problems, attitudes and behaviors that are disruptive to the caregiver.<br><br>**Goal:** Facilitate analytic skills in caregiver that would help them understand contingencies of care recipient behaviors and methods for regulating behaviors.<br><br>**Examples:** Care recipients may exhibit varied cognitive deficits such as excessive, burdensome worrying, intolerance, and low motivation. Caregiver learns antecedents of problem behaviors and methods for dealing with them. Caregiver may acquire skills for enhancing cognitive functioning of the care recipient. The caregiver may impart cognitive skills training to enhance care recipient functioning. | **Problem:** Negativistic attitudes toward caregiver from social environment of caregiver.<br><br>**Goal:** Change attitudes to be more neutral or positive toward caregiver.<br><br>**Examples:** Cognitive coping skills aimed at helping the caregiver deal with negative attitudes and interpersonal and communication skills aimed at generating positive attitudes from social environment. |

*(continued)*

**TABLE 2.1** *(continued)*

Primary Entity Targeted

| Primary domain targeted | Caregiver | Care recipient | Family/social and physical environment |
|---|---|---|---|
| **Behavior** | **Problem:** Unable to implement behavioral strategies to regulate their own behaviors.<br><br>**Goal:** Acquire behavioral skills that would enable caregiver to better monitor and regulate their own behavior.<br><br>**Examples:** Skills on how to assess one's own behavior in relation to the care recipient and other persons in the social environment are demonstrated and practiced. | **Problem:** Unable to implement behavioral strategies to diminish disruptive behaviors of care recipient or facilitate desired behaviors of care recipient.<br><br>**Goal:** Acquire behavioral skills to monitor and regulate behavior of the care recipient.<br><br>**Examples:** Caregiver engages in role-play of behavior modification methods aimed at decreasing repetitive questions by the care recipient. | **Problem:** Unable to implement behavioral strategies to appropriately/adequately respond to the needs of caregiver/care recipient in social and physical environments.<br><br>**Goal:** Acquire behavioral skills to monitor and regulate the social and physical environment.<br><br>**Examples:** Practice of behavioral skills aimed at changing behavior of persons in the social environment such as other family members. Demonstration and practice on how to assess the physical environment. Practice of behavioral scripts that might be followed to access existing services for changing environment. |

**TABLE 2.1** *(continued)*

Primary Entity Targeted

| Primary domain targeted | Caregiver | Care recipient | Family/social and physical environment |
|---|---|---|---|
| **Affect** | **Problem:** Caregiver experiences too much negative affect (distress, depression) and too little positive affect.<br><br>**Goal:** Acquire knowledge and/or skills for regulating affect in the caregiver (e.g., decrease negative affect and increase positive affect). Participate in activities aimed at directly enhancing affect (e.g., counseling, support groups).<br><br>**Examples:** Learn to identify and engage in pleasant activities. Skills training for affect regulation. Joining groups for emotional support. | **Problem:** Care recipient exhibits negative affect (e.g., anxiety and/or depression).<br><br>**Goal:** Develop methods for regulating the affect of the care recipient.<br><br>**Examples:** Provide pleasant diversion when care recipient becomes distressed. | **Problem:** Negative affect directed at caregiver from social environment of caregiver.<br><br>**Goal:** Acquire skills for monitoring affect in the social environment and learning communication skills to change affect in social environment. Understanding how others in environment affect caregiver emotionally.<br><br>**Examples:** Teaching communication skills designed to change affect in social environment. Learning behavioral strategies that maximize |

Note: The problems, goals, examples identified are not intended to be definitive, they merely serve as examples.

**TABLE 2.2  Interventions Classified by Delivery System Characteristics**

| Attribute | Definition of attribute | Dimension |
|---|---|---|
| Frequency | How frequently is intervention delivered | Higher frequency = higher intensity |
| Duration | How long does each encounter last | Longer duration = higher intensity |
| Individual (yes/no) | Does contact occur on a one-to-one basis | High personalization |
| Group (yes/no) | Does contact occur in group context | Low personalization |
| Face-to-face (yes/no) | Does contact occur face-to-face | High personalization |
| Telephone (yes/no) | Does contact occur via tele-communication device | Low personalization |
| Caregiver initiated contact (yes/no) | Does caregiver initiate contact | High personalization |
| Interventionist initiated contact (yes/no) | Does interventionist initiate contact | Low personalization |
| Highly structured | Highly structured, scripted intervention | Low personalization |
| Open ended | Unstructured, flexible intervention | High personalization |

Note: Delivery characteristics can be used to derive an intensity measure for each intervention.

ize the way in which an intervention is delivered to the participant. It includes the frequency and duration of the intervention (*intensity level*), whether it is delivered at the individual level or as a group intervention, whether it occurs face to face or via technological devices, such as telephones or microcomputers, whether contact is initiated by the interventionist or the caregiver, whether it is completely standardized or individualized to the participant, whether it is proscriptive and highly structured or open-ended (*personalization level*). Using the parameters in this table, one could test hypotheses linking intensity or dose to the effectiveness of an intervention. For example, interventions that are highly individualized and are delivered with high frequency and face to face on an individual basis are likely to be more effective than interventions that are standardized, delivered infrequently, and in a group context.

Theoretically, all four of these dimensions can be orthogonal to each other. Thus, one could create a four-dimensional space and locate components of any intervention in that space. Given the complexity of thinking about different interventions in terms of a four-dimensional space with multiple levels for each dimension, it is convenient to characterize interventions first in terms of two dimensions—the *entity* and *domain* being targeted—and then consider separately the delivery system used to implement the intervention (i.e., intensity and personalization). Combining the entity and domain dimensions yields a 3 (entities) by 4 (domains) matrix. Definitions and examples for each cell of this matrix are provided in Table 2.1. The number of potential delivery system characteristics is large. Key dimensions of methods of delivery are provided in Table 2.2.

Elements of this classification system can be linked to the stress-process model in the following way. We would argue that interventions targeting the care recipient or the social and physical environment represent attempts to alter the environmental stressors. For example, the environmental skills building intervention would fall into this category because it is aimed at altering the physical environment of the caregiver and care recipient. As shown in Figure 2.3, such interventions target the primary source of stress in the sequential model. Similarly, interventions targeting caregiver cognitions about their abilities as caregivers should have their primary impact on the appraisal of demands and adaptive capacities. Interventions targeting caregiver affect such as feelings of depression and anxiety are aimed at altering the emotional response of the caregiver, and finally, interventions targeting caregiver behavior should have direct effects on the behavioral response of the caregiver. Thus, interventions can be conceptualized as primarily targeting a specific component of the stress-health sequential model. Because of the multiple feedback loops in the sequential model, an intervention targeting one component of the model should over time affect other components as well.

Our approach to conceptualizing interventions has several advantages. First, it provides a common framework for characterizing many different approaches to interventions for caregivers. This should facilitate comparisons across studies and enable meta-analyses of caregiver intervention research. Second, the identification of discrete components of multifaceted interventions may help us identify

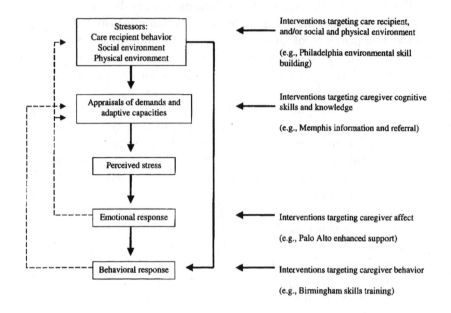

**FIGURE 2.3   REACH intervention strategies and their role in a stress model.**

key features of an intervention that contribute to positive outcomes. Finally, the inclusion of delivery system characteristics, which are often overlooked and are rarely systematically measured in caregiver intervention research, helps us explore how the content and delivery methods interact to produce desired outcomes. In general, we would expect interventions high on all four dimensions—high intensity, highly personalized, targeting multiple domains and targets—would be more effective than interventions low on these dimensions.

Our goal in this chapter was to provide a framework for thinking about the caregiving experience and for characterizing intervention approaches used with caregivers. Although we would not claim to be exhaustive in presenting existing perspectives on caregiving, we have described the dominant themes and issues that are of concern to researchers and practitioners. No doubt new perspectives and even more challenging issues will emerge as research in this area progresses.

# REFERENCES

Axelrod, R.M. (1984). *The evolution of cooperation.* New York: Basic Books.

Bandura, A. (1977). *Social learning theory.* Englewood Cliffs, NJ: Prentice-Hall.

Barker, J.C. (1997). Between humans and ghosts: The decrepit elderly in a Polynesian society. In J. Sokolovsky (Ed.), *The cultural context of aging, Second edition* (pp. 407–424). New York: Bergin and Garvey.

Barash, D.P. (1982). *Sociobiology and behavior* (2nd ed.). New York: Elsevier.

Batson, C.D., & Coke, J.S. (1983). Empathic motivation of helping behavior. In J.R. Cacioppo & R.E. Petty (Eds.), *Social psychophysiology: A sourcebook.* New York: Guilford Press.

Baumann, D.J., Cialdini, R.B., & Kendrick, D.T. (1981). Altruism as hedonism: Helping and self-gratification as equivalent responses. *Journal of Personality and Social Psychology, 40,* 1039–1046.J.

Berkowitz, L. (1972). Social norms, feelings, and other factors affecting helping and altruism. In L. Berkowitz (Ed.), *Advances in experimental social psychology, Vol 6.* New York: Academic Press.

Biegel, D.E., Sales, E., & Schulz, R. (1991). *Family Caregiving in Chronic Illness: Family Caregiver Applications Series, Vol. 1.* Newbury Park, CA: Sage Publications, Inc.

Bourgeois, M.S., & Schulz, R. (1996). Interventions for caregivers of patients with Alzheimer's disease: A review and analysis of content, process, and outcomes. *International Journal of Aging and Human Development, 43(1),* 35–92.

Bowan, M. (1966). The use of family theory in clinical practice. *Comprehensive Psychiatry, 7(5),* 345–374.

Brickman, P., Rabinowitz, B.C., Karuza, J., Coates, D., Cohn, E., & Kidder, L. (1982). Models of helping and coping. *American Psychologist, 37,* 38–384.

Brody, E.M. (1985). Women in the middle and family help to older people. *The Gerontologist, 21(5),* 471–480.

Brody, S.J., Poulshock, S.W., & Masciocchi, C.F. (1978). The family caring unit: A major consideration in the long-term support system. *The Gerontologist, 18,* 556–561.

Bruhn, J.G. (1977). Effects of chronic illness on the family. *The Journal of Family Practice, 4(6),* 1057–1060.

Cantor, M.H. (1983). Strain among caregivers: A study of experience in the United States. *The Gerontologist, 23,* 597–604.

Cassileth, B., & Hamilton, J. (1979). The family with cancer. In B. Cassileth (Ed.), *The cancer patient: Social and medical aspects of care* (pp. 233–247). Philadelphia: Lee & Febiger.

Cohen S. (1988). Psychosocial models of the role of social support in the etiology of physical disease. *Health Psychology, 7,* 269–297.

Cohen, S., Kessler, R.C., & Gordon, L.U. (1995). *Measuring stress.* New York: Oxford University Press.

Cohler, B., Groves, L., Borden, W., & Lazarus, L. (1989). Caring for family members with Alzheimer's disease. In E. Light & B. Lebowitz (Eds.), *Alzheimer's disease treatment and family stress: Directions for research* (pp. 50–105). Washington, DC: National Institute of Mental Health.

Coppel, D.B., Burton, C., Becker, J., & Fiore, J. (1985). The relationship of cognitions associated with coping reactions to depression in spousal caregivers of Alzheimer's disease patients. *Cognitive Therapy and Research, 9,* 253–266.

Dunkin, J.J., & Anderson-Hanley, C. (1998). Dementia caregiver burden: A review of the literature and guidelines for assessment and intervention. *Neurology, 51*(Suppl. 1), S53–S60.

Eliott, G.R., & Eisdorfer, C. (1982). *Stress and human health.* New York: Springer.

Forsyth, D.R. (1987). *Social psychology.* Monterey, CA: Brooks/Cole.

Giacquinta, G. (1977). Helping families face the crisis of cancer. *American Journal of Nursing, 77,* 185–188.

Gray-Price, H., & Szczesny, S. (1985). Crisis intervention with families of cancer patients: A developmental approach. *Topics in Clinical Nursing, 11,* 58–70.

Greenberg, M.S. (1980). A theory of indebtedness. In K.J. Gergen, M.S. Greenberg, & R.H. Willis (Eds.), *Social exchange: Advances in theory and research* (pp. 3–26). New York: Plenum.

Haley, J., & Ranson, D.C. (1976). Development of a theory: A history of a research project. In C.E. Sluzki & D.C. Ransom (Eds.), *Double bind: The foundations of the communication approach to the family.* New York: Grune & Stratton.

Haley, W.E., Han, B., & Henderson, J.N. (1998). Aging and ethnicity: Issues for clinical practice. *Journal of Clinical Psychology in Medical Settings, 5,* 393–409.

Haley, W.E., Levine, E.G., Brown, S.L., & Bartolucci, A.A. (1987). Stress, appraisal, coping, and social support as predictors of adaptational outcome among dementia caregivers. *Psychology and Aging, 2,* 323–330.

Hamilton, W.D. (1964). The genetical evolution of social behaviour, I and II. *Journal of Theoretical Biology, 7,* 1–52.

Hatfield, E., Walster, G.W., & Piliavin, J.A. (1978). Equity theory and helping relationships. In L. Wispe (Ed.), *Altruism, sympathy, and helping* (pp. 115–139). New York: Academic Press.

Herz, F., & McGoldrick, M. (1980). The impact of death and serious illness on the family life cycle. In E. Carter & M. McGoldrick (Eds.), *The family life cycle: A framework for family therapy* (pp. 223–240). New York: Gardner Press.

Hoffman, M G. (1982). Development of prosocial motivation: Empathy and guilt. In N. Eisenberg (Ed.), *The development of prosocial behavior* (pp. 281–313). New York: Academic Press.

Horowitz, A. (1985). Family caregiving to the frail elderly. In M.P. Lawton & G. Maddox (Eds.), *Annual review of gerontology and geriatric: Vol. 5* (pp. 194–246). New York: Springer.

Kaplan, D. (1982). Intervention strategies for families. In J. Cohen, J. Cullen, & L. Martin (Eds.), *Psychosocial aspects of cancer* (pp. 221–233). New York: Raven Press.

Knight, B.G., Lutzky, S.M., & Macofsky-Urban, F. (1993). A meta-analytic review of interventions for caregiver distress: Recommendations for future research. *The Gerontologist, 33*(2), 240–248.

Leventhal, H., Leventhal, E.A., & Nguyen, T.V. (1985). Reactions of families to illness: Theoretical models and perspectives. In D.C. Turk & R.D. Kerns (Eds.), *Health, illness and families: A life-span perspective* (pp. 108–145). New York: John Wiley.

Mailick, M. (1979). The impact of severe illness on the individual and family: An overview. *Social Work in Health Care, 5,* 117–128.

Minuchin, S. (1974). *Families and family therapy.* Cambridge, MA: Harvard University Press.

Moen, P., Robison, J., & Fields, V. (1994). Women's work and caregiving roles: A life course approach. *Journal of Gerontology: Social Sciences, 49,* S176–S186.

Montgomery, R.J.V., Stull, D.E., & Borgatta, E.F. (1985). Measurement and the analysis of burden. *Research on Aging, 7,* 137–152.

Pagel, M., Becker, J., & Coppel, D. (1985). Loss of control, self-blame, and depression: An investigation of spouse caretakers of Alzheimer's disease patients. *Journal of Abnormal Psychology, 94,* 169–182.

Parsons, T. & Bales, R. (1955). *Family socialization and interaction.* Glencoe, IL: Free Press.

Pearlin, L.I., Mullan, J.T., Semple, S.J., & Skaff, M.M. (1990). Caregiving and the stress process: An overview of concepts and their measures. *The Gerontologist, 30*(5), 583–594.

Quinn, W., & Herndon, A. (1986). The family ecology of cancer. *Journal of Psychosocial Oncology, 4*(1/2), 45–49.

Reis, H.T., & Gruzen, J. (1976). On mediating equity, equality, and self-interest: The role of self-presentation in social exchange. *Journal of Experimental Social Psychology, 12,* 487–503.

Schulz, R., O'Brien, A.T., Bookwala, J., & Fleissner, K. (1995). Psychiatric and physical morbidity effects of dementia caregiving: Prevalence, correlates, and causes. *The Gerontologist, 35,* 771–791.

Schulz, R., Tompkins, C.A., & Rau, M.T. (1988). A longitudinal study of the psychosocial impact of stroke on primary support persons. *Psychology and Aging, 3,* 131–141.

Schulz, R., Tompkins, C.A., Wood, D., & Decker, S. (1987). The social psychology of caregiving: Physical and psychological costs to providing support to the disabled. *Journal of Applied Social Psychology, 17,* 401–428.

Singer, B.A. (1983). Psychosocial trauma, defense strategies and treatment considerations in cancer patients and their families. *American Journal of Family Therapy, 11*(3), 15–21.

Skinner, J.H. (1995). Ethnic/racial diversity in long-term care use and services. In Z. Harel & R. Dunkle (Eds.), *Matching people with services in long-term care.* (pp. 49–72). New York: Springer.

Szapocznik, J., & Kurtines, W.M. (1989). *Breakthroughs in family therapy with drug-abusing problem youth.* New York: Springer Publishing Company.

Thompson, S.C., & Pitts, J.S. (1992). In sickness and in health: Chronic illness, marriage, and spousal caregiving. In S. Spacapan, S. Oskamp, et al. (Eds.), *Helping and being helped: Naturalistic studies. The Claremont Symposium on Applied Psychology* (pp. 115–151). Newbury Park, CA: Sage Publications, Inc.

U.S. House of Representatives. (1987). *Exploding the myth: Caregiving in America.* (Select Committee on Aging Publication No. 99–611). Washington, DC: Government Printing Office.

Vettese, J. (1981). Family stress and mediation in cancer. In P. Ahmed (Ed.), *Living and dying with cancer* (pp. 273–284). New York: Elsevier.

von Bertalanffy, L. (1968). *General systems theory.* New York: George Braziller.

Wellisch, D. (1985). Family therapy and cancer: Keeping house in a foundation of quicksand. In M. Lansky (Ed.), *Family approaches to major psychiatric disorders.* Washington, DC: American Psychiatric Press.

Wilson, E.O. (1998). *Consilience: The unity of knowledge.* New York: Alfred A. Knopf.

# 3

# Interventions for In-Home Caregivers: A Review of Research 1990 to Present

*Joel Kennet, Louis Burgio, and Richard Schulz*

## INTRODUCTION

Intervention studies for family caregivers have been a mainstay in the gerontological literature for more than two decades. Existing reviews of the caregiver intervention literature focus primarily on the outcomes of intervention studies and general methodological limitations of individual studies (i.e., sampling and recruitment issues, adequacy of outcome measures, and generalization issues) (Toseland & Rossiter, 1989; Knight, Lutzky, & Macofsky-Urban, 1993; Zarit & Teri, 1992). A more recent review by Bourgeois, Schulz, and Burgio (1996) examined studies published between 1980 and 1992 with a focus on the therapeutic process of interventions, including the intensity and integrity of the interventions used. The intent of the present chapter is to update and extend earlier reviews of this literature in order to set the stage of subsequent chapters of this book which focus on issues of theory, measurement, treatment implementation, and public policy regarding dementia caregiver intervention research.

This chapter begins with a brief summary of conclusions reached in prior reviews of the intervention studies. This section is followed by examples of intervention approaches representing key substantive domains within the intervention literature. We conclude with general summaries of the literature and suggestions for future directions.

## OVERVIEW OF PRIOR REVIEWS

Although anecdotal reports of early intervention efforts were generally positive, the first critical reviews of the literature were considerably more sobering. Toseland and Rossiter's (1989) review of 29 studies concluded that while caregivers evaluated interventions positively there was "no clear link . . . between participants' satisfaction (with group interventions) and other important outcomes for caregivers such as improving coping skills, preventing psychological disturbances, increasing caregiver support systems, or improving caregivers' ability to care for themselves" (p. 438). Similarly, "time-limited psychoeducational interventions have modest therapeutic benefits as measured by global ratings of well-being, mood, stress, psychological status, and caregiving burden" (p. 481). Focusing exclusively on interventions aimed at alleviating caregiver distress, Knight, Lutszky, and Macofsky-Urban (1993) concluded that individual psychosocial interventions and respite programs are moderately effective, though psychosocial interventions with groups are less effective. Zarit and Teri (1992), in describing the available intervention literature as the "first generation" of studies, point out that interpretation of this preliminary work should be tempered by the fact that expectations for particular intervention outcomes and the malleability of caregivers have been overly optimistic, and that some intervention effects may be underestimated because of methodological limitations of the studies.

Bourgeois, Schulz, and Burgio (1996) organized their review of the literature around six broad categories, including support groups, individual and/or family counseling, case management, respite and day care services, skills training, and various combinations of these strategies. Detailed assessments of the complex literature in each of these areas are contained in the original review. However, a number of general conclusions can be derived from their analysis of the literature. First, the complexity and rigor of intervention studies continues to improve with an increasing emphasis on randomized designs. Second, the literature on the whole supports the conclusion that more is better. Multicomponent interventions that blanket caregivers with a diversity of services and supports in the hopes that a combination of components will impact on a caregiver's unique needs tend to generate larger effects than narrowly focused interventions. Similarly, single component interventions with higher intensity (frequency and duration) also have a greater positive impact on the caregiver than similar interventions with lower intensity. Third, achieving generalization of effects beyond the specific target of an intervention has been difficult. Thus, for example, a skills training intervention may effectively enhance a caregiver's ability to manage the patient but may not necessarily reduce their sense of subjective burden. Based on their review, Bourgeois, Schulz, and Burgio (1996) conclude that future intervention research needs to address three recurrent themes. First, caregiver characteristics need to be considered more systematically in tailoring interventions to individual needs. Without a thorough knowledge and understanding of individual caregivers and their unique personal and psychological histories and circumstances, interventions can only continue to be designed for the "average" caregiver, with average results. Second, treatments need to be described, measured, and monitored to insure that caregivers are receiving the treatment as prescribed and to permit replication of treatment effects with similar groups. Without a complete understanding of what comprises an efficacious treatment and how subject characteristics interact with treatment factors, caregivers and professionals may waste their time in efforts that yield only mediocre outcomes. Finally, the desired outcomes of interventions need to be more clearly articulated. What constitutes a reasonable outcome for a given intervention and how might it vary for different caregivers, patients, families, and professionals? The remainder of this chapter provides a more updated view of the literature on caregiver interventions. In order to provide some structure to our review, we use the conceptual framework articulated in chapter 2 to organize the presentation of the recent literature.

## INCLUSION CRITERIA FOR THIS REVIEW

Computerized searches were carried out to identify journal articles and book chapters on the topic of in-home caregiving of elders, published between 1990 and late 1997. Additionally, a mailing was sent to a number of leading researchers in the field (identified by a CRISP search of current grant recipients), asking them to provide any recent, unpublished results, or articles that may have been missed in the library searches. Most of the studies included focus on interventions for dementia patients; however, several studies are based on caregiving interventions with other patient populations. Although our goal was to find numerous examples of randomized trials, we include in this review all studies reporting results of one or more interventions aimed at improving outcomes of caregivers, regardless of the design of the study. Thus, a full range of methodologies is represented among these studies, including case studies, quasi-experimental designs, panel studies, and true experiments or randomized trials. It should be noted that the 40 manuscripts included in this review do not represent 40 separate studies. A number of investigators published separately different results from the same study.

In chapter 2 we provided a conceptual framework for characterizing elements of dementia caregiver intervention studies. Briefly, in a 3 × 4 matrix we describe interventions based on two dimensions: the primary target of the intervention (caregiver, patient, or social/physical environment) and the primary domain being targeted (cognitive skills, knowledge, behavior, or affect). With the exception of a few highly focused interventions such as the provision of respite, virtually all caregiving interventions fall into multiple cells of this matrix and are therefore best viewed as multicomponent interventions. We use this framework to organize the intervention research literature to be reviewed, and present below examples of interventions that fall predominantly into a single cell as well as examples of multicomponent interventions. We begin with interventions organized by domain targeted.

## EXAMPLES OF INTERVENTIONS ORGANIZED
## BY SUBSTANTIVE DOMAINS TARGETED

### Knowledge

Virtually all caregiving interventions attempt to enhance the caregiver's knowledge about the disease, caregiving challenges and solutions, and/or service options available to caregivers and patients. For example, Brennan, Moore, and Smyth (1991) installed computers in caregivers homes which permitted access to an electronic database on caregiving. Brodaty, Roberts, and Peters (1994) implemented an intensive training program totaling 18 hours in which caregivers learned about disease processes, communication problems, behavioral disorders, physical and emotional impact on the carer, etc. Unfortunately, treatment effects in both of these studies on health-related outcomes were not observed, suggesting that a strong emphasis on knowledge alone may have limited impact.

### Cognitive Skills

Several of the interventions included in this review involved strategies aimed at improving the cognitive skills of caregivers. Typically, cognitive skills interventions include efforts to teach everyday problem solving techniques or time management methods, as well as teaching participants to alter dysfunctional thoughts (Gallagher-Thompson & Steffen, 1994). Teaching caregivers coping skills is another example of cognitive skills training, although such interventions may also include elements of affect management and behavioral training. The expectation is that the combination of knowledge with generalized problem solving skills will enable the caregiver to evaluate and deal with new problems associated with patient decline. Specific examples of cognitive skills training include studies with support groups that emphasize problem solving (Labrecque, Peak, & Toseland, 1992), cognitive-behavioral therapy, and coping skills training (Castle, Wilkins, Heck, Tanzy, & Fahey, 1995; Gallagher-Thompson & DeVries, 1994; Gallagher-Thompson & Steffen, 1994).

A unique variation of this type of intervention involves memory retraining for the care-recipient (e.g., Brodaty & Peters, 1991) along with other methods aimed at enhancing the cognitive functioning of the AD patient in the hopes that this will have beneficial effects on the caregiver. On the whole, these intervention approaches are associated with moderate success in some studies in terms of delayed institutionalization or improved psychological well-being of the caregiver. However, each of these studies has methodological limitations making it difficult to draw firm conclusions regarding causal relations between interventions and outcomes.

## Behavior

Interventions intended to modify caregiver behavioral skills have been carried out with some success. One promising example of a behavioral intervention involved teaching caregivers skills in communicating with their care recipients (Ripich & Wykle, 1997). The intervention involved four weekly 2-hour sessions, in which participants read, held discussions, watched videotapes, and engaged in role-playing activities designed to enhance communication skills. This study had an added dimension in that a fairly large proportion of the participants were African-Americans, who were particularly well served by the intervention as evidenced by increases in positive affect and decreases in reported hassles. Both African-American and Caucasian participants improved in knowledge and satisfaction with their communications with care recipients.

In two studies, Bourgeois and colleagues (1990, 1997) taught caregivers targeted communication skills. Bourgeois (1990) taught caregivers to conduct between 8 and 21 structured treatment sessions with three spouse care recipients using communication wallets. Use of these wallets, which contained personally relevant sentences and pictures, was encouraged through the caregivers' use of graduated prompting and praise reinforcement. Data from direct observational recording showed that all three care recipients increased on-topic speech during the training sessions. The investigator also reported increases in conversation involving untrained topics. Results maintained at a 3- and 6-week follow-up.

Bourgeois, Burgio, Schulz, Beach, and Palmer (1997) taught seven caregivers to use prosthetic memory aids to decrease care recipient repetitive verbalization. Prosthetic memory aids involve the use of simple statements written on cue cards or erasable tablets that are intended to cue care recipients' memory for everyday events (e.g., "Carol gets home from work at 6 p.m."). It was hypothesized that the presence of these cues would decrease the need for repeated questioning from the care recipient. Compared to seven matched controls, care recipients in the treatment group showed reductions in repetitive verbalizations that maintained up to 6-months posttreatment. Increases in caregiver self-efficacy were also reported at the 6-month follow-up.

## Affect

Almost all interventions focus on some aspect of managing negative affect or enhancing positive affect in the caregiver. A number of studies view this as one of the primary goals of their intervention and use strategies such as counseling, emotional support, and teaching affect management skills as a means for achieving these goals. For example, Toseland, Rossiter, Peak, and Smith (1990) carried out a large-scale (n = 154) study of daughters and daughters-in-law of frail elders, comparing the efficacy of individual versus group counseling. Both types of counseling were based on an environmental systems framework, relying heavily upon validation and confirmation of caregiving experiences, encouragement and praise for providing care, affirmation of participants' ability to cope, and support and understanding for struggling with difficult situations. Individually counseled participants had greater reductions in burden and psychiatric symptoms than did group counseling participants. Not surprisingly, the latter group was more improved in social support received, while both counseling groups enjoyed improvement in their relationships with care recipients relative to control participants.

The interventions carried out by Whitlatch and her colleagues (Whitlatch, Zarit, & von Eye, 1991; Whitlatch, Zarit, Goodwin, & von Eye, 1995) were designed to reduce caregiving stress through individual and family counseling. The earlier of these two studies consisted of a reanalysis of data from an investigation conducted during the previous decade (Zarit, Anthony, & Boutselis, 1987). Whitlatch et al. (1991) employed a statistical technique known as

Prediction Analysis in order to account for initial differences among caregivers on the outcome measures. Since some caregivers reported low depression at baseline, floor effects were obtained in the initial study as a result of these individuals being unable to improve. By dividing caregivers on the basis of their initial scores on outcome measures, and providing differential definitions of success on the basis of those scores, these investigators were able to demonstrate that caregivers enrolled in individual and family counseling were more likely to have successful outcomes than participants in support groups or on a waiting list. The latter study (Whitlatch et al., 1995) consisted of a one-year follow-up of the participants from the 1987 study. Here it was found that the likelihood of placement a year after the intervention could be predicted on the basis of the success-fulness of the intervention as defined in the earlier (Whitlatch et al., 1991) study.

Finally, Teri and Uomoto (1991) reported case studies (n = 4) wherein all participants received eight hours of training on strategies for decreasing depression through increasing participation in pleasant activities. Depression, as measured by HDRS and Beck Depression Inventory scores, was reduced among participants who initially scored high.

In summary, interventions targeting the affect of the caregiver have yielded positive outcomes, particularly in reducing sense of burden and in delaying institutionalization. Several studies have concentrated on affect in combination with knowledge and other target areas, and these will be discussed in the section on multifaceted interventions.

## EXAMPLES OF INTERVENTIONS ORGANIZED BY ENTITY TARGETED

### Caregiver

Almost all interventions include the caregiver. Even when the primary goal of an intervention is to effect changes in the physical or social environment or changes in the behavior of the care-recipient, the intervention is often delivered through the caregiver. This is to be expected since the goals of most interventions are to achieve desirable changes in the behavior or affect of the caregiver. As the examples above illustrate, this can be achieved in a wide variety of ways including enhancing caregivers' knowledge, teaching cognitive or behavioral skills, or providing emotional support or counseling.

## Care Recipient

Interventions whose primary goal is to change the behavior or affect of the care recipient fall into this category. This approach is based on the rationale that desirable changes in the care recipient will have a positive impact on the caregiver. Two strategies serve as good examples of this approach: one approach targets the patient directly while the other uses the caregiver as means for achieving patient change.

Studies in which medications are given to patients to maintain or enhance cognitive function, eliminate disruptive behaviors, or enhance patient affect are good examples of the first approach. Although such studies are usually not viewed as caregiving intervention studies, they clearly represent an important means for reducing caregiver distress and can be used as an adjunct to more traditional caregiver interventions. Another direct approach involves interventions such as memory re-training, memory wallets, reality orientation, etc., which can also be delivered directly to the care recipient. Only a handful of the studies found in our search explicitly employed interventions designed to improve the functioning of the care recipient. In two of the studies conducted by Brodaty and his colleagues (Brodaty & Peters, 1991; Brodaty, McGilchrist, Harris, & Peters, 1993), the investigators provided memory retraining for demented participants. Carers for individuals in the memory retraining group were used as a control for comparison against caregivers who had received a comprehensive, multifaceted battery of therapeutic and educational interventions. Since the objective was to test the efficacy of the comprehensive intervention program in terms of survival and time until nursing home admission, data on the effects of the memory retraining on caregiver status were not reported. Hinchliffe, Hyman, Blizard, and Livingston, 1992; Hinchliffe, Hyman, Blizard, & Livingston, 1995) also targeted care recipients to some extent in their comprehensive intervention program. These investigators provided psychotherapeutic drugs and engaged care recipients in a variety of activities to provide stimulation. Since the overall intervention program included multiple components, it is impossible to determine the unique effects of the procedures used to improve the status of care recipients.

The second approach is to teach behavior management skills to the caregiver who then applies them to the care recipient. Good examples of this approach include the work of Bourgeois and colleagues (Bourgeois, 1990; Bourgeois et al., 1997) and Ripich and Wykle (1997) which are described above. Recent findings suggest that these approaches may be effective treatments for care recipients and their caregivers.

## Social/Physical Environment

Some interventionists advocate an even broader focus for their interventions and target the social environment of the caregiver which might include other family members or an extended support system. Examples of physical environment changes include alterations in the home that might make caregiving easier or removing the care recipient from the home altogether for brief or extended periods of time as might be the case with respite interventions. For example, Pynoos and Ohta (1991) conducted a small-scale panel study wherein participant caregivers were allowed to choose environmental interventions from a list of possible changes generated by a team of experts. Typically the interventions chosen targeted specific problem behaviors, such as unsafe use of stairs, losing or misplacing things, or incontinence. The interventions provided quick, inexpensive, and effective countermeasures, such as a handrail for stair usage, a locked security box for frequently lost items, or adult diapers. This overall strategy proved to be successful in most cases. At the 7-month follow-up, 89% of the interventions employed were still considered to be effective by the caregivers.

A number of studies in our review examined the effects of providing various forms of respite to caregivers. Deimling (1992) divided participants *post hoc* on the basis of the cognitive and physical stability of the care recipient over the course of the study. Caregivers either received home health aides or placed their charges in temporary care for approximately 20 hours per month over a 4-month period. Carers for stable elders appeared to benefit from the respite in terms of depression, physical health, and relationship strain, while those caring for declining elders appeared not to benefit. Since this was not a randomized trial we should be cautious in attributing causality to the interventions.

Another study investigating the effects of brief respite periods provided over a long term was conducted by Theis, Moss, and Pearson (1994). These investigators found that up to 4 hours per week of in-home respite, along with short-term institutional stays provided over the course of a year, was insufficient to bring about positive changes in mood, quality of life, or responses to caregiving. Zarit, Greene, Ferraro, Townsend, and Stephens (1996) also chose a long-term perspective in their comparison of caregivers in New Jersey and Ohio, with adult day care up to two days per week as the treatment (day-care facilities were not available for the Ohio sample). Over the course of 3 months, the New Jersey caregivers were improved on measures of overload, worry and strain, depression, and anger.

Other studies have examined the short-term effects of temporarily placing a disabled elder into a care facility. For example, Larkin and Hopcroft (1993) studied the effects of a 2-week inpatient placement on caregiver physical health, activities of daily living (ADLs), and other measures, finding improvement on the Brief Symptom Inventory and a reported improvement in sleep. Finally, Caradoc-Davies and Harvey (1995) utilized measures of ADLs, physical health, depression, stress, social adjustment, and social supports, before and after an unspecified period of institutional respite. In this study, improvement was found in ADLs, physical health, and personal distress.

As a whole, respite appears to have improved the well-being of caregivers in the majority of cases, whether the respite periods were brief and repeated or simply a temporary, one-time arrangement. However, readers should be cautioned that most of these investigations of respite utilization are panel studies. A well-known randomized trial carried out by Lawton, Brody, and Saperstein (1989) found effects for delayed institutionalization among those persons assigned to the respite condition, but no effects for caregiver well-being.

However, only 58% of participants offered respite actually took advantage of it.

## MULTICOMPONENT INTERVENTIONS

Given the multiple challenges of caregiving and the wide variability in individual resources, it should not be surprising to find that virtually all caregiver interventions are multifaceted. Since caregiving for an elderly relative can affect virtually all facets of an individual's life, it is likely that distress is experienced by caregivers along a variety of dimensions. In the following sections, examples of multifaceted intervention studies are reviewed in order of increasing complexity in terms of the number of domains and targets included in the intervention.

### Behavioral and Cognitive Skills

Toseland and Smith (1990) administered weekly one-hour individual counseling sessions to female caregivers. The counseling emphasized problem solving, time management, and stress reduction techniques, and was carried out over an 8-week period. In addition, the design of this study enabled a comparison of the efficacy of professional versus peer counseling. Both treatment groups were improved relative to controls on measures of psychiatric symptomatology and relationships with care recipients; professionally counseled participants also improved in subjective well-being.

### Knowledge and Affect

Most of the multifaceted interventions in this review were classified as targeting the knowledge and affective state of the caregiver. Goodman and Pynoos (1990) compared a knowledge intervention with one targeting affect, both being delivered by telephone. In this study, the group receiving the knowledge intervention listened to 12 lectures on Alzheimer's disease over a 12-week period, while participants in the network group were divided into smaller groups with calls among members scheduled throughout the intervention period. Both groups in this study gained information and reported increases in social supports as well as satisfaction with supports. The group receiving lectures had greater gains in information and social support, while the telephone network group reported less support from friends and family, suggesting that the networks provided a substitute for such support.

The target areas of affect and knowledge were also addressed in a study conducted by Ingersoll-Dayton, Chapman, and Neal (1990). In this study all participants attended seven one-hour seminars, conducted at the workplace, covering the following topic areas: normal physical aging; common emotional problems of elderly people; communication with elderly family members; community services for older people; financial and legal concerns of Medicare, Medicaid, and long-term care insurance; residential options; and caregiver wellness or juggling work and family obligations. Upon completion of the lecture series, participants were offered one of three treatment options: care planning, support groups, or a buddy system. The care planning option appeared to be largely a knowledge intervention, wherein a social worker met with caregivers and helped them to assess their situations and suggest possible resources. In support groups, caregivers met with each other, along with two facilitators, and discussed their caregiving situations. Both of these treatment options were associated with a decrease in negative affect, while attendance at the lecture series resulted in increased knowledge of aging services and an increase in absenteeism at the workplace. None of the caregivers opted for the buddy system option.

The series of studies conducted by Mittelman and her colleagues (Mittelman, Ferris, Steinberg, Shulman, Mackell, Ambinder, & Cohen, 1993; Mittelman, Ferris, Shulman, Steinberg, Ambinder, Mackell, & Cohen, 1995; Mittelman, Ferris, Shulman, Steinberg, & Levin, 1996) also appeared to employ intervention techniques aimed at improving affect and enhancing knowledge. In the 1993 study, individual and family counseling was provided, along with an effort to educate caregivers and their family members about the effects of Alzheimer's Disease. Initially (Mittelman et al., 1993), the intervention was found to be associated with a lower rate of institutional placement after one year. Mittelman and colleagues (1995) reported that the intervention was also successful in preventing caregivers from increasing in depressive symptoms, since this trend was evident among controls but not among experimental participants. The most recent report (Mittelman et al., 1996) suggests that the intervention program was also successful in delaying placement over the long term. Using survival analysis, median time from baseline to placement was 329 days longer for participants receiving the intervention than for control participants.

## Knowledge and Affect Targeting Caregiver and Social/ Physical Environment

A pair of studies conducted in Ontario, Canada, by Mohide and her colleagues (Mohide, Pringle, Streiner, Gilbert, Muir, & Tew, 1990; Drummond, Mohide, Tew, Streiner, Pringle, & Gilbert, 1991) also employed techniques to enhance knowledge and improve affect, but had a third component, namely altering the physical and social environment by providing respite. Their intervention consisted of weekly visits from caregiver support nurses who provided educational materials and individually tailored programs of support based on needs, along with four hours per week of scheduled, in-home respite. An optional monthly support group was also offered, as was additional respite in case of need. This intervention program did not yield statistically significant positive change on any outcome variables, although quality of life was somewhat improved for the treatment group and somewhat worsened among those receiving conventional care. The latter study (Drummond et al., 1991) demonstrated that although the change in quality of life was not significant (20% difference between treatment and control following intervention), the ratio of cost of implementation to improvement in quality of life was low enough to compare favorably with other health care interventions existing in Canada.

Oktay and Volland (1990) also focused on affect, knowledge, and respite. In this large study (n = 191), caregivers of frail elders recently discharged from a hospital received counseling, referrals, education, support groups, and respite services. Control group participants had access to these services as well, but were not required to participate in them. Treatment group participants reported a small reduction in stress, as measured by the General Health Questionnaire (GHQ), and a substantial reduction in subsequent days spent in the hospital.

## Affect, Behavior, and Cognitive Skills

Gallagher-Thompson and DeVries (1994) targeted affect through training in cognitive and behavioral skills. In this article, the authors described a training program for caregivers, specifically females, wherein participants learned relaxation techniques, cognitive techniques for dealing with dysfunctional thoughts, and assertiveness skills. Decreases in hostility were found between pre- and posttesting occasions, and high usage rates were reported by participants 18 months following completion of the training program. Gallagher-Thompson and Steffen (1994) reported on an experimental study comparing a cognitive-behavioral therapy somewhat similar in content to that described above, although delivered individually, with a brief psychodynamic intervention. In the psychodynamic intervention, the focus was on understanding past losses and conflicts in separation and individuation through their reenactment in the therapeutic relationship. Both of these interventions were successful in relieving caregiver depression. However, psychodynamic therapy was more effective when the caregiver had been in the caregiving role for less than 42 months, while cognitive behavioral therapy was more effective when the caregiver/care recipient relationship was of a greater duration.

Two case studies were also published describing interventions of this type. Kaplan and Gallagher-Thompson (1995) provided treatment to a 72-year-old clinically depressed wife caregiver. The authors conducted 17 sessions of individual counseling spanning 8.5 months. Therapy consisted of cognitive-behavioral therapy for depression. With the use of the Beck Depression Inventory and other standardized depression measures, the authors reported full remission of major depression. In the other case study, Gwyther (1990) utilized a focused "social work intervention" with a 68-year-old wife caregiver of a patient with Alzheimer's disease. Although the article described only one case, the author stated that an unspecified number of caregivers was receiving this intervention in an ongoing study. Therapy consisted of two face-to-face counseling sessions followed by therapeutic telephone calls at 1-week postintervention and at 6-month intervals for 18 months. The therapeutic contacts involved assisting the caregiver to utilize formal and informal caregiver services. In addition, the caregiver was taught behavior management strategies that were then incorporated into a written service plan. The service plan could be modified in response to a caregiver-initiated contact or during a scheduled social worker contact. Revised service plans were written and mailed to the caregiver. The author reported that after intervention, the caregiver experienced improvements in feelings of conflict.

## Affect, Knowledge, and Cognitive Skills

Demers and Lavoie (1996) provided a support group intervention focusing on providing information and support, and teaching problem solving skills. Treatment group participants attended 10 weekly two-and-a-half hour meetings, while control group participants did not have resources of this type readily available to them. In the meetings, participants held discussions on problems they were experiencing, explored potential solutions, and received information on specific topics. Results were mixed: burden actually increased among treatment group participants while depression remained stable; in the control group, burden remained stable while depressive symptoms increased. At the 3-month follow-up, this pattern persisted.

## Knowledge, Cognitive and Behavioral Skills

The series of studies conducted by Brodaty and colleagues (Brodaty & Peters, 1991; Brodaty, McGilchrist, Harris, & Peters, 1993; Brodaty, Roberts, & Peters, 1994) appeared to focus on teaching problem solving and coping skills while increasing caregiver knowledge. The earliest of these (Brodaty & Peters, 1991) was a follow-up of an intervention study (Brodaty & Gresham, 1989) wherein treatment group participants received training, a second group received respite over the same duration of time, and a third group was put on a waiting list. This initial study demonstrated that the intervention was effective in reducing stress and delaying institutional placement. The follow-up (Brodaty & Peters, 1991) conducted 39 months after the intervention, found that participants in the training conditions were much less likely to place their relatives than controls, and that their care recipients had a higher rate of survival. Brodaty, McGilchrist, Harris, and Peters (1993) reported the results of a 5-year follow-up of the same participants, with similar results. The most recent study (Brodaty, Roberts, & Peters, 1994) was a quasi-experimental design, wherein support group attendees were offered a training program, and those accepting and completing the training were compared with noncompleters and with those accepting training to be offered at a later date (wait list). The training program consisted of a full-day workshop in addition to five monthly sessions held during the usual support group time slot. Attendees were provided with didactic information, experiential exercises, reading materials, and training in stress management and problem solving techniques, among others. In this study, the intervention failed to yield differences in stress, burden, life satisfaction, well-being, or knowledge. The authors concluded that interventions had a higher likelihood of success when they were individually tailored to meet the needs of caregivers.

## Affect, Knowledge, Cognitive and Behavioral Skills

Labrecque, Peak, and Toseland (1992) and Toseland, Labrecque, Goebel, and Whitney (1992) adopted this multifaceted approach in attempting to assist their female participants. In both studies, participants met in support groups that focused on education, problem solving, stress reduction, and support. Meetings were for two hours, and were held weekly for eight weeks. Labrecque and colleagues (1992) reported improvement in caregivers' perceptions of care recipients' health, with no other significant effects. Toseland and colleagues (1992) reported that treatment group participants had higher marital satisfaction, used more active behavioral strategies, had more knowledge of community resources, and had fewer pressing problems. Control group participants estimated they spent more hours caregiving and reported greater subjective burden.

## Affect, Knowledge, Cognitive and Behavioral Skills, and Respite

The most comprehensive intervention program among the studies in this review was undertaken by Hinchliffe and her colleagues. Hinchliffe and colleagues (1992) described a pilot study which demonstrated that reducing distressing behavior on the part of care recipients was an effective means of improving caregiver mental health. Hinchliffe and colleagues (1995) described a study which initially appeared to primarily target care recipient behavior, but which, on closer inspection, targeted many facets of caregivers' status as well. Participant caregiver/care recipient dyads underwent a thorough assessment, results of which were presented to a team of experts, who devised an individualized package designed to reduce the most bothersome behaviors exhibited by the care recipient. Following assessment, pairs were randomly assigned to treatment-first or treatment-last conditions.

The interventions took place in-home, and involved drug therapy for care recipients, in order to manage such problems as aggression, night disturbances, restlessness, and sexual disinhibition. These and other problems were also managed through a variety of other means. For example, repetitive questioning was handled by encouraging the carer to involve the care recipient in activities he/she enjoyed, and suggesting that the carer allow the patient to discover, through concrete means, the answers to his/her questions by replying with instructions to do so; night disturbance was handled by instructing the carer in maintaining a variety of daytime activities and discouraging the taking of naps, etc. Regarding the caregiver, respite was incorporated into the intervention to a considerable extent, as was training in coping skills, psychological support, and drug therapy in cases of depression. Education on dementia was also provided, as was training in cognitive skills, such as time management, and behavioral skills such as relaxation techniques. The intervention took place over a 16-week period, in 1-hour visits, the actual number of visits depending on need. This intervention program was successful in improving mental health for the treatment-first participants; no improvement was found among those awaiting treatment.

## GENERAL CONCLUSIONS ABOUT THE RECENT
## INTERVENTION LITERATURE

Anyone expecting to find a silver bullet solution to alleviating care-giver distress will clearly be disappointed by the intervention litera-ture reviewed here. There is no single, easily implemented and consistently effective method for eliminating the stresses of care-giving. This is not surprising given the complexity of the caregiving experience, the variability in caregiver resources, and the variety of outcomes examined. The literature clearly points to one overriding conclusion, namely that interventions which are comprehensive, in-tensive, and individually tailored are likely to be more effective than those that are not.

Virtually all interventions studies examined in this review reported some level of success and as a group they provide valuable insights about different methods for achieving caregiver impact as well as the pitfalls of conducting intervention research in this complex area. Because the needs of caregivers are multiple and diverse, they can be assisted in varied ways. There exists strong consensus among researchers that all caregivers are likely to benefit from enhanced knowledge about the disease, the caregiving role, and resources available to caregivers. Once the informational needs have been met, the caregiver may additionally benefit from interventions that train the caregiver in general problem solving skills as well as more specific skills in areas such as managing patient behaviors or their own affect. The current group of intervention studies also suggest that there may be important synergies achieved by simultaneously treating the care recipient (e.g., giving medications or memory re-training) and/or altering the social and physical environment of the caregiver/care recipient dyad. These latter strategies are rela-tively new and promising.

The existing literature also points to a rich array of methods for delivering interventions to caregivers including microcomputers, the telephone, and individual and group sessions. As sophisticated com-munication technologies become more available to individuals, the treatment delivery options will increase further. Although new tech-nology has the potential of overwhelming already stressed caregivers,

**TABLE 3.1 Published Caregiver Intervention Studies, 1990–1997**

| Authors, year | Sample | Design | Intervention procedure, duration, measurement points | Control Condition Description | Dependent variables | Effects |
|---|---|---|---|---|---|---|
| Bayer-Feldmann & Greifenhagen (1995) | 2 caregiver-patient dyads. | Case study. | Psycho-educational intervention with family systems therapy aimed at broadening the support system and improving interaction between patient and caregiver. Multiple sessions led by psychologist and physician. | None. | Open-ended evaluation of intervention. | Intervention evaluated positively by caregivers; reduced stress of caregiving. |

**TABLE 3.1 (continued)**

| Authors, year | Sample | Design | Intervention procedure, duration, measurement points | Control Condition Description | Dependent variables | Effects |
|---|---|---|---|---|---|---|
| Berry, Zarit, & Rabatin (1991) | 40 daughters or wives of dementia patients, ≥ 3 uses of respite services per month. | Participants self-assigned to in-home respite or day care conditions prior to study. | Home care users vs. adult day care users; data collected in a single face-to-face interview and five subsequent telephone interviews; measurement timepoints not published. | None. | Time spent caregiving with and without patient, noncaregiving time; Burden Interview, MBPC, Support Network Checklists. | Home care users had more time freed by respite than day care users; day care users' free time was spent working or catching up on household chores; home care users had higher life satisfaction ratings. |

*(continued)*

**TABLE 3.1** *(continued)*

| Authors, year | Sample | Design | Intervention procedure, duration, measurement points | Control Condition Description | Dependent variables | Effects |
|---|---|---|---|---|---|---|
| Bourgeois (1990) | 3 dyads, female care recipients with AD, and spouse CGs. | Intrasubject multiple baseline across conversational topics. | Caregiver training in use of communication wallets, 8–21 CG-controlled/staged treatment sessions with CR, graduated prompting and praise reinforcement. Multiple measurements during 2–4 week baseline, 2 week intervention period, 3 and 6 week follow-up assessments. | Dyads served as their own controls. | Direct observation of 11 conversational categories (# of statements per 5 minutes), CG perception of change, naive judges = ratings of conversations (social validation). | CGs learned to use memory wallets, all 3 CRs increased ontopic speech, generalization of effect to untrained topics, naive judges reported postintervention conversation improved, effects maintained at 3 and 6 week FU. |

**TABLE 3.1** (*continued*)

| Authors, year | Sample | Design | Intervention procedure, duration, measurement points | Control Condition Description | Dependent variables | Effects |
|---|---|---|---|---|---|---|
| Bourgeois, Burgio, Schulz, Beach, & Palmer (1997) | 7 trained CGs of dementia patients and 7 matched controls. | Hybrid design: Treatment vs. matched control comparison; within group multiple baseline across subjects. | CGs taught various written cuing procedures (e.g., memory boards, index cards) to decrease CRs repetitive vocalizations. 2–8 week baseline period in interventions groups, 4–10 week intervention with 11, 1-hour weekly home visits, one 3-hour workshop. 3- and 6-month follow-up. | Groups of 7 CGs matched on gender and MMSE scores. CGs tracked repetitive vocalizations, no intervention. | CG recording daily frequency of vocalization, CG self-efficacy and satisfaction. | Compared with controls, treatment group showed reduction of repetitive vocalization that persisted over time. Intrasubject: all treatment CGs showed reduction from baseline. CGs in intervention group showed slight increase in self-efficacy at follow-up. CGs reported very satisfied with program. |

*(continued)*

**TABLE 3.1** *(continued)*

| Authors, year | Sample | Design | Intervention procedure, duration, measurement points | Control Condition Description | Dependent variables | Effects |
|---|---|---|---|---|---|---|
| Brennan, Moore, & Smyth (1991) | 22 CGs of AD patients, 13F, 9M. | Study of usage patterns of computer-link system. | Computers installed in homes and networked to an electronic database on caregiving, a decisional support system, and a communication pathway among CGs in the network and professional staff; data collected over a 7-day period, with CGs having been online for 1 week to 4 months. | Controls given a monthly telephone call, but results are not discussed in this article. | Usage rates, usage purposes. | 68% used system during the observed week, average log-on duration 13 minutes; 67% of time spent in communication area, 11% in electronic encyclopedia, 9% in private mail, 5% in decision support. |

**TABLE 3.1** *(continued)*

| Authors, year | Sample | Design | Intervention procedure, duration, measurement points | Control Condition Description | Dependent variables | Effects |
|---|---|---|---|---|---|---|
| Brodaty, McGilchrist, Harris, & Peters (1993) | 91 CGs, 43M, 48F, of mildly demented CRs. | Sequential assignment into 3 groups: immediate training, delayed training, respite (memory training for CR). | 10-day intensive residential training program, involving memory retraining, reminiscence therapy, and environmental reality orientation, aimed at alleviating psychological distress, providing information, increasing coping skills, reducing isolation, and improving self care; 10-day respite for third group; measurement timepoints at 0 and 12 months, annual phone contact to establish date of placement and/or death. | AB vs. BA vs. C design, delayed training group received treatment 6 months after admission into study; specifics of respite condition not provided. | CR: time to Nursing Home Admission, time to death, CG: GHQ, Duke University North Carolina Health Status Profile (DUNC), trait neuroticism scale from Eysenck Personality Inventory, satisfaction with contacts received. | Training of caregivers significantly associated with delayed nursing home admission and reduced mortality, CG psychiatric morbidity associated with decreased CR survival time. |

*(continued)*

85

**TABLE 3.1** (*continued*)

| Authors, year | Sample | Design | Intervention procedure, duration, measurement points | Control Condition Description | Dependent variables | Effects |
|---|---|---|---|---|---|---|
| Brodaty & Peters (1991) | 96 dementia CGs, 52F, 44M, follow-up of Brodaty & Gresham (1989). | 3 groups: Dementia carers, memory retraining, and wait list (delayed treatment). | Carers received training in coping with care-giving difficulties. In memory re-training group, only CRs received memory retraining; survival analysis for death and placement, conducted at 39 months after intervention. | Memory retraining and wait list groups served as controls. | Cost of institutionalization, health care costs, survival, survival at home. | Treatment group subjects had significantly higher survival and fewer placements; cost analysis revealed significant savings as a result of treatment; no differences in health care usage among CGs. |

**TABLE 3.1** *(continued)*

| Authors, year | Sample | Design | Intervention procedure, duration, measurement points | Control Condition Description | Dependent variables | Effects |
|---|---|---|---|---|---|---|
| Brodaty, Roberts, & Peters (1994) | 81 CGs, 19M, 62F, of demented CRs. | 3 groups: training completers, training non-completers, and controls. | Training sessions totaling 18 hours, covering disease process, communication problems, and behavioral disorders: physical and emotional impact on the caregiver; the nature of stress and stress management techniques; problem-solving techniques and management of specific behavioral problems; 4-month duration; measurement timepoints at 2 weeks prior to training onset and up to 1 month after training offset. | Controls on waiting list. | Family Burden Interview, GHQ, Satisfaction with Life Scale (SWLS), Positive and Negative Affect Scales (PANAS), Happiness Scale, knowledge of dementia. | No significant change on any variables. |

*(continued)*

**TABLE 3.1** *(continued)*

| Authors, year | Sample | Design | Intervention procedure, duration, measurement points | Control Condition Description | Dependent variables | Effects |
|---|---|---|---|---|---|---|
| Caradoc-Davies & Harvey (1995) | 39 CGs, 28F, 11M, of disabled elderly patients, who regularly used respite services. | All participants received treatment (panel study). | Institutional respite of unspecified duration; measurement timepoints within 1 week prior to admission and 1 week after discharge. | No control group. | Barthel ADL, GHQ, Zung depression, Greene Scale (stress), social adjustment (SAS-SR scale), social supports. | ADL scores significantly improved, no difference in overall stress, but significant improvement in personal distress subscale, significantly improved GHQ scores, no other differences were significant. |

**TABLE 3.1** *(continued)*

| Authors, year | Sample | Design | Intervention procedure, duration, measurement points | Control Condition Description | Dependent variables | Effects |
|---|---|---|---|---|---|---|
| Castle, Wilkins, Heck, Tanzy, & Fahey (1995) | 11 wives of dementia patients. | Panel study. | Eight sessions, 1 1/2 hours weekly support group therapy, focused on building coping skills through education, shared experience, and a supportive environment to address each caregiver's current concerns; measurement timepoints at baseline, 8 weeks, and 12 weeks. | No control group. | Beck Depression & Anxiety scales, Hamilton Depression Scale, Geriatric Depression Scale, MMSE, Zarit Burden Scale, Lubbens Social Network Scale, UCLA Domain of Caregiver Appraisal, Symptom Checklist-90-Revised; immunological analysis of blood samples. | Change in scores on psychological inventories is not reported; however, study establishes a link between caregiving stress and physical health by quantifying immunological correlates of CG depression and stress. |

*(continued)*

**TABLE 3.1** *(continued)*

| Authors, year | Sample | Design | Intervention procedure, duration, measurement points | Control Condition Description | Dependent variables | Effects |
|---|---|---|---|---|---|---|
| Deimling (1992) | 78 CGs (gender not reported) of highly physically and mentally impaired elders. | Panel study, divided into 4 groups on the basis of cognitive and physical stability or decline of the CR. | Respite from home health aides (averaging 18 hours per month) or institutional respite (averaging 22 hours per month), for the 4-month course of the study; measures taken at entry (personal interview) and 4–6 months after start of service (telephone follow-up). | No control group. | CES-D, self-perceived health, relationship strain, activity restriction, ADL, CG assessment of CR cognitive function. | Significant decreases in depression in CGs of stable CRs; significant improvement in reported physical health in stable CR group, but decline in group where CR was experiencing cognitive decline; similar finding for relationship strain; respite did not alleviate activity restriction for CGs in the stable groups. |

**TABLE 3.1** *(continued)*

| Authors, year | Sample | Design | Intervention procedure, duration, measurement points | Control Condition Description | Dependent variables | Effects |
|---|---|---|---|---|---|---|
| Demers & Lavoie (1996) | 120 CGs of frail elders, 89F, 31M, French-speaking, no restriction on age, relation to CR, or cohabitation. | Treatment subjects recruited from organizations offering support groups; controls through community health centers not offering support groups. | 10 weekly 2 1/2-hour meetings of support groups; information/support/problem solving skills focus; measurements pre- and postintervention and subsequently at 3 months. | Due to quasi-experimental design, at T1, treatment subjects were higher than controls in % female, use of day care, CR memory and behavior problems, and depression. | Zarit Burden Interview, Generalized Contentment Scale (GCS), MBPC, Rapid Disability Rating Scale (RDRS), informal support, self-perceived health and change in health. | Burden increased in treatment group and decreased in control; depression remained stable in treatment group while increasing in control; burden and depression effects persisted at the 3-month timepoint. |

*(continued)*

**TABLE 3.1** *(continued)*

| Authors, year | Sample | Design | Intervention procedure, duration, measurement points | Control Condition Description | Dependent variables | Effects |
|---|---|---|---|---|---|---|
| Drummond, Mohide, Tew, Streiner, Pringle, & Gilbert (1991) | 42 CGs, gender not specified, of demented relatives. | Block randomization into treatment or conventional care groups. | Home visits from Community Support Nurses (CSNs), health assessments, education on dementia and caregiving, 4 hours weekly of in-home respite, additional respite on demand, optional monthly 2-hour support group session; measurements at 0, 3, and 6 months. | Conventional care, focused on patient. | CES-D, STAI, Caregiver Quality of Life Instrument (CQLI). | No effects on CES-D or STAI, some improvement in CQLI, but not statistically significant. |

**TABLE 3.1** (*continued*)

| Authors, year | Sample | Design | Intervention procedure, duration, measurement points | Control Condition Description | Dependent variables | Effects |
|---|---|---|---|---|---|---|
| Ferrell, Grant, Chan, Ahn, & Ferrell (1995) | 50 CGs of elderly cancer patients, 38F, 12M, 46 in-home. | Panel study. | Three 1-hour sessions of instruction in pain management, $50 allowance for non-drug intervention equipment; measurement timepoints prior to intervention, and 1 and 3 weeks after last session. | No control group. | Quality of Life Tool, Family Pain Questionnaire (Ferrell, et al., 1993), Caregiver Burden Tool. | Significant improvement in QOL at 1 week, and knowledge (no timepoint given). |

(*continued*)

**TABLE 3.1** *(continued)*

| Authors, year | Sample | Design | Intervention procedure, duration, measurement points | Control Condition Description | Dependent variables | Effects |
|---|---|---|---|---|---|---|
| Fritz, Farver, Hart, & Kass (1996) | 244 AD CGs, 174F, 70M, 124 pet owners, 120 no pets. | Study of effects of pet ownership on CG psychological health; nonrandom selection, with possible bias. | No intervention; recruitment included a letter describing the study (article does not say whether study topic was revealed), therefore, pet owners may have differentially responded. | Control group consisted of respondents who did not own pets. | Lexington Attachment to Pets Scale, MBPC, ZBI, Life Satisfaction Index-Z, GDS. | Men who were attached to dogs scored somewhat better on depression, life satisfaction, and burden than nonpet-owning males. Women under age 40 who were attached to cats had markedly better scores on the above measures than nonpet-owning females younger than 40. |

**TABLE 3.1** (*continued*)

| Authors, year | Sample | Design | Intervention procedure, duration, measurement points | Control Condition Description | Dependent variables | Effects |
|---|---|---|---|---|---|---|
| Gallagher-Thompson & DeVries (1994) | 48 wives or daughters of frail elderly. | Description and preliminary data from one of three treatment groups. | Eight weekly 2-hour training classes followed by booster sessions 1 and 2 months post-treatment; goal of teaching coping skills for feelings of anger and frustration related to caregiving; measurement time-points prior to and after treatment, and at follow-up (18 months post-treatment). | No control group. | Hostility items from Multiple Affect Adjective Checklist (MAAC), CG satisfaction reports, follow-up survey. | Significant decrease in hostility as measured by MAAC; follow-up survey indicated high levels of use of acquired skills at home. |

(*continued*)

**TABLE 3.1** *(continued)*

| Authors, year | Sample | Design | Intervention procedure, duration, measurement points | Control Condition Description | Dependent variables | Effects |
|---|---|---|---|---|---|---|
| Gallagher-Thompson & Steffen (1994) | 66 depressed CGs of frail elders, 61 F. | Random assignment into cognitive-behavioral or brief psychodynamic intervention. | Cognitive-behavioral (CB) group received instruction in challenging dysfunctional thoughts and adaptive problem solving; in brief psychodynamic (PD) group, therapy focused on understanding past losses and conflicts in separation and individuation through their reenactment; both groups received 16–20 sessions, two per week for 4 weeks, once per week afterward; assessments at 0, 10 weeks, immediately after treatment, 3, and 12 months post-treatment. | No control group. | Schedule for Affective Disorders and Schizophrenia (SADS), Hamilton Depression Scale, GDS, Beck Depression Inventory (BDI), health rating. | Overall, no differences between groups (both treatments successful). Time spent caregiving interacted with treatment method, such that PD was most helpful if caregiver was in role for less than 3 1/2 years, CB more effective after 3 1/2 years of caregiving. |

**TABLE 3.1** *(continued)*

| Authors, year | Sample | Design | Intervention procedure, duration, measurement points | Control Condition Description | Dependent variables | Effects |
|---|---|---|---|---|---|---|
| Goodman & Pynoos (1990) | 66 family CGs; lecture group: n = 31, 24F; network group: n = 35, 29F. | Matched groups design. | Lecture group assigned to hear 12 telephone-accessed lectures about AD over a 12-week period; Network group was divided into smaller groups of 4–5 CGs, who called each other in rotation over the 12-week period; measurements prior to and after treatments. | No control group. | Zarit Burden Interview, MBPC, Caregiver-Elder Relationship Scale, Mental Health Scale (Vleit & Ware, 83), Social Networks (Vaux & Harrison, 85), Perceived Social Support for Caregiving (Goodman), AD knowledge test. | Both groups improved in knowledge, perceived social support, and satisfaction with support. Lecture group gained more knowledge and more frequent emotional support from family and friends, as well as satisfaction with support. Network group had less frequent emotional support from family and friends. |

*(continued)*

**TABLE 3.1** *(continued)*

| Authors, year | Sample | Design | Intervention procedure, duration, measurement points | Control Condition Description | Dependent variables | Effects |
|---|---|---|---|---|---|---|
| Gwyther (1990) | 1 wife of an AD patient. | Case study. | "Social work intervention" of two face-to-face counseling sessions followed by therapeutic telephone calls at one week and then at 6-month intervals for 18 months. | None. | Feelings of conflict. | Unspecified improvement as a result of intervention. |

**TABLE 3.1** (*continued*)

| Authors, year | Sample | Design | Intervention procedure, duration, measurement points | Control Condition Description | Dependent variables | Effects |
|---|---|---|---|---|---|---|
| Hinchliffe, Hyman, Blizard, & Livingston (1995) | 40 pairs, 11M, 29F CGs, not receiving psychiatric services, demented CRs, CGs GHQ ≥ 4 (probable psychiatric morbidity). | Block randomized into treatment-first and delayed treatment groups. | Comprehensive therapy for both CG and CR, including psychotherapeutic drugs, activity involvement, respite, education, support groups, instruction in time management, and relaxation techniques; 16 week duration; measures at baseline, 16, and 32 weeks. | AB vs. BA design, control consisted of delay of intervention for 16-week duration. | General Health Questionnaire (GHQ). | Improvement for treatment-first group, no improvement for delayed treatment group. |

(continued)

**TABLE 3.1** *(continued)*

| Authors, year | Sample | Design | Intervention procedure, duration, measurement points | Control Condition Description | Dependent variables | Effects |
|---|---|---|---|---|---|---|
| Hinchliffe, Hyman, Blizard, & Livingston (1992) | 16 CGs, 12F, 4M, of day-care attenders with dementia. | Panel study. | No description published, but appears to be multifaceted. | No control group. | General Health Questionnaire (GHQ28). | Reduction in GHQ scores between baseline and time 2 measurement. |

**TABLE 3.1** *(continued)*

| Authors, year | Sample | Design | Intervention procedure, duration, measurement points | Control Condition Description | Dependent variables | Effects |
|---|---|---|---|---|---|---|
| Ingersoll-Dayton, Chapman, & Neal (1990) | 256 employee CGs (23%) and anticipated CGs (37%), 37 M, CR ailments not furnished. | One of 3 treatments offered to all participants. | 7 weekly 1-hour seminars presented by professionals, at the workplace, followed by one of three 8-week treatment options: care planning, support groups, or buddy system; measurements at entry, 7 weeks, and 15 weeks. | No control group. | Helpfulness and impact questionnaire (derived from Emlen & Koren, 84), stress and strain items from Stewart & Archbold, 88, affect items from Bradburn, 69. | Attendance at seminars associated with increases in knowledge and absenteeism; buddy system group was not attended; attending other 2 groups yielded decreases in negative affect. |

*(continued)*

**TABLE 3.1** (*continued*)

| Authors, year | Sample | Design | Intervention procedure, duration, measurement points | Control Condition Description | Dependent variables | Effects |
|---|---|---|---|---|---|---|
| Kaplan & Gallagher-Thompson (1995) | 1 clinically depressed wife caregiver. | Case study. | Cognitive-behavioral therapy for depression; 17 individual counseling sessions over 8 1/2 months. | None. | Beck Depression Inventory. | Full remission of major depression due to counseling. |

**TABLE 3.1** (*continued*)

| Authors, year | Sample | Design | Intervention procedure, duration, measurement points | Control Condition Description | Dependent variables | Effects |
|---|---|---|---|---|---|---|
| Kosloski & Montgomery (1995) | 181 CG/CR dyads, gender not reported, CR physically or mentally impaired. | Subjects were in treatment group of Montgomery & Borgatta, 1989, and are examined for factors leading to placement. | Free respite services were made available to all subjects ($882 Medicare waiver), with actual usage monitored; measurement timepoints at baseline and 1 year. | No control group; study contrasts CGs who placed their relative with those who did not. | CR health and function, CG health, time spent caregiving, CG anxiety, CR income, CG attachment to CR, outside service use, respite use. | Age and AD were significant predictors of placement, adding respite use to the model yielded significant improvement of fit (increasing respite use associated with delayed placement). |

*(continued)*

**TABLE 3.1** *(continued)*

| Authors, year | Sample | Design | Intervention procedure, duration, measurement points | Control Condition Description | Dependent variables | Effects |
|---|---|---|---|---|---|---|
| Labrecque, Peak, & Toseland (1992) | 66 wives of frail elderly veterans, recruited on the basis of self-perceived need for intervention. | Single-blind, randomized into control or support-group intervention conditions; long-term effects examined. | 8 weekly 2-hour support group sessions, focusing on education and discussion, support, problem-solving, and stress reduction; measurement timepoints: within 2 weeks prior to intervention, within 2 weeks after, 6 months, 1 year. | Control group subjects given assistance only if they requested it. | CG/CR health, burden, service use & knowledge, informal support, depression, anxiety, interpersonal competence, pressing problems, marital relationship, satisfaction with intervention. | CG's perception of CR's health positively affected by intervention; no other effects attributable to support group participation. |

**TABLE 3.1** *(continued)*

| Authors, year | Sample | Design | Intervention procedure, duration, measurement points | Control Condition Description | Dependent variables | Effects |
|---|---|---|---|---|---|---|
| Larkin & Hopcroft (1993) | 21 AD CRs and 22 CGs, 19F, 3M. | Panel study. | 2-week inpatient stay, VA copayment; measurement timepoints at 3 days prior to admission (T1) and discharge (T2), and 14 days after discharge (T3). | No control group. | Brief Symptom Inventory (BSI), ADL, formal and informal supports. | Significant reduction in BSI scores between T1 and T2; 86% of CGs reported improvement in sleep; increase in CG receptivity to long-term placement noted over the course of the study. |

*(continued)*

**TABLE 3.1** (*continued*)

| Authors, year | Sample | Design | Intervention procedure, duration, measurement points | Control Condition Description | Dependent variables | Effects |
|---|---|---|---|---|---|---|
| Mittelman, Ferris, Steinberg, Shulman, Mackell, Ambinder, & Cohen (1993) | 206 (120F, 86M) spousal pairs, AD diagnosis for CR. | Random assignment into treatment or control group. | Individual and family counseling, support groups, education, ad hoc counseling; 12-month duration; measures at baseline, 4, 8, and 12 months, and every 6 months afterward. | Support and counseling resources available, but not mandatory, assistance in obtaining services not provided. | Formal care usage, Short Psychiatric Evaluation Scale (SPES), Geriatric Depression Scale (GDS), Burden Interview, MBPC, physical health (OARS), family cohesiveness (FACES III). | Lower placement rate at 1 year. |

**TABLE 3.1** *(continued)*

| Authors, year | Sample | Design | Intervention procedure, duration, measurement points | Control Condition Description | Dependent variables | Effects |
|---|---|---|---|---|---|---|
| Mittelman, Ferris, Shulman, Steinberg, Ambinder, Mackell, & Cohen (1995) | Same as above. | Same as above. | Same as 1993 study. | Same as above. | Geriatric Depression Scale | Controls more depressed than treatment subjects, who remained stable. |
| Mittelman, Ferris, Shulman, Steinberg, & Levin (1996) | Same as 1993 study. | Same as 1993 study. | Same as 1993 study. | Same as 1993 study. | Time until placement over 8-year period. | Greater time until placement in treatment group; treatment most effective in delaying placement when CR had mild to moderate dementia. |

*(continued)*

**TABLE 3.1** (*continued*)

| Authors, year | Sample | Design | Intervention procedure, duration, measurement points | Control Condition Description | Dependent variables | Effects |
|---|---|---|---|---|---|---|
| Mohide, Pringle, Streiner, Gilbert, Muir, & Tew (1990) | 60 dementia CGs, 43F, 17M. | Random assignment into treatment and control groups. | Weekly home visits by specially trained caregiver support nurses (CSNs), providing educational materials, and individually tailored programs of support, 4 hours per week scheduled in-home respite, on-demand respite; optional monthly 2-hour support group; duration 6 months; measurement timepoints at entry, 3 months, and 6 months; 12–18 month follow-up interview also conducted. | Conventional community nursing care. | CES-D, STAI, Caregiver Quality of Life Instrument (CQLI), health self-rating, Cantril Self-Anchoring Striving Scale. | No significant change on any variables; trend toward increase in CQLI scores in treatment group, and decrease in control group. |

**TABLE 3.1** *(continued)*

| Authors, year | Sample | Design | Intervention procedure, duration, measurement points | Control Condition Description | Dependent variables | Effects |
|---|---|---|---|---|---|---|
| Oktay & Volland (1990) | 191 CG/CR pairs, hospital-discharged frail elderly, 116F, 75M, 76% African-American. | Assignment to treatment or control group on the basis of date of discharge (quasi-experimental design). | Coordinated program of medical and social support, including assessment, case management, skilled nursing, counseling, referrals, respite, education, support group, medical backup, and on-call help; minimum 1 nurse and 1 social worker visit per month; measurement timepoints at 1, 3, 6, 9, and 12 months after discharge. | Control group had access, but was not required to receive services. | GHQ (CG stress), physical health, Negative Impact of Caregivers Scale, health service use, CR: ADL/IADL, Mental Status Questionnaire, health service use. | Small reduction in stress and substantial reduction in days spent in hospital for treatment group. |

*(continued)*

**TABLE 3.1** *(continued)*

| Authors, year | Sample | Design | Intervention procedure, duration, measurement points | Control Condition Description | Dependent variables | Effects |
|---|---|---|---|---|---|---|
| Pynoos & Ohta (1991) | 12 CGs, 7F, 5M, of AD patients. | Panel study. | List of problems and proposed physical/environmental interventions generated by a team comprised of a clinical gerontologist, an occupational therapist, and a psychologist. CG was allowed to choose up to $100 worth of interventions from the list; measurement timepoints at baseline and 7 months after implementation of intervention. | No control group. | CG's perception of effectiveness and safety of the interventions. | 66% of interventions were initially effective; of those, 89% continued to be effective at follow-up; ineffective interventions failed mainly due to failures to implement on the part of the CG. |

**TABLE 3.1** *(continued)*

| Authors, year | Sample | Design | Intervention procedure, duration, measurement points | Control Condition Description | Dependent variables | Effects |
|---|---|---|---|---|---|---|
| Ripich & Wykle (1997) | 28 AD CGs, 18F, 10M, 8AA (7F), 20 white (11F). | Panel study. | Four weekly 2-hour sessions in groups of 8–10; instruction on communication with AD patient, including readings, discussions, videotape, and role-playing. | No control group. | Positive and Negative Affect (PANAS), 12 items from CES-D, perceived health, Caregiver Hassles Scale, knowledge assessment, satisfaction with communication. | AA subjects had significant increase in positive affect following treatment and significant decrease in hassles; both groups had significant increase in knowledge and satisfaction with communication. |

*(continued)*

**TABLE 3.1** *(continued)*

| Authors, year | Sample | Design | Intervention procedure, duration, measurement points | Control Condition Description | Dependent variables | Effects |
|---|---|---|---|---|---|---|
| Teri & Uomoto (1991) | 4 CGs, 2M, 2F, of AD and depressed CRs. | Case study; all 4 subjects received treatment, order of treatment, and control varied. | Eight 60-minute sessions teaching behavioral strategies for decreasing depression by increasing pleasant events; varied duration of intervention; varied measurement timepoints. | Cases 1 and 2 used first week as baseline; case 3 used AB design, case 4 used ABAB design. | CG depression (HDRS and BDI scores). | Subjects with high initial depression were less depressed with treatment. |

**TABLE 3.1** (*continued*)

| Authors, year | Sample | Design | Intervention procedure, duration, measurement points | Control Condition Description | Dependent variables | Effects |
|---|---|---|---|---|---|---|
| Theis, Moss, & Pearson (1994) | 130 pairs, 14M, 116F CGs of demented and nondemented elderly. | Panel study. | In-home respite up to 4 hours/week and institutional respite (short-term stays in long-term facility); 12-month duration; measurement timepoints at 0, 6, and 12 months. | No control group. | Profile of Mood States (POMS), Quality of Life Index (QOL), Response to Caregiving (Feelings about Caregiving and Impact on Family subscales, and Burden Interview). | No significant effects on any outcome variables at either timepoint, downward trends evident. |

(*continued*)

**TABLE 3.1** (*continued*)

| Authors, year | Sample | Design | Intervention procedure, duration, measurement points | Control Condition Description | Dependent variables | Effects |
|---|---|---|---|---|---|---|
| Toseland, Labrecque, Goebel, & Whitney (1992) | 89 CG wives of frail elderly veterans, highly burdened. | Random recruitment into control and support groups, participants blind to existence of other condition. | Eight weekly 2-hour sessions; sessions consisted of support, education and discussion, problem solving, and stress reduction; measurement time-points within 2 weeks before and after intervention. | Differential recruitment of control vs. treatment participants (script differed such that controls only agreed to be interviewed, treatment subjects agreed to interviews and support group attendance). | CG physical health, CR health and function (Patient Assessment Tool for Home Care; PATH), burden (Montgomery & Borgatta Burden Scale; MBBS), depression (Beck Depression Inventory and GDS), anxiety (STAI), self-efficacy, help-seeking and coping, service use, social support. | After treatment, controls estimated higher # of hours spent caregiving and greater subjective burden; no difference in service usage; treatment group had higher marital satisfaction, use of active behavioral coping strategies, knowledge of community resources, and fewer pressing problems. |

## TABLE 3.1 (continued)

| Authors, year | Sample | Design | Intervention procedure, duration, measurement points | Control Condition Description | Dependent variables | Effects |
|---|---|---|---|---|---|---|
| Toseland, Rossiter, Peak, & Smith (1990) | 154 daughters and daughters-in-law of frail elders. | Subjects assigned into individual counseling, group counseling, or control conditions on the basis of time of recruitment. | Group counseling: 8 weekly 2-hour sessions; individual counseling: 8 weekly 1-hour sessions; both interventions based on an ecological systems framework, focusing on validation and confirmation of caregiving experiences, encouragement and praise, and affirmation of coping ability; measurement timepoints within 2 weeks before and after intervention | Control subjects were informed of no-treatment status, and given funds for respite; minimal support (information and referral). | Bradburn Affect Balance Scale (BABS), burden (ZBI), psychiatric symptoms (BSI), social supports, CG-CR relations (Personal Change Scale), project satisfaction. | Individually counseled group had greater reduction in burden and severity of psychiatric symptoms than group participants; group participants had greater increases in social support; both interventions produced positive changes in CG-CR relations; satisfaction with treatment greater for intervention than control subjects. |

(continued)

**TABLE 3.1** *(continued)*

| Authors, year | Sample | Design | Intervention procedure, duration, measurement points | Control Condition Description | Dependent variables | Effects |
|---|---|---|---|---|---|---|
| Toseland & Smith (1990) | 87 daughters and daughters-in-law of frail elders. | Random assignment into professional, peer, or no counseling conditions. | Weekly 1-hour individual counseling sessions, using action-oriented model of intervention, including problem identification, problem solving, stress reduction, and time management (see Toseland 88 for description); duration 8 weeks; pre-test and post-test data collected within 2 weeks of first and last counseling sessions. | Control group recruitment occurred 6 months prior to study. | Bradburn Affect Balance Scale (BABS), Zarit Burden Interview (ZBI), Brief Symptom Inventory (BSI), social supports: number, satisfaction, and perceived change; knowledge of service availability (Community Resource Scale); CG-CR relations: Self-Appraisal of Change Scale, satisfaction with intervention. | Both peer and professionally counseled groups improved in psychiatric symptomatology and relationships with care recipients; professionally counseled group improved in subjective well-being. |

**TABLE 3.1** (*continued*)

| Authors, year | Sample | Design | Intervention procedure, duration, measurement points | Control Condition Description | Dependent variables | Effects |
|---|---|---|---|---|---|---|
| Vernooij-Dassen, Felling, Huygen, & Persoon (1995) | 138 dementia CGs, gender info. not furnished. | Random assignment into control or intervention group. | Emotional and practical support from home health aides, 4 hours/week; 10-month duration; measurement timepoints not specified. | No information given. | Sense of competence, as measured by newly developed questionnaire; likelihood of placement. | No overall effect on sense of competence, but female, in-home caregivers in treatment group were more improved than those in control group. Reduced likelihood of placement in treatment group. |

(*continued*)

**TABLE 3.1** (*continued*)

| Authors, year | Sample | Design | Intervention procedure, duration, measurement points | Control Condition Description | Dependent variables | Effects |
|---|---|---|---|---|---|---|
| Whitlatch, Zarit, & von Eye (1991) | 113 dementia CGs, 63% daughters and wives, 30% husbands and sons, 7% other. | Random assignment into counseling, support, or wait list group. | Counseling focused on CGs and their families, support groups utilized interactions among CGs to reduce stress (full description of interventions is in Zarit, Anthony, & Boutselis, 1987; this study consists of a reanalysis of existing data). | Control group on waiting list. | Brief Symptom Inventory, personal strain, role strain; Prediction Analysis is used to specify direction and amount of change expected for individuals based on initial scores and group assignment. | Improvement on BSI and other measures more likely with treatment than without; improvement more likely with counseling than with support groups. |

**TABLE 3.1** (*continued*)

| Authors, year | Sample | Design | Intervention procedure, duration, measurement points | Control Condition Description | Dependent variables | Effects |
|---|---|---|---|---|---|---|
| Whitlatch, Zarit, Goodwin, & von Eye (1995) | 132 dementia CGs, no gender data published, sample overlaps study above. | Same as above. | Same as above; this study examines data obtained in a 1-year follow-up of Zarit, et al., (1987). | Same as above. | Same measures as above, but treatment success in above analysis is related to dichotomous variable: placed or not placed. | Successful treatment response on BSI and personal strain measures related to lower placement likelihood. |

*(continued)*

## TABLE 3.1 *(continued)*

| Authors, year | Sample | Design | Intervention procedure, duration, measurement points | Control Condition Description | Dependent variables | Effects |
|---|---|---|---|---|---|---|
| Zarit, Greene, Ferraro, Townsend, & Stephens (1996) | 323 dementia CGs, approximately 60% F. | Treatment group consisted of NJ CGs entering day care; controls were OH CGs for whom day care was not available. | ≥ 2 days per week of day-care use; 3 months duration; baseline and 3-month measurement timepoints. | Neither controls nor treatment subjects receiving more than 8 hours per week of other paid help; controls expressed willingness to use day care. | Role captivity, overload, worry, and strain, depression (CES-D), anger, positive affect (PANAS). | Treatment group had less overload, worry and strain, depression, and anger; role captivity and positive affect unaffected. |

it can be used effectively if introduced in a graduated step-wise fashion.

Although there are clearly many challenges remaining for caregiving intervention researchers, two deserve special emphasis. One concerns the choice of outcomes and the other concerns methods for identifying the optimal mix of intervention components for a particular caregiver. The studies reviewed here focused on a wide range of outcomes including caregiver distress, physical and mental health, care-recipient behavior, and care recipient institutionalization. In selecting an appropriate outcome for an intervention we think it useful to clearly identify the expected proximal and distal outcomes. Proximal outcomes are those that the interventions are directly intended to have an effect upon while distal outcomes are typically contingent on first achieving the proximal outcomes. As an example, the proximal outcome for an intervention aimed at changing patient problem behaviors would be a reduction in unwanted behaviors. A distal outcome may include a reduction in caregiver distress. Too often interventions fail to assess relevant proximal outcomes making it difficult to understand how or why an intervention did or did not work. In addition, interventionists frequently focus on distal outcomes such as time to institutionalization without considering the relationship between the proximal goals of the intervention (e.g., enhancing knowledge of the caregiver) and the distal outcomes. For example, an intervention designed to delay institutionalization by providing a caregiver with information about resources options may have the unintended effect of facilitating institutionalization.

A recurrent theme of this review has been that caregivers have multiple needs that interventionists need to address in order to maximize impact. Finding the optimal mix of program elements for a given caregiver/care recipient dyad at a particular point in the disease trajectory should be a major goal of intervention researchers. However, achieving this goal is virtually impossible with studies of limited sample size and limited intervention approaches. What is needed are large studies with diverse populations that would enable one to fully explore the complex interactions among caregiver and care recipient characteristics, treatment components, and methods of delivery.

# REFERENCES

Bayer-Feldmann & Greifenhagen (1995). Gruppenarbeit mit Angehorigen von Alzheimer-Krankenein systemischer Ansatz. *Psychotherapie Psychosomatik Medizinische Psychologie, 45,* 1–7.

Berry, G.L., Zarit, S.H., & Rabatin, V.X. (1991). Caregiver activity on respite and nonrespite days: A comparison of two service approaches. *The Gerontologist, 31*(6), 830–835.

Bourgeois, M. (1990). Enhancing conversation skills in patients with Alzheimer's disease using a prosthetic memory aid. *Journal of Applied Behavior Analysis, 23,* 31–64.

Bourgeois, M.S., Schulz, R., & Burgio, L. (1996). Interventions for caregivers of patients with Alzheimer's Disease: A review and analysis of content, process, and outcomes. *International Journal of Aging and Human Development, 43*(1), 35–92.

Bourgeois, M., Burgio, L., Schulz, R., Beach, S., & Palmer, B. (1997). Modifying repetitive verbalization of community dwelling patients with AD. *The Gerontologist, 37*(1), 30–39.

Brennan, P.F., Moore, S.M., & Smyth, K.A. (1991). ComputerLink: Electronic support for the home caregiver. *Advances in Nursing Science, 13*(4), 14–27.

Brodaty, H., & Gresham, M. (1989). Effect of a Training Programme to Reduce Stress in Carers of Patients with Dementia. *British Medical Journal, 299,* 1375–1379.

Brodaty, H., McGilchrist, C., Harris, L., & Peters, K.E. (1993). Time until institutionalization and death in patients with dementia. *Archives of Neurology, 50,* 643–650.

Brodaty, H., & Peters, K.E. (1991). Cost effectiveness of a training program for dementia carers. *International Psychogeriatrics, 3*(1), 11–22.

Brodaty, H., Roberts, K., & Peters, K. (1994). Quasi-experimental evaluation of an educational model for dementia caregivers. *International Journal of Geriatric Psychiatry, 9,* 195–204.

Caradoc-Davies, T.H., & Harvey, J.M. (1995). Do social relief admissions have any effect on patients or their caregivers? *Disability and Rehabilitation, 17*(5), 247–251.

Castle, S., Wilkins, S., Heck, E., Tanzy, K., & Fahey, J. (1995). Depression in caregivers of demented patients is associated with altered immunity: impaired proliferative capacity, increased CD8+, and a decline in lymphocytes with surface signal transduction molecules (CD38+) and a cytotoxicity marker (CD56+ CD8+). *Clinical Experimental Immunology, 101,* 487–493.

Deimling, G.T. (1992). Respite use and caregiver well-being in families caring for stable and declining AD patients. *Journal of Gerontological Social Work, 18*(1/2), 117–134.

Demers, A., & Lavoie, J. (1996). Effect of support groups on family caregivers to the frail elderly. *Canadian Journal on Aging, 15*(1), 129–144.

Drummond, M.F., Mohide, E.A., Tew, M., Streiner, D.L., Pringle, D.M., & Gilbert, J.R. (1991). Economic evaluation of a support program for caregivers of demented elderly. *International Journal of Technology Assessment in Health Care, 7*(2), 209–219.

Ferrell, B.R., Grant, M., Chan, J., Ahn, C., & Ferrell, B.A. (1995). The impact of cancer pain education on family caregivers of elderly patients. *Oncology Nursing Forum, 22*(8), 1211–1218.

Fritz, C.L., Farver, T.B., Hart, L.A., & Kass, P.H. (1996). Companion animals and the psychological health of Alzheimer patient caregivers. *Psychological Reports, 78*, 467–481.

Gallagher-Thompson, D., & DeVries, H.M. (1994). Coping with frustration classes: Development and preliminary outcomes with women who care for relatives with dementia. *The Gerontologist, 34*(4), 548–552.

Gallagher-Thompson, D., & Steffen, A.M. (1994). Comparative effects of cognitive-behavioral and brief psychodynamic psychotherapies for depressed family caregivers. *Journal of Consulting and Clinical Psychology, 62*(3), 543–549.

Goodman, C.C., & Pynoos, J. (1990). A model telephone information and support program for caregivers of Alzheimer's patients. *The Gerontologist, 30*(3), 399–404.

Gwyther, L. (1990). Letting go: Separation-individuation in a wife of an Alzheimer's patient. In R.J. Kastenbaum & J. Hendricks (Eds.), *The International Journal of Aging and Human Development.* Amityville, NY: Baywood.

Hinchliffe, A.C., Hyman, I., Blizard, B., & Livingston, G. (1992). The impact on carers of behavioural difficulties in dementia: A pilot study on management. *International Journal of Geriatric Psychiatry, 7*, 579–583.

Hinchliffe, A.C., Hyman, I.L., Blizard, B., & Livingston, (1995). Behavioural complications of dementia—can they be treated? *International Journal of Geriatric Psychiatry, 10*, 839–847.

Ingersoll-Dayton, B., Chapman, N., & Neal, M. (1990). A program for caregivers in the workplace. *The Gerontologist, 30*(1), 126–130.

Kaplan, C.P., & Gallagher-Thompson, D. (1995). The treatment of clinical depression in caregivers of spouses with dementia. *Journal of Cognitive Psychotherapy: An International Quarterly, 9*, 35–44.

Knight, B.G., Lutzky, S.M., & Macofsky-Urban, F. (1993). A meta-analytic review of interventions for caregiver distress. *The Gerontologist, 33*, 240–248.

Kosloski, K., & Montgomery, R.J.V. (1995). The impact of respite use on nursing home placement. *Gerontologist, 35*(1), 67–74.

Labrecque, M.S., Peak, T., & Toseland, R.W. (1992). Long-term effectiveness of a group program for caregivers of frail elderly veterans. *American Journal of Orthopsychiatry, 62*(4), 575–588.

Larkin, J.P., & Hopcroft, B.M. (1993). In-hospital respite as a moderator of caregiver stress. *Health & Social Work, 18*(2), 133–138.

Lawton, M.P., Brody, E.M., & Saperstein, A.R. (1989). A controlled study of respite service for caregivers of Alzheimer's patients. *The Gerontologist, 29*(1), 8–16.

Mittelman, M.S., Ferris, S.H., Shulman, E., Steinberg, G., Ambinder, A., Mackell, J.A., & Cohen, J. (1995). A comprehensive support program: Effect on depression in spouse-caregivers of AD patients. *The Gerontologist, 35*(6), 792–802.

Mittelman, M.S., Ferris, S.H., Steinberg, G., Shulman, E., Mackell, J.A., Ambinder, A., & Cohen, J. (1993). An intervention that delays institutionalization of Alzheimer's Disease patients: Treatment of spouse-caregivers. *The Gerontologist, 33*(6), 730–740.

Mittelman, M.S., Ferris, S.H., Shulman, E., Steinberg, G., & Levin, B. (1996). A family intervention to delay nursing home placement of patients with Alzheimer Disease. *Journal of the American Medical Association, 276*(21), 1725–1731.

Mohide, E.A., Pringle, D.M., Streiner, D.L., Gilbert, J.R., Muir, G., & Tew, M. (1990). A randomized trial of family caregiver support in the home management of dementia. *Journal of the American Geriatrics Society, 38*, 446–454.

Oktay, J.S., & Volland, P.J. (1990). Posthospital support program for the frail elderly and their caregivers: A quasi-experimental evaluation. *American Journal of Public Health, 80*(1), 39–46.

Pynoos, J., & Ohta, R.J. (1991). In-home interventions for persons with Alzheimer's Disease and their caregivers. *Physical and Occupational Therapy in Geriatrics, 9(3-4)*, 83–92.

Ripich, D.N., & Wykle, M. (personal communication, 1997). Maintaining communication in persons with Alzheimer's Disease: Effects of a training program on African-American and White caregivers.

Teri, L., & Uomoto, J.M. (1991). Reducing excess disability in dementia patients: Training caregivers to manage patient depression. *Clinical Gerontologist, 10*(4), 49–63.

Theis, S.L., Moss, J.H., & Pearson, M.A. (1994). Respite for caregivers: An evaluation study. *Journal of Community Health Nursing, 77*(1), 31–44.

Toseland, R.W., Labrecque, M.S., Goebel, S.T., & Whitney, M.H. (1992). An evaluation of a group program for spouses of frail elderly veterans. *The Gerontologist, 32*(3), 382–390.

Toseland, R.W., & Rossiter, C.M. (1989). Group interventions to support family caregivers: A review and analysis. *The Gerontologist, 29,* 438–448.

Toseland, R.W., Rossiter, C.M., Peak, T., & Smith, G.C. (1990). Comparative effectiveness of individual and group interventions to support family caregivers. *Social Work, 35*(3), 209–217.

Toseland, R.W., & Smith, G.C. (1990). Effectiveness of individual counseling by professional and peer helpers for family caregivers of the elderly. *Psychology and Aging, 5*(2), 256–263.

Vernooij-Dassen, M., Huygen, F., Felling, A., & Persoon, J. (1995). Home care for dementia patients. *Journal of the American Geriatrics Society, 43*(4), 456–457.

Whitlatch, C.J., Zarit, S.H., Goodwin, P.E., & von Eye, A. (1995). Influence of the success of psychoeducational interventions on the course of family care. *Clinical Gerontologist, 16*(1), 17–30.

Whitlatch, C.J., Zarit, S.H., & von Eye, A. (1991). Efficacy of interventions with caregivers: A reanalysis. *The Gerontologist, 31*(1), 9–14.

Zarit, S.H., Anthony, C.R., & Boutselis, M. (1987). Interventions with caregivers of dementia patients: Comparison of two approaches. *Psychology and Aging, 2*(3), 225–232.

Zarit, S.H., Greene, R., Ferraro, E., Townsend, A., & Stephens, M.A.P. (1996, November). Adult day care and the relief of caregiver strain: Results of the adult day care collaborative study. Symposium presented at the annual meetings of the Gerontological Society of America, Washington, D.C.

Zarit, S.H., & Teri, L. (1992). Interventions and services for family caregivers. In K.W. Schiae & M. Powell Lawton (Eds.), *Annual Review of Gerontology and Geriatrics, Vol. 11* (pp. 287–310). New York: Springer.

# 4

# The Pragmatics of Implementing Intervention Studies in the Community

*Linda O. Nichols, Charlotte Malone,*
*Barbara Tarlow, and David Loewenstein*

## INTRODUCTION AND OVERVIEW

An intervention is the product of three interdependent and intersecting forces—theory, the culture and nature of research, and the culture of the setting/community. Once a theoretical framework for an intervention has been selected, consideration must be given to the myriad aspects of implementing the intervention. It is possible to organize a discussion of intervention implementation by using the same headings research proposals and articles do—subjects, sites, intervention format, recruitment, retention. However, an alternative approach is to examine the pragmatics of intervention implementation by assessing the failure or success of an intervention based on how well researchers understand and work with the culture of the community.

This chapter addresses the major cultural considerations of implementation, the major elements to be considered in matching an intervention to a community, and the marketing strategies to be considered in "selling" an intervention. In discussing the various factors involved in intervention implementation, the reader should keep in mind that these issues must be addressed in the research design and planning stage, as well as considering them individually during implementation. Flexibility in design and implementation is necessary to maximize the fit between intervention and community, which is one of the most critical factors in the successful implementation of the intervention (Zakus, 1998).

## UNDERSTANDING THE CULTURAL CONTEXT OF THE COMMUNITY

In practice, theory and research most often have the strongest influence on initial design of the intervention. However, community forces determine the success or failure of the intervention. Because the community setting can exert an ex post facto design effect, any successful implementation should consider the community, as well as the theory and nature of research, when designing an intervention. To be successful, every aspect of the design and implementation of an intervention must mesh with the culture of the community. If the community does not participate, the intervention will not be successful (Zakus, 1998).

The cultural context of a community might be defined as all the "historical, economic, social, political, and geographical elements" that influence individuals within a given community (Helman, 1994, p. 5)—the norms, beliefs, attitudes, and behaviors a group shares. These elements themselves are layered structures, containing many subcomponents. It also is important to understand that cultural context is dynamic, changing over time as the lives of individuals within the community intersect with the lives of others (Helman, 1994). For example, the social setting of an intervention may include the interaction between various participants, the interaction between participants and research investigators, the interaction between investigators and research sponsors, as well as the interaction between participants and sponsors. Some or all of these relationships likely will change over the course of an intervention.

To understand and work with the community culture is to gain cultural competence. Cultural competence is an understanding of the culture and its role as the context for behavior and is often used in health care delivery systems when the cultures of provider and patient are dramatically or obviously different (Downs, Bernstein, & Marchese, 1997; Kagawa-Singer, 1997). However, cultural differences frequently are present between researchers and participants, even those from the same communities. One of the most basic approaches to understanding the cultural context for an intervention is to begin by researching, observing, and analyzing the culture of the community. Given the caveat that, by definition, communities are comprised of heterogeneous subpopulations, identifying a community culture is an arduous task.

What constitutes the cultural environment of an intervention study? Certainly, the culture is more than the sum totals of a community's historical, economic, social, political, and geographical elements or its norms, beliefs, and attitudes. For interventions, such as REACH, where multiple sites, multiple levels of intervention, and multiple investigators are involved, the intervention environment can, indeed, be a complex concept. To be effective, an intervention must be designed with these various layers of environment in mind, and the researcher's cultural competence must encompass each of these multiple layers.

Cultural competence requires that the researcher assess the attitudes, beliefs, behaviors, and ideology of individuals within the community. One must consider how these perceptions will effect implementation of the study. Will the community view the study as beneficial or harmful? Does the intervention process respect community taboos and values? Could the intervention be modified to accommodate community taboos without jeopardizing the integrity of the research? (Chapter 5 further explores issues of cultural diversity in research populations.)

Researchers must be experienced in and capable of identifying leaders within a community. However, they also need to be skilled at determining whether community leaders are speaking for the welfare of the community, or if, perhaps, they are protecting self-interests, furthering personal/political aspirations, or attempting to avert a change in the status quo (Fals-Borda & Rahnema, 1991; Zakus, 1998). By contrast, marginal citizens or individuals functioning on the fringe of a community may be eager to participate in the research process to elevate their standing within the community. Yet these individuals may be no more representative of a community than are the acknowledged community leaders. Also to be considered is whether any perceived benefits to be gained by the community as an aggregate outweigh any risks incurred by individuals. Again, issues such as these can be minimized by conducting thorough investigations during the design phase of a research project.

Under certain conditions, cultural factors also can play a significant role in facilitating intervention implementation. Congruence between the basic beliefs, attitudes, and values of the interventionists and those of the community and research participants help minimize conflicts during implementation (Majumdar & Roberts, 1998). For example, REACH interventionists at the Memphis site encountered a case in which a care recipient's behaviors were viewed by the spouse as "works of the devil" rather than as manifestations of Alzheimer's disease. The interventionist's familiarity with similar beliefs (expressed across America's Bible belt) allowed her to respond to the caregiver appropriately.

By the same token, however, cultural factors can and do become barriers to intervention implementation. For example, in working with primary caregivers for Cuban-American persons with dementia, recruiters and interventionists must be not only knowledgeable about issues of caregiving but also fluent in the Spanish language and familiar with the customs of the Cuban-American family unit (Arguelles & Loewenstein, 1997). Cuban-American extended families often live together, and different family members provide different levels of care: instrumental and social support. Daughters and daughters-in-law often are the primary caregivers of a parent with dementia, even when the nonaffected parent is living in the home (Mintzer et al., 1992). However, automatically assuming that the primary caregiver is a spouse or child would be erroneous. In-laws, nieces, siblings, or grandchildren actually may provide the majority of care to a patient. A similar pattern has been demonstrated among African-American caregivers where there often is an extended network of family members (Lawton, Rajagopal, Brody, & Kleban, 1992). These variations in caregiving patterns must be thoroughly explored.

## UNDERSTANDING THE CULTURAL CONTEXT OF RESEARCH

Just as communities evince a cultural context, research as an endeavor also develops a cultural context within which it operates. The culture of research is complex and pluralistic. There are general beliefs and practices which guide the scientific community at any time and influence the implementation of interventions. These beliefs are the result of evolution in scientific thinking and methodology and reflect current thinking about best practices. For example, the current standard for study design is the randomized clinical trial. These research beliefs and practices interact with theoretical constructs and constraints in the design of the intervention. The large-scale, multisite dementia study most recently funded by NIA, REACH, is a longitudinal randomized clinical trial.

Like the cultural context of a community, the cultural context of research is a multilayered and dynamic entity that changes over the course of the research. The disciplines, personal beliefs, values, ideologies, and behaviors of all the individual research team members are a part of this context. These attributes and values may or may not be visible or obvious. However, there are other attributes that usually are not visible but also constitute a part of the cultural context of research. These include the researchers' perceptions—of themselves as researchers, of the research process as a method of scientific inquiry, of what is an acceptable problem to study, of the community as a setting for intervention, and of the potential community members as subjects.

The cultural factors within the research milieu also can facilitate or hinder research efforts. When other organizations or professionals not involved in the study serve as referral sites, the cultures and politics of the research organization and the referring organization may conflict. This issue is discussed in depth below. Within the study team itself, cultures also may be different. For example, in interdisciplinary caregiving studies, the terms used to describe study participants can be a clue to the different cultures of the researchers (e.g., client, patient, consumer, care recipient). In implementing an intervention study, these differences can influence the researchers' perception of and interactions with study subjects. Even the use of the terms "participant" or "subject" may imply a different degree of collaboration and/or collegiality between those who study and those who are studied. The issue of collaboration between researcher and participant is being increasingly recognized as a critical success factor, although in most cases, the researcher still controls the study and the intervention (Schwab & Syme, 1997).

As with aspects of community culture, congruence between the aspirations of the researchers and the goals of the community, whether visible or obscure, play a substantial role in either facilitating or hindering the research process. Researchers may have biases toward participants that influence their willingness to treat participants as collaborators (Beisecker, Murden, Moore, Graham, & Nelmig, 1996; Downs et al., 1997). It is important to know who the investigators are and if they are part of the community or outside it (town versus gown). If the investigators differ from the community (e.g., in cultural, racial, ethnic, or other differences), it is important to establish credibility, both for the investigators and for their institution. Chapter 5 explores in detail some of the factors which can facilitate or hinder research in a culturally diverse community setting.

## MARKETING THE STUDY—THE USE OF SOCIAL MARKETING THEORY

One basic aspect of cultural competence is understanding how to market a study to the community. Although researchers often assume that participants should readily embrace the opportunity to participate in intervention studies, research studies are more likely to be successful if an effort is made to market them to communities and individuals. Marketing an intervention is a critical research strategy even when communities and/or individuals have expressed a desire to participate and have iterated needs or wants they wish to achieve as an outcome of the study.

The principles of social marketing can help the researcher implement an intervention in the community. Social marketing has been defined as

> . . . the application of commercial marketing technologies to the analysis, planning, execution and evaluation of programs designed to influence the voluntary behavior of target audiences in order to improve their personal welfare and that of society. (Andreason, 1995, quoted in Brown, 1997 p. 27)

In other words, social marketing allows researchers to determine whether the intervention is one the community wants and whether the community will participate in the intervention. It helps researchers design interventions that are consistent with what the participants, as well as the researchers, need and want (Brown, 1997). An application of social marketing theory can be seen in the 1998 ad campaign from Partnership for a Drug Free America. These ads include age appropriate casting, handheld camera shots, music and quick editing, MTV techniques designed to appeal to teenagers and young adults. To successfully market an intervention or a behavioral change, it is necessary to reach and recruit the targeted audience.

Reaching and recruiting the targeted audience is one of the most challenging phases of the research process, frequently plagued by inadequate planning and insufficient resource allocation. Problems associated with inadequate sample size are commonplace in the conduct of clinical research, but often go unreported in the literature (Dowling & Wiener, 1997; Graham et al., 1991; Thompson, Heller, & Rody, 1994). Investigators are cautioned that:

> It is safe to assume in planning a study that the number of subjects who meet the entry criteria and agree to enter the study will be fewer, often by several fold, than the number projected at the outset. The solutions to this problem are to estimate the magnitude of the recruitment problems empirically with a pretest, to plan the study with an accessible population that is larger than believed necessary, and to make contingency plans should the need arise for an even larger source of subjects. (Hulley & Cummings, 1988, p. 26)

Social marketing theory focuses on attracting the targeted audience (potential participants) by meshing what the audience needs and wants with activities, attitudes, and/or behaviors that will benefit the audience. Applying the four "P"s of commercial marketing—product, price, place, promotion—to intervention studies allows a researcher to examine the intervention from the perspective of the consumer and to identify potential problems with attracting participants and keeping them interested in the study (recruitment and retention). The Bayer Institute for Health Care Communication has developed nine questions about the "mysteries of health" (i.e., What is going to happen? Why are you doing this rather than something else?). They suggest clinicians assume patients have these questions about every health care encounter and that they be answered as a matter of course (Bayer Institute, 1995). In like fashion, the researcher must anticipate the questions consumers will be asking about the feasibility of participating in the intervention and answer them as a matter of course. These questions can be summarized as the four P questions—questions consumers (potential participants) ask about the product (research intervention) being marketed to them.

## Product—Is This Something I Need or Want or Care About?

There are two major considerations in evaluating the community's response to the product (research intervention)—the research problem or need and the intervention designed to address the problem or need.

*Do I Care About This Problem?* Does the community care about the problem? How serious is it? Researchers and the community may differ on their definitions of what constitutes an important problem. For example, Winslow (1997) found that, for caregivers of Alzheimer's patients, neither formal support nor coping strategies mediated primary stressors (e.g., ADL and IADL dependency, problematic behaviors) in the directions hypothesized. In addition, different communities may perceive problems differently. Many studies have identified feelings of anger, isolation, and financial burden as problems common among groups of caregivers. However, in a study of factors associated with caregiver burden among Hispanic families caring for AD patients, these factors were absent. Instead, Cox and Monk (1993) identified the belief that one could be a better caregiver, lack of time for oneself, and the dependency needs of the care recipient as important issues for this group of caregivers.

Research in other areas of health care has shown that the driving force of acceptance is the "consumer's" interest or needs (Brown, 1997; Green & Kreuter, 1991). On an individual practitioner level, one of the most important predictors of patient adherence to a treatment regime is the *patient's* perception of the severity of the illness rather than the physician's (Meichenbaum & Turk, 1987). In designing health care systems, organizations must take into account community needs and perceptions (Davis, 1997). For example, consumers often do not select heath care plans based on the parameters health care professionals believe are important, such as health care quality; or, they may define the parameters differently (Dranove, White, & Wu, 1993; McGlynn, 1997). Quality to a health care professional may mean Joint Commission on Accreditation of Healthcare Organizations (JCAHO) accreditation; quality to a health care consumer may mean having phone calls returned quickly or the convenience of a close location.

The research problem may be serious to both researchers and the community, but it may be taboo, frightening, stigmatized, or embarrassing. For example, although aggressive sexual behavior by dementia care recipients, or sexual intimacy between caregiver and care recipient, may be relevant issues, older caregivers may feel uncomfortable talking about them. The research problem also may be political or politicized. For instance, interventions and funding for the reduction of teen pregnancy and HIV/AIDs have become part of a larger liberal/conservative political agenda and battleground.

Other considerations when evaluating the importance of the problem to the community are its visibility and length of time it has been a problem. The duration of the problem for the participant negatively affects adherence to a treatment regimen (Meichenbaum & Turk, 1987). Research has shown that "invisible" problems such as asymptomatic health care conditions have treatment adherence rates of 30–35% (Marston, 1970). If the problem is invisible or esoteric, researchers must make it more accessible and important to the community. The basic marketing strategy to counter this problem is to create demand.

The attitudes of family caregivers toward therapeutic interventions provide an excellent example of a targeted group caring about a problem. First, most family caregivers of dementia patients are accustomed to research studies that target the patient. By involving a loved one in a drug efficacy study or novel nonpharmacological intervention, the family caregiver often derives comfort from the fact that he/she is accessing every potential resource to enhance the patient's cognitive status and quality of life.

In contrast, research studies that focus on caregivers may be perceived differently. Researchers often implicitly assume that family caregivers can be easily recruited because of the stress inherent in the caregiver role. Unfortunately, family caregivers may be reluctant to participate in such studies because of their unwillingness to acknowledge to themselves or others that they require any emotional support or assistance. Caregivers may believe that difficulty coping with their own distress is tantamount to failing to be an "effective caregiver." Caregivers may need services but view their needs for therapeutic support as being "selfish" when compared to the needs and/or distress of a loved one diagnosed with AD. Among male spousal caregivers, denial and minimization of distress to others may be particularly prominent, partly due to limited expectations of their children (Harris, 1993).

*Do I Care About This Intervention?*   The most visible part of the product is the intervention itself. No matter how important the problem is, the intervention itself must be a product the community wants and needs. Many of the same questions about the community's perception of the problem can be asked about their perception of the intervention. The major question is whether the community needs or wants the intervention. One of the factors most highly correlated with treatment adherence is the patient's perception of treatment efficacy (DiMatteo, Reiter, & Gambone, 1994)—whether participants believe this intervention will help. However, belief in an intervention's efficacy is not related to the form of the intervention. The intervention may be a modification or adaptation of something the community already feels comfortable with and understands, or it may be experimental and controversial.

Furthermore, other factors may influence whether the research consumer will "buy" an intervention. The same questions must be asked about the intervention as about the problem. Is any aspect of it taboo, frightening, stigmatized, or embarrassing? Longer interventions, both per session and over time, and complex interventions are more likely to negatively influence adherence (Meichenbaum & Turk, 1987). The intervention, as well as the problem, may be politicized. For example, part of the political agenda of interventions for teen pregnancy has focused on the appropriateness of using government funds or public schools to teach methods of birth control besides abstinence.

In the final analysis, developing successful research products may need to mirror the design of successful consumer products. One of the "new" professions to arise this century has been that of the trend spotter or forecaster. These individuals pick up on ideas, fashions, and products that are already popular in some segment of society. These trends are then commercialized and mass marketed, but at least some portion of the consumer audience was involved in the development of the product.

In a parallel analogy, Schwab and Syme attribute the failure of several well-funded, highly publicized, multisite trials to a lack of "community participation—the involvement of people in designing and implementing research and interventions intended to benefit them" (Schwab & Syme, 1997, p. 2049). They argue for a new form of public health and epidemiology that focuses on the ecological reality of the participants and their participation. In this new paradigm of intervention study, culturally competent scientists, like trend spotters, work with the potential research population in defining studies, developing instruments, and creating data collection methods that reflect the lives of the population.

## Price—Is the Price Too High?

In a consumer-based society like that in the U.S., individuals are accustomed to a return (usually immediate or rapid) on their investments. With commercial marketing, consumers can easily determine if a price is too high for a product. As has been shown by the Beanie Baby phenomenon of the late 1990s, if the consumer's desire/demand is great enough, he/she will purchase the product even if the price is high. In social marketing, where the goal is to change behavior or influence participation, the return on investment is less clear. In addition, the return may not be immediate or may not even be a direct return to the participant. For example, the return on investment or benefit for control group participants frequently is described as some variant of "helping others in the future." Unless participants have an altruistic, social (e.g., others are participating) or emotional (e.g., family member) reason for participating, this somewhat dubious benefit is difficult to sell in a consumer-based culture.

Exchange theory suggests that people will pay the price they consider a product or benefit to be worth (Brown, 1997). The "exchange" must be equal. The price for participating in an intervention may be measured in time, risks, inconvenience, embarrassment, or emotional or physical distress. For example, barriers to recruiting family caregivers into intervention studies are the considerable time and effort involved in attending multiple treatment sessions, making arrangements for someone to supervise the patient, and guilt stemming from leaving the patient with others while they address their own concerns. In essence, the perceived benefits may not seem to outweigh the costs of being a participant.

Issues of unequal exchange (real or perceived) may arise in the recruitment process. Some caregivers may question the extent to which their participation is to their benefit as compared to the benefit of academic research investigators. When a research recruiter offers a caregiver the opportunity to receive free services, which were formerly rare or nonexistent in the community (e.g., family therapy for care providers), caregivers may be skeptical of the legitimacy of the study or feel it sounds "too good to be true." This issue is particularly relevant when recruiting by telephone since these perceived solicitations may be viewed as an invasion of privacy and may elicit concerns regarding "scams" against older persons, which have been increasingly publicized by the media.

Some issues of unequal exchange are unique to randomized clinical trials. Most caregivers have no idea what "randomized" means in the description of a study. When this distinction is made clear, it can foster a reluctance to participate on the part of those persons randomized to the control group. Resistance to participation may be the result of an intervention being too highly promoted in the recruitment process, or it may result from an individual's perception that he/she will be cheated if assigned to the control group. Strategies can be incorporated into the research design to help prevent this misconception and avoid participation refusal. For example, control group participants might be offered access to the intervention at the end of their control group participation, or they might be given generic resource materials and information to pursue additional support on their own. Some intervention studies attempt to equalize the exchange and lower the price of participation by offering monetary compensation for participation (e.g., at data collection points). However, the monetary value of incentives generally is not the main driving force for participation in a research study, especially one that is longitudinal, time-consuming, or complex. To ensure adequate participation, researchers must determine the real price participants are expected to pay and lower it, if it is too high.

## Place—Is It Convenient for Me to Get This Product?

That consumers are willing to be inconvenienced and travel long distances for certain reasons, such as for a scarce resource (e.g., for discontinued Beanie Babies), or perceived value (e.g., bypass the corner store for Wal-Mart) is a well-known marketing axiom. However, in general, research interventions are not perceived as a scarce, desirable resource. Most research studies fall into the category of "buyer's market," and researchers must make the study as convenient for participants as possible. Convenience is definitely a factor in the perceived price of research participation. If an intervention can be made part of a participant's usual routine, ensuring participation will be easier. For example, as a convenience, the Memphis REACH site sees caregivers and care recipients at their usual, scheduled physicians' appointments. Other aspects of convenience include availability of parking, distance from the parking lot, ability to drive, and access to public transportation. For many lower income older persons, transportation is the most common constraint to participation in activities (Transportation Research Board, 1988).

While convenience is an important aspect of place, the symbolic meaning of place is equally important. Would one segment of the community feel uncomfortable, frightened, or out-of-place at the intervention site? Researchers must look for any positive or negative community associations with intervention sites. These associations may be obscure but still present. In one rural Southern community, for example, a building proposed as an intervention site had been a hardware store in the 1960s owned by a rabid supporter of segregation who advertised ax handles as weapons against Civil Rights workers. Although the building had changed owners and functions several times, older African-American members of the community did not feel comfortable in the building and participation in the study was low. Only after a key member of the African-American community became a supporter of the study was this history revealed. The intervention site was changed and participation increased to expected levels.

## Promotion—Do I Know About This Product?

Promotion is the most difficult, most time- and labor-intensive, and most costly part of a study's marketing. While commercial marketing campaigns can cost millions of dollars and utilize the skills of highly creative advertising agencies, research study marketing often must rely on a more minimal approach. University media relations, public service announcements, brochures, and word-of-mouth are more often the tools of recruitment for research studies. These methods are used because they are available and, more importantly, fairly inexpensive. In fact, significant impediments to successful recruitment are the cost of recruiting and the lack of planning and budgeting for the resources needed to meet recruitment and retention goals. Despite their importance to success, little has been published on intervention costs, in general, or recruitment costs, specifically.

Earlier studies have reported on the effectiveness of a variety of recruitment strategies employed for enrolling older adults, particularly minority recruitment, but did not include a cost analysis (Stoy et al., 1995; Williams, Vitiello, Ries, Bokan, & Prinz, 1988). More recent published works are beginning to address research costs. An article by Anderson, Fogler, and Dedrick (1995) reports the cost of seven strategies employed to recruit community-based older adults. Press releases and advertisements produced 80% of their sample at a cost of $37 per enrollee, while posters and brochures produced only 3% of the sample at a cost of $904 per enrollee. In sharp contrast is an article by Patrick, Pruchno, and Rose (1998) that reports a snowball technique as being their most successful recruitment strategy—producing 37% of their sample at a cost of $20 per enrollee. Health care costs have become an important area of concern for federal agencies, including the National Institutes of Health and the Agency for Health Care Policy and Research. Researchers should anticipate increased attention to the inclusion and reporting of cost analysis and cost benefit of recruitment by funding agencies (Russell, Gold, Siegel, Daniels, & Weinstein, 1996).

In marketing a study, researchers must train themselves to think like marketers (or hire an advertising agency, something which no study will ever have money to do!). What is the first lesson in thinking like an advertising executive? The message needs to grab the audience's attention. For example, in an article about the Miami REACH site, reporter Stephen Smith (1998) succinctly and powerfully captured the essence of Alzheimer's caregiving—"a disease so greedy it steals more than one life at a time, demanding more hours than a day has to yield." Researchers must interest the media in some aspect of the study that will encourage media promotion.

What is the second important lesson in promotion? The audience needs to hear the message. Researchers must go to where participants are. There are three general environments where researchers may find participants: a) "in house" (people already known to the research team, sometimes known as recruiting from within a closed system); b) cooperating agencies and professionals (referrals); and c) the community (direct or self-referrals by community-based individuals). Each environment presents unique challenges to and opportunities for cultural competence.

*In-House Promotion.*    In this promotion and recruitment strategy, the potential participants, such as family caregivers who accompany an Alzheimer's disease patient to a memory loss clinic, are accessible and can be easily approached by clinician/researchers to participate. An advantage to recruiting in this environment is that the response rate of persons recruited into studies by researchers who are also their health care providers is high, and this method is inexpensive compared to other recruitment sources (Anderson et al., 1995). Investigators drawing a sample from within their own institution need to be objective in their size estimates of potential study subjects. Unexpectedly low sample sizes can be avoided by specifically inquiring into the actual numbers of dementia patients in the facility and objectively estimating the numbers of eligible caregivers who may agree to participate. With in-house recruiting and promotion, researchers must be alert to hidden pitfalls; it is not always possible to be objective about one's own culture. For example, the caregiver population may not be generalizable. The culture of the organization may make it difficult for potential participants to refuse, thus raising ethical issues of coercion. Finally, politics, biases, and hidden agendas may cause unanticipated difficulties.

*Cooperating Agencies or Professionals Promotion.*    Recruitment for dementia caregiving studies frequently requires contacting prospective participants through referrals from cooperating agencies or professionals. It is important to draw on the professional networks of each investigator when attempting to identify and contact possible referral sites for the recruitment of caregivers. Investigators need to visit and solicit the cooperation of several referral sources during the design phase, always contacting more sites than what is expected to be needed to generate an adequate sample size. Institutional administrations need to be informed of the research collaboration and their cooperation secured. Gaining access to the patient/client population of another agency requires not only an understanding of the culture of the referring agency but also much time and effort, including project presentations to administrators and staff, personal contacts, the exchange of necessary documentation, and numerous phone calls. Making application for Institutional Review Board approval at a cooperating site can easily take two to three months to complete.

Obtaining the cooperation of another health care institution is a complex and many layered process that can involve policies and politics outside the purview of the investigators. Having a well-respected and influential advocate at the institution being approached for cooperation is an important advantage. In large metropolitan areas, where several major teaching medical centers coexist, a competitive climate may stifle or prohibit cooperative research efforts. Entry into another institution may be denied, not on the merits of the proposed research project, but on the basis of the needs of the other institution's gatekeepers who wish to keep intact an accessible, ready pool of subjects for their own research agendas (Dowling & Weiner, 1997).

After entree into a cooperating site is complete, meeting with those persons who actually will be making the referrals is critical. A liaison who will serve as point of contact for the research team in generating referrals should be chosen for each cooperating site. The site liaison and other key staff need to be familiar with the general nature of the study and with the recruitment process specifically. In today's tightly run health care environment, staff may see the request for study referrals as one more task to accomplish in an already busy day. The labor-intensive efforts of securing the cooperation of the administration of an institution may be undermined by resistance to a project from informal gatekeepers at the point of clinical referral (McNeely & Clements, 1994). Researchers should keep referral forms short and easy to use, remembering that the important step is getting the name of someone who is likely to be eligible for the study.

If the referral process is seen as burdensome by the cooperating agency, researchers may want to consider reimbursing the staff for their time spent on the study, if reimbursement is an allowable expense of the granting and research agency. Arranging for members of the research team to do some of the screening work is another option, but one that can be complicated by issues of patient confidentiality. If the agency can benefit in any way from cooperating with the study, that advantage should be highlighted in conversations with personnel who are being asked to cooperate. Additional avenues of reciprocity can be explored, such as shared publication opportunities or promotional or educational talks at the cooperating sites by members of the research team.

Remember that a research study is being marketed. If participants are being recruited through cooperating agencies or professionals, find out what marketing tactics are routinely used to reach those intermediaries. For example, the Memphis REACH intervention is based in primary care and the source of referrals is primary care physicians and their staffs. Professional letters and phone calls are not the best way to "sell" physicians. The Memphis staff implemented the most successful physician marketing strategy known to them, the pharmaceutical representative strategy. REACH staff visit the providers' offices often enough to be remembered but not often enough to be annoying. At each visit, staff take something for recruitment and educational sessions for staff and caregivers—sticky notes, magnets, brochures and holders to place in the waiting rooms, and small seasonal treats (e.g., candy for Halloween with a REACH sticker on it). Fax back forms are faxed every week, to make it easy for staff to jot down a referral and send it back without writing out a separate fax form. One advantage to continuing contact is the opportunity for research staff to learn the culture—the norms, attitudes, behaviors, and values—of the referring agencies and how best to work within that culture.

*Community Promotion.*    If a study is being marketed directly to the public, the public has to hear about it. Public service announcements late at night (often the favorite time for community service, free advertising to be aired) are useful only if the study is designed for television-watching insomniacs. Promotion (recruitment) in the community often demands the most flexible and creative recruitment strategies. Community-based caregivers can be targeted for public promotional recruitment activities. Public advertising through television, radio, newspapers, special interest bulletins, mass mailings, workplace newsletters, WebPage announcements, professional and lay e-mail networks, special interest groups, and public lectures are all potential avenues for informing other professionals and dementia caregivers about research opportunities. The cost and effectiveness of these strategies varies according to the methods employed and the potential subjects targeted for enrollment.

The literature consistently shows that the best recruitment strategy is a multipronged effort (Carter, Elward, Malmgren, Martin, & Larson, 1991; Patrick et al., 1998; Stoy et al., 1987; Whelton et al., 1997). Recruitment efforts can begin with promotional activities; radio and newspaper announcements can herald the advance of a particular study, fostering expectation of the study and generating a favorable recruitment climate. Additionally, persons identified at cooperating referral sites may respond more favorably when a specific request for participation is preceded by a public announcement. The number of times adults must hear a message to remember it ranges from 3–50. Repeated public advertising during the recruitment period is important to keep the project visible in the community. Repeated messages function also as "just-in-time" marketing. The potential participant may not need the information the first time it is presented; but when it is needed, it should be available in a convenient location. The use of labor-intensive techniques such as snowballing (asking known individuals for the names of additional potential participants), using outreach workers, and gaining the cooperation of respected neighborhood leaders can be critical components in reaching minority and underserved populations. Approaches tailored to the recruitment and retention of targeted subpopulations, as detailed in chapter 5, need to be implemented early in the recruitment process.

A productive source of referrals for dementia caregivers may be community-based support groups. Associations comprised of both lay and professional persons, such as the Alzheimer's Association, which has national, state, and regional divisions, can be a significant resource in locating potential research participants. Networking with organization professionals and volunteers can lead to opportunities to meet and directly recruit caregivers of persons with dementia. The Alzheimer's Association and other groups frequently cooperate in announcing research projects in organization mailings and newsletters.

*Ongoing Promotion and Marketing.*  Marketing does not cease once a participant is in the study. Interventionists are an integral part of an intervention's continued marketing. The interventionists' ability to establish rapport with clients is a significant factor in keeping participants in the study. Research on clinician/patient communication has shown that the relationship with the clinician is one of the most important factors in adherence to treatment (Meichenbaum & Turk, 1987). Interventionists must be more than technically proficient. Their communication and interpersonal skills are important predictors of adherence (DiMatteo et al., 1993, 1994; Donovan & Blake, 1992; Squire, 1990). An interventionist's bicultural/bilingual experience or common backgrounds may make participants feel more comfortable (Majumdar & Roberts, 1998), but cultural competency in the participants' culture is a necessity for interventionists regardless of their backgrounds (Kagawa-Singer, 1997).

## IMPLEMENTATION PRAGMATICS—WHAT ELSE IS NEEDED?

With an understanding of cultural competence and social marketing theory, it is clear that several additional strategies not routinely used in research studies would help research teams implement their interventions more successfully. Some are simple to implement; others are more controversial and could require a change in regulations and/or mindset on the part of researchers, institutions, and funding agencies.

One useful generic recruitment strategy which has been suggested by others is to build into the research design resources to support a recruitment coordinator (Anderson et al., 1995; Dowling & Wiener, 1997; McNeely & Clements, 1994). Having an identified recruitment coordinator can greatly facilitate entree into cooperating institutions and the community and the ongoing management of recruitment activities. An experienced recruitment coordinator can focus time, personnel, and resources on intensive and multifaceted recruitment activities. The recruitment coordinator can assume responsibility for tracking recruitment and enrollment progress from the very start of the enrollment period and compare the results of ongoing recruitment efforts with recruitment goals in order to initiate new strategies when enrollment falls below expectation. Early attention to flagging enrollment leaves time to initiate new strategies and recruit new referral sites if needed. Extending time in the field to recruit participants is costly and delays the start of later sequential research activities.

Research teams also should consider hiring a marketing professional or contracting with a marketing firm. Marketing professionals have the skills to design unique, memorable print and promotional materials that convey the study message in the simplest and most effective manner possible. A marketing professional can serve as the study liaison with the media, packaging the study in a way that gets it noticed and publicized. Hiring an in-house person could be cost efficient if there are multiple studies being conducted simultaneously by the same research team, organization, or department. Input by a marketing professional during the proposal writing phase also can strengthen arguments for adequate funding of recruitment strategies.

The issue of appropriate promotional materials and marketing strategies is a difficult one. Social marketing theory would suggest that a research study market an intervention to its target audience in the same way a more commercial entity would market to the same audience. Granting agencies and grantee agencies have developed rules and regulations to govern the conduct of research to avoid lapses in ethics and coercion of participants. These rules and regulations were developed in a climate that values research and research participation (the furthering of science) as an end in itself. This culture of valuing research may be at variance with the culture of the community, especially in a consumer-oriented society. Moreover, many of the rules governing research practices were developed during a time when research funding was abundant and health care was predominantly fee-for-service, with more staff and more flexibility in scheduling patients (potential participants) for longer or multiple visits.

Recruitment in lean health care and research environments with fewer staff and shorter times for recruitment may signal the need for a reexamination of research rules and regulations, while still keeping the protection of participants foremost. For example, the American College of Physicians statement on fee splitting is used appropriately by many health care universities to protect patients from coercion into research studies by their physicians. However, movie tickets given to office staff for submitting names for referrals (with the concurrence of the physician) also are considered fee splitting. As discussed earlier, staff in busy offices or agencies may see the request for referrals as one more task that cannot be accommodated during their day.

Issues surrounding how research should be conducted will be difficult to resolve and may evoke strong emotional responses from researchers, their organizations, and sponsors. One key to their resolution is cultural competence—understanding the multiple cultures of research, grantee agencies, sponsors, researchers, and referral organizations, as well as the community culture. However, the most important means to a realistic and pragmatic implementation strategy is community participation, " . . . embracing the experience and partnership of those we are normally content simply to measure" (Schwab & Syme, 1997, p. 2050). As researchers operating in an increasingly dynamic and diverse environment, perhaps we need to expand the focus of our responsibility to include not only "protecting our subjects" but also actively collaborating with them to develop better research methodologies consistent with community realities and expectations.

## REFERENCES

Anderson, L., Fogler, J., & Dedrick, R. (1995). Recruiting from the community: Lessons learned from the diabetes care for older adults project. *The Gerontologist, 35*, 395–401.

Andreason, A. (1995). *Marketing social change: Changing behavior to promote health, social development, and the environment.* San Francisco: Jossey Bass.

Arguelles, T., & Lowenstein, D. (1997). Research says "si" to development of culturally appropriate cognitive assessment tools. *Generations, 21*, 30–31.

Bayer Institute for Health Care Communication, Inc. (1995). Clinician/patient communication to enhance health outcomes [workbook]. West Haven, CT.

Beisecker, A.E., Murden, R.A., Moore, W.P., Graham, D., & Nelmig, L. (1996). Attitudes of medical students and primary care physicians regarding input of older and younger patients in medical decisions. *Medical Care, 34,* 126–137.

Brown, C.A. (1997). Anthropology and social marketing: A powerful combination. *Practicing Anthropology, 19,* 27–29.

Carter, W., Elward, K., Malmgren, J., Martin, M., & Larson, E. (1991). Participation of older adults in health programs and research: A critical review of the literature. *The Gerontologist, 31,* 584–592.

Cox, C., & Monk, A. (1993). Hispanic culture and family care of Alzheimer's patients. *Health & Social Work, 18,* 92–100.

Davis, R. (1997). Community caring: An ethnographic study within an organizational culture. *Public Health Nursing, 14,* 92–100.

DiMatteo, M., Sherbourne, C., Hays, R., Ordway, L., Kravitz, R., McGlynn, E., Kaplan, S., & Rogers, W. (1993). Physician characteristics influence patients' adherence to medical treatment: Results from the medical outcomes study. *Health Psychology, 12,* 93–102.

DiMatteo, M., Reiter, R., & Gambone, J. (1994). Enhancing medication adherence through communication and informed collaborative choice. *Health Communication, 6,* 253–265.

Donovan, J., & Blake, D. (1992). Patient noncompliance: Deviance or reasoned decision-making? *Social Science & Medicine, 34,* 507–513.

Dowling, G., & Wiener, C. (1997). Roadblocks encountered in recruiting patients for a study of sleep disruption in Alzheimer's disease. *Image: Journal of Nursing Scholarship, 29,* 59–64.

Downs, K., Berstein, J., & Marchese, T. (1997). Providing culturally competent primary care for immigrant and refugee women. A Cambodian case study. *Journal of Nurse-Midwifery, 42,* 499–508.

Dranove, D., White, W.D., & Wu, L. (1993). Segmentation in local hospital markets. *Medical Care, 31,* 52–64.

Fals-Borda, O., & Rahnema, M. (Eds.). (1991). *Action and Knowledge: Breaking the monopoly with participatory action research.* New York: Apex.

Graham, S., Hellmann, R., Marshall, J., Freudenheim, J., Vena, J., Swanson, M., Sielezny, M., Nemoto, T., Stubbe, N., & Raimondo, T. (1991). Nutritional epidemiology of postmenopausal breast cancer in western New York. *American Journal of Epidemiology, 134,* 552–566.

Green, L.W., & Kreuter, M.W. (Eds.). (1991). *Health promotion planning: An educational and environmental approach* 2nd ed. Mountain View, CA: Mayfield.

Harris, P.B. (1993). The misunderstood caregiver? A qualitative study of the male caregiver in Alzheimer's disease victims. *Gerontologist, 33,* 551–556.

Helman, C.G. (1994). *Culture, health and illness: An introduction for health professionals*, 3rd ed. Oxford: Butterworth-Heinemann Ltd.

Hulley, S., & Cummings, S. (1988). *Designing clinical research*. Baltimore: Williams and Wilkins.

Kagawa-Singer, M. (1997). Addressing issues for early detection and screening in ethnic populations [review]. *Oncology Nursing Forum, 24*, 1705–1711.

Lawton, M.P., Rajagopal, D., Brody, E., & Kleban, M.H. (1992). The dynamics of caregiving for a demented elder among black and white families. *Journal of Gerontology, 47*, S156–S164.

Majumdar, B., & Roberts, J. (1998). AIDS awareness among women: The benefit of culturally sensitive educational programs. *Health Care for Women International, 19*, 141–153.

Marston, M.V. (1970). Compliance with medical regimens: A review of the literature. *Nursing Research, 10*, 312–323.

McGlynn, E.A. (1997). Six challenges in measuring the quality of health care. *Health Affairs*, May/June,7–21.

McNeely, E., & Clements, S. (1994). Recruitment and retention of the older adult into research studies. *Journal of Neuroscience Nursing, 26*, 57–61.

Meichenbaum, D., & Turk, D.C. (1987). *Facilitating treatment adherence: A practitioner's guidebook*. New York: Plenum Press.

Mintzer, J.E., Rubert, M.P., Loewenstein, D., Gamez, E., Millor, A., Quinteros, R., Flores, L., Miller, M., Rainerman, A., & Eisdorfer, C. (1992). Daughters caregiving for Hispanic and non-Hispanic Alzheimer patients: Does ethnicity make a difference? *Community Mental Health Journal, 28*, 293–303.

Patrick, J., Pruchno, R., & Rose, M. (1998). Recruiting research participants: A comparison of the costs and effectiveness of five recruitment strategies. *The Gerontologist, 38*, 295–302.

Russell, L., Gold, M., Siegel, J., Daniels, N., & Weinstein, M. (1996). The role of cost-effectiveness analysis in health and medicine. *Journal of the American Medical Association, 276*, 1172–1177.

Schwab, M., & Syme, S.L. (1997). On paradigms, community participation, and the future of public health. *American Journal of Public Health, 87*, 2049–2051.

Smith, S. (February 5, 1998). Helping the helpers. Miami Herald [online]. Available at: http://www.herald.com/liv_art/docs/050886.htm.

Squire, R.W. (1990). A model for empathic understanding and adherence to treatment regimens in practitioner/patient relationships. *Social Science & Medicine, 30*, 325–339.

Stoy, D., Curtis, C., Dameworth, K., Dowdy, A., Hegland, J., Levin, J., & Sousoulas, B. (1995). The successful recruitment of elderly black subjects in a clinical trial: The CRISP experience. *Journal of the National Medical Association, 87,* 280–286.

Transportation Research Board, National Research Council. (1988). Transportation in an aging society: Improving mobility and safety for older persons, Vol 1, Special Report 218. Washington, D.C.

Thompson, M., Heller, K., & Rody, C. (1994). Recruitment challenges in studying late-life depression: Do community samples adequately represent depressed older adults? *Psychology and Aging, 9,* 121–125.

Whelton, P., Bahnson, J., Appel, L., Charleston, J., Cosgrove, N., Espeland, M.A., Folmar, S., Hoagland, D., Krieger, S., Lacy C., Lichtermann, L., Oates-Williams, F., Tayback, M., & Wilson, A.C. (1997). Recruitment in the trial of nonpharmacologic intervention in the elderly (TONE). *Journal of the American Geriatrics Society, 45,* 185–193.

Williams, D., Vitiello, R., Ries, R., Bokan, J., & Prinz, P. (1988). Successful recruitment of elderly community-dwelling subjects for Alzheimer's disease research. *Journal of Gerontology: Medical Sciences, 43,* M69–M74.

Winslow, B.W. (1997). Effects of formal supports on stress outcomes in family caregivers of Alzheimer's patients. *Research in Nursing and Health, 20,* 275–287.

Zakus, J.D.L. (1998). Resource dependency and community participation in primary health care. *Social Science & Medicine, 46,* 475–494.

# 5

# Development and Implementation of Intervention Strategies for Culturally Diverse Caregiving Populations

*Dolores Gallagher-Thompson, Patricia Aréan, David Coon, Ana Menéndez, Kellie Takagi, William E. Haley, Trinidad Argüelles, Mark Rubert, David Lowenstein, and Jose Szapocznik*

## INTRODUCTION

The purpose of this chapter is to discuss issues related to the development and implementation of intervention programs for caregivers of culturally diverse backgrounds who are caring for a relative with Alzheimer's disease or another form of dementing illness. Culturally appropriate interventions are needed in order to encourage family members to actively participate in programs that could be of practical assistance to them in coping with the everyday stress of caregiving. However, until very recently, most caregiving research (in general) and caregiver intervention research (specifically) focused almost exclusively on Caucasians. Regarding the former: a recent review article by Schulz, O'Brien, Bookwala, and Fleissner (1995) that summarized the negative impact of caregiving on the caregivers' mental and physical health across a variety of studies concluded that few studies investigated potential associations between psychiatric symptomatology and demographic variables such as ethnicity and socioeconomic status. Those few studies found conflicting results (e.g., in some, non-White ethnicity was associated with greater self-reported depression, but not in others), leading these authors to conclude that more research is needed to address even the most basic questions about how both ethnicity and cultural identification may impact on caregivers.

Related papers by Aranda and Knight (1997) and Connell and Gibson (1997) specifically focus on analyzing empirical research published in the last decade that did examine the impact of culture and/or ethnicity on the dementia caregiving experience. Connell and Gibson found that the majority of studies they reviewed (10 of 12 studies) examined differences between Black and White caregivers; one compared Black and Hispanic caregivers, and one compared White and Hispanic caregivers. In general they found that the non-White caregivers were more likely to be an adult child, friend, or family member other than a spouse. Black caregivers, when compared to the other groups, tended to report lower levels of distress, burden, and depression, held strong beliefs about filial support, and were more likely to use prayer, faith, or religion as coping mechanisms. Similar conclusions were drawn by Aranda and Knight, who focused on caregiving in the Latino population. While they did not limit their review to caregivers of dementia patients only, but rather included data from family members caring for relatives with severe diabetes and other chronic, debilitating health problems, their conclusions seem appropriate to dementia caregivers as well. Note that they caution the reader that the term "Latino" is somewhat problematic given the intragroup differences that do exist (for example, between Mexican Americans, Puerto Rican Americans, Cuban Americans and those from Central and South America) in both culture and everyday language usage. Aranda and Knight concluded that caregivers of older Latinos face special challenges because they care for family members at higher risk for specific physical illnesses who are disabled at earlier ages and who have more functional disabilities. Perhaps more importantly, they also point out that cultural factors can influence the appraisal of ongoing stressful events (such as dementia caregiving) and in turn, the types of coping behaviors that are used to modulate stress, as well as the perception and use of family supports. Thus, even within the Latino community, service delivery programs need to be sensitive to differences that may be present between groups; for example, within the Latino community, Mexican Americans and Cuban Americans may perceive and respond to caregiving differently. This may, in turn, be related to such other important contextual variables as immigration status, length of time in this country, educational background, facility in use of the English language, and current socioeconomic status. However, these relationships have only begun to be explored in studies featuring caregivers of various ethnic backgrounds.

Now, if we specifically focus on intervention research with family caregivers of varying ethnicity (not just a description of the caregiving experience per se), we find even less information. An excellent recent review and critique of caregiver intervention research was published by Bourgeois, Schulz, and Burgio (1996). This paper includes over 100 references, most of which describe studies (of varying quality and extent of experimental control) in which caregivers received different kinds of interventions (e.g., support groups, skill training packages, individual and family counseling, etc.). A wide range of outcome measures were reported on as well, but of particular relevance to this chapter is the fact that very little attention has been paid to the role of ethnic and cultural background, beliefs, and values in the entire field of caregiver intervention research. Even in this well-done review, the authors do not highlight these factors, despite the fact that they discuss a myriad of other factors that can influence how caregivers respond to interventions. These include adequacy of outcome measures, the intensity and integrity of the interventions used, the changing needs of caregivers throughout their caregiving career, and other important individual differences (e.g., gender and relationship to the care receiver). In fact, a thorough review of the current published literature indicates that there are very few intervention studies of any kind that are geared specifically toward ethnic minority caregivers. Those few that do exist will be discussed below, including the REACH project itself, which of course is in progress and does not yet have data to report.

Despite this paucity of information about the response of ethnically diverse family caregivers to interventions designed to improve their quality of life, there is a rich background of literature that can be drawn upon to assist in conceptualizing the kinds of interventions that may prove to be culturally sensitive and appropriate for caregivers of different ethnic and cultural backgrounds. In the remainder of this chapter this literature will be discussed, grouped under the following conceptual headings: 1) how dementia is understood by different ethnic groups (that is, their explanatory models for this disease); 2) cultural beliefs and attitudes about caregiving for a demented elder; and 3) specific issues related both to designing and implementing interventions for caregivers of specific ethnic and cultural groups. The chapter will close with a section describing how at least some of these conceptual and practical issues have been addressed in the REACH project.

## EXPLANATORY MODELS FOR ILLNESS AMONG DIFFERENT ETHNIC AND CULTURAL GROUPS

Over 20 years ago, Kleinman, Eisenberg, and Good (1978) introduced into medicine and health care a long-held notion in the field of anthropology: namely, that culture strongly affects how one constructs reality and how one thinks about physical illness. They made a critical distinction between disease (abnormalities in the structure and function of bodily organs and systems) and illness (the patient's experience of sickness) which they posited did not have a one-to-one relationship to one another. Rather, it is generally accepted that similar degrees of organ pathology may generate quite different reports of pain and distress, and illness may occur in the absence of documented disease. They go on to comment that illness is culturally shaped in the sense that how we perceive, experience, and cope with disease is based on our explanations of sickness, which are specific to the systems of meaning that we employ.

According to health psychologists Landrine and Klonoff (1992), most White Americans assume that illness can be described and treated without reference to family, community, or the gods. In contrast, countless anthropological studies have found that many ethnic/cultural groups construe illness as a process caused by natural, interpersonal, and/or supernatural causes; thus, these cultural groups have their own cures for illness and (often) their own indigenous healers. Among these groups common causes for illnesses in general include: violations of the demands and expectations of social roles or moral and religious taboos, and/or belief in the agency of quasi-natural agents (such as hot/cold foods or weather, and various "states" of one's blood such as weak or thin). According to a review about the causes of illness in 189 cultures around the world (done by Murdock, 1980, and cited in Landrine & Klonoff, 1992, p. 268), the majority believe that illness is supernaturally caused. This includes mystical retribution (punishment by the gods or other forces for rule violations) and magical causation (witchcraft, sorcery, and the "evil eye" used against the person by others). In fact, Landrine and Klonoff (1992) conclude that new diseases about which little may be known initially from a scientific perspective (such as AIDS and possibly dementia) are especially likely to be understood in terms of preexisting culturally determined health-related schemas. This suggests that members of certain cultural and ethnic minority groups may understand their symptoms in terms that are radically different from those used by health care professionals, who are most typically trained in Western medicine and are often members of the majority culture.

Since it is true that some patients' beliefs about the causes and cures of their illnesses will therefore be at odds with Western biomedical training, some authors have proposed guidelines for understanding health perceptions, behaviors, and expectations. Buchwald, Caralis, Gany, et al. (1994) describe specific ways to elicit explanatory models of illness from patients of varying ethnic backgrounds, and recommend that responses be listened to in a nonjudgmental manner, so that progress can be made collaboratively in diagnosing and treating the illness. Their paper lists several predictors of what they term "behavioral ethnicity" including: emigration from a rural area, little formal education, frequent returns to the country of origin, and major differences in diet and preferred language. The more common these background variables are, the more likely it is that cultural factors will be an important element that can either help or hinder the care provided. Furthermore, Buchwald et al. (1994) suggest the importance of negotiating treatment options with the patient and family whenever possible, so that optimal treatment can be provided that is also culturally consistent. They present the LEARN model as a set of guidelines for fostering cross-cultural communication about health care issues: Listen with empathy and understanding to the patient and family's perception of the problem; Explain your perceptions of the problem; Acknowledge and discuss similarities and differences; Recommend treatments and treatment options; and finally Negotiate treatments and gain agreement as to what will be done, and when (1994, p. 120). Use of a simple model such as this has been described as very helpful to facilitate compliance with treatment recommendations across cultures, for most illnesses. This model suggests that clinicians should avoid labeling diverse explanatory models of illness as simply reflecting ignorance and lack of information that should be addressed solely through education; rather, the clinician should strive to provide assistance so that it can be accepted within the world view of the patient and the family. To the authors' knowledge, it has not been applied to the care of dementia victims.

The past decade has seen an explosion of information and knowledge about Alzheimer's disease (AD) and related forms of dementia, such as dementia due to multiple strokes, or end-stage Parkinson's disease, or AIDS. A number of popular self-help books have appeared, such as an updated edition of the 36-Hour Day (Mace & Rabins, 1991) which describes many of the behavioral problems encountered in the later stages of caregiving for a family member with AD, along with practical coping suggestions. Other works describe very personal accounts of the caregiving process, such as Davidson's moving volume about several years in her life with her very demented husband, a former university professor (Davidson, 1997). These and similar books reveal the extent to which dementia is understood as a physical disease, much like heart disease or diabetes. It is also clear that the writers understand that its basic cause is unknown and adequate treatments are recognized as not yet available. This information appears to have been widely disseminated to and accepted by many Americans of European ancestry, among whom the dementias are generally not regarded as mental illnesses or as caused by supernatural or interpersonal forces; rather the disease model is firmly held. The reader is referred to a recent comprehensive review chapter by Peskind and Raskind (1996) which discusses a host of features to be assessed when diagnosing dementia and deciding upon possible interventions, such as cognitive status, certain morphological changes in the brain, behavioral problems, medical history, and results of blood tests, head scans, and other biological measures. Clearly, no attribution to supernatural or magical causation is made among most Western practitioners for any kind of dementia.

Given these potentially radically different starting points for understanding and treating dementia, it is understandable that conflicts may exist between health care providers and their patients, particularly when patients maintain culturally rooted beliefs and practices that may be difficult to ascertain and to work with (Kato, 1996). In addition, when it comes to dementia, unfortunately, very few anthropological studies have been done specifically addressing beliefs about this illness. Yet it is fair to conclude, on the basis of what has been presented so far, that ethnicity will affect how families approach the care of relatives with AD (Haley, Han, & Henderson, 1998). In some cases ethnicity may lead to dramatically different culturally prescribed views about dementia, such as the belief among some Oklahoma Choctaws that dementia is not due to brain disease at all, and that symptoms can reflect a connection with spirits (Haley et al., 1998). In other instances ethnicity may lead to more subtle differences in the degree to which certain values or expectations are held (such as the extent to which daughters are expected to be caregivers). Although we have much less empirical information to inform us than is the case with other illnesses, there are some clinical reports and case studies, as well as several literature reviews and a small number of empirically based studies, to guide our thinking in this regard. In the sections that follow, we will review what is known about how dementia is viewed and understood by the major racial and ethnic groups in the U.S. today. We will do this by assembling information according to the four major groups designated by the U.S. Bureau of the Census. These are: Black or African Americans, Hispanic Americans, Asian/Pacific Islander Americans, and American Indian/Alaska Native Americans. Before proceeding, we need to formally recognize the limitations of our approach, given the heterogeneity within each of these groupings (Yeo, 1996). For example, included within the category of Asian/Pacific Islanders are persons of Japanese, Chinese, Korean, Vietnamese, Filipino, Laotian, Hmong, Thai, and Asian Indian backgrounds. Most assuredly, these individuals do not share the same language, diet, customs, or religious and cultural beliefs; rather, each has its own unique cultural heritage. Similarly, included among Hispanics are those from South and Central America, Mexico, and some Caribbean islands such as Cuba and Puerto Rico. While they more often will share a common language, their political and socio-cultural experiences vary widely. In all cases, health care beliefs and practices are heavily influenced by immigration status (number of years in the U.S.) and by a related factor termed acculturation, or the extent to which individuals have taken on the beliefs and practices of the dominant culture (Green, 1995). Acculturation has been found to be a very significant factor in explaining health beliefs and practices; however, it is a difficult concept to measure, since it is widely recognized as a dynamic process that varies according to content area. For example, a person may be highly acculturated in terms of language (for employment purposes) but maintain many beliefs and practices of the culture of origin when it comes to family values, diet, religiosity, and the like (Green, 1995). When treating ethnic minority elders, clinicians must make a correct assessment of the patient's and family's location along the acculturation continuum, to understand correctly how they view and cope with stress of caregiving (Valle, 1989).

We will also relate this information to what is known about specific caregiving beliefs, expectations, and behavioral patterns in the four major groups noted above. In the final sections we will discuss the design and implementation of culturally sensitive and appropriate interventions for caregivers of different ethnic and cultural backgrounds, as they have been undertaken in the REACH project.

## Cultural Beliefs about Dementia and Implications for Caregiving among African Americans

Previous writing on African Americans and dementia suggests both similarities and differences in comparison with White Americans. African Americans have higher rates of hypertension, stroke, and vascular dementia than Whites (Baker, 1996). However, recent epidemiological research also suggests that African Americans have much higher incidence of Alzheimer's disease than Whites (Tang et al., 1998), perhaps due in part to lower levels of educational attainment (a risk factor for dementia). In terms of cultural differences, an excellent review chapter by Lewis and Ausberry (1996) highlights a number of important points to keep in mind when working with Black or African-American families in the U.S. at the present time. First is their history of slavery which led, among other things, to the development of the family as the primary support institution, followed by the church (often referred to as the "church family"). African-American families are often described in terms of the concept of consanguinity (kinship that is biologically based and rooted in blood ties) as well as in terms of "fictive kin" or persons with whom one is close and who function as a member of the family, although no blood ties are present. (This is also seen in the Latino culture: godmothers, for example, may be very close friends who are regarded as family). Both are important in the family structure. Second, in terms of the aging process, a growing body of literature describes aging as a survival process rather than as an adaptive process (Burton, 1992). Consistent with this view, African-American families have described aging as a time of "overcoming life's hurdles" although "surviving the day-to-day struggles isn't easy," reflecting the view that movement into old age is a transition, not a crisis. We see this as well in the fact that African-American families are far less likely than White families to present their impaired relatives at specialized clinics for a dementia workup, and when they do, dementia is typically more severe (Ballard, Nash, Raiford, & Harrell, 1993). Third, multiple infarcts (silent small strokes) or transient ischemic attacks have been found by some to be prominent features in dementia in African Americans, and may thus complicate the diagnostic picture (Baker, 1996). Because of the pattern of deterioration that results from these small vascular accidents, the situation may in fact go relatively unnoticed, and/or any related failings be regarded as "normal aging," until a more dramatic change in function is noted (e.g., following a major stroke). At that time cognitive loss may be acknowledged by the family, although its significance may be minimized, as long as the elder can partake in some family activities and can function in some capacity within the family system (Lewis & Ausberry, 1996). Caregiving is more likely to be viewed as a normal expectation rather than a disruption of the life course in African-American families (Haley et al., 1996).

Dementia may therefore be a less negative diagnosis for many African Americans compared to White Americans because of this and related attitudes. According to Gaines (1989), role performance is valued much more highly than cognitive ability among African Americans, so that if an elder can function in some way and perform some role in and for the family, he or she will still be valued and can maintain a sense of self-worth. Several studies have found less distress (e.g., fewer symptoms of depression and greater satisfaction with the caregiving role) among African Americans compared to Anglo caregivers including the work of Hinrichsen and Ramirez (1992), Haley et al. (1995), Lawton, Rajagopal, Brody, and Kleban (1992), and Mui (1992), although this is not a totally uniform finding in the literature (see Wood & Parham, 1990). However, relatively little is known about the cultural mechanisms that may underlie such differences.

In terms of coping strategies, African-American caregivers were more likely to report use of cognitive strategies such as reframing the situation and use of positive self-statements reflecting their determination to survive. They were also more likely to use prayer than their Anglo counterparts (Segall & Wykle, 1988–89; Wood & Parham, 1990; Wykle & Segall, 1991). However, contrary to common assumptions about African Americans, Haley et al. (1996) found no differences in use of prayer, church-related caregiving assistance, or levels of social supports between White and African-American caregiving families. In addition, placement of the care receiver was a rare event when family was still available (Lockery, 1991). Haley et al. (1996) also found that African-American caregivers appraised caregiving problems as less stressful than White families, and had higher self-efficacy in coping with caregiving problems. Previous experience with adversity may help African-American caregivers to reframe difficult life circumstances such as caregiving that cannot be readily changed (Wood & Parham, 1990; Gibson, 1992).

Taken together, these studies suggest that, in contrast to findings with Anglo caregivers where high levels of depression, stress, and burden are common (cf. Gallagher-Thompson, 1994, and Gallagher-Thompson, Coon, Rivera, et al., 1998, for reviews of this literature), African-American caregivers may experience the situation quite differently. The considerable strengths of the African-American community in the face of caregiver burden have implications for the kinds of interventions that will be helpful to them. Lockery (1991), for example, has suggested that interventions for African Americans that relieved some of the economic burdens of caregiving, or those aimed at capitalizing on strengths by maximizing the involvement of family and church in the care of the demented person, should be developed and evaluated, along with programs to reduce the behavior problems often associated with dementia in its later stages (regardless of etiology). In addition, interventions should attend to other differences which are relevant to caregiving. African-American caregivers (and noncaregivers) are generally in poorer health than Whites (Haley et al., 1996) and thus interventions including some emphasis on health promotion may be of value.

## Cultural Beliefs about Dementia and Implications for Caregiving among Hispanic Americans

According to many Hispanic cultural traditions, good physical and mental health are viewed as the result of balance. It is the combination of faith, nutrition, and how one lived one's life that brings an illness about (Gallagher-Thompson, Talamantes, Ramirez, & Valverde, 1996). In the process of identifying a family member as demented, the family may for years deny the severity of the memory and behavioral impairments that they observe because the person always ate well and was very religious. On the other hand, for a person with a history of improper behavior, dementia may be viewed as a punishment from God for past sins, or as the result of *el mal de ojo* (the evil eye), which means a curse placed on one person by another. Yet another belief is that the brain "dries up" leading to behaviors *como un niño* (childlike).

Among Hispanic Americans, there is considerable social stigma associated with Alzheimer's disease and other forms of dementia, since dementia is regarded as a form of mental (not physical) illness, and mental illnesses are, at the very least, embarrassing and bring shame to the family (Sanchez, 1992). Although there are differences among Hispanic caregivers (based on the heterogeneity noted earlier in this chapter), there are several commonalities, including: limited knowledge about dementia as a disease process; limited access to resources for support; limited availability of trained bilingual and/

or bicultural health care providers in this field; and finally, increased levels of depression, burden, and stress among the family caregivers (Valle, 1989).

Several key cultural values that impact on the understanding and care of dementia victims and their families have been described by Villa, Cuellar, Gamel, and Yeo (1993). The first of these is *familismo,* which refers to the primary importance of family over the individual, or family pride, which is instilled early and nurtured throughout the person's life and used as the context within which values such as mutual assistance versus individual problem solving are taught. The second major value is called *personalismo* and refers to the fact that Hispanics value interpersonal relations and social interactions in which individuals deal with one another as caring, compassionate persons rather than as impersonal players of specific roles. The third major value is termed *espiritismo* and this refers to a belief system in which the world is inhabited by both good and evil spiritual beings who can affect humans, particularly their health and well-being, in positive and negative ways (Villa et al., 1993, pp. 37–39). As noted above, this can lead to a set of beliefs about the dementia coming from God. If so, it is only God who can change things, thus leaving Hispanic families to believe that this is their cross to bear, and by suffering with the burdens of caregiving, they will redeem themselves.

Additional information about how Latinos view dementia and caregiving can be found in Henderson and Gutierrez-Mayka (1992) who were among the first social scientists to talk directly with Hispanics about this topic. They interviewed Cuban American caregivers in the Tampa region, and found clear patterns of gender role responsibility for caregiving, requiring females to be the primary caregivers, so that wives, daughters, and daughters-in-law were most commonly found. In fact, it is expected within the culture that daughters become the primary caregiver. Furthermore, a stigma of "craziness" related to dementia was reported; it was thought to extend to the entire family, especially if deviant behavior was shown by the elder (e.g., wandering, being unable to eat properly around people, etc.). These findings were essentially supported in the work of Orona and Alkayyali (1992) who conducted open-ended interviews with Mexican Americans living in San Jose, CA. In addition, they found that most caregivers had extremely limited knowledge of dementia, were not given adequate information by their physicians, and, contrary to expectations (given the value of *familismo* described above), were receiving minimal to no assistance from extended family members living in the area. Further corroboration was found in the work of Cox and Monk (1993) who interviewed a predominantly Puerto Rican sample of family caregivers in New York and Baltimore. Their respondents scored very high on a self-report measure of depression. This was found to be positively correlated with adherence to the cultural norm of filial support, obligating adult children to take care of their aging parents, and not to use professional (outside) help because of the shame it would bring upon the family. Often these adult children are also employed outside the home, and have their own families to raise with young children and/or teenagers requiring their care as well. This apparent conflict between expectations and current roles (which are highly influenced by, and reflective of, the acculturation process) may reflect changing values, as described by Lacayo (1993). It may be that with increasing acculturation, less adherence will be paid to traditional values (including family responsibility for caregiving), thus strongly encouraging caregivers to seek and to utilize outside services for their demented relative. But in order to do this effectively, some of the traditional beliefs about dementia will have to be challenged.

Several other recent studies have shown that high levels of distress, and particularly high self-reported depressive symptoms, are common among Latino caregivers. For example, Mintzer, Rubert, Loewenstein, et al. (1992) found high levels of dysphoria among both Cuban American and Anglo daughters who were caregiving for their demented mothers; about one-third of each group scored above a traditional cut-off score that suggested clinical depression, although there was no significant difference between groups. Kemp and Adams (1996) conducted one of the largest studies of ethnic differences among caregivers, in the Los Angeles area. They compared the responses of Japanese American (N=31), Hispanic American (N=45), African American (N=49), and Anglo caregivers (N=67) who were interviewed about their experiences and were specifically asked about depressive symptoms. They found that the Hispanic caregivers reported the most distress of the four groups: they were in fact significantly higher than each of the other three on the depression measure, with the average score suggesting major depression. The other three groups were equivalent, and substantially lower, but still in the range indicating clinically significant symptoms. A similar pattern was found on measures of distress (more generally) and physical complaints. Also, Mexican-American caregivers reported more lack of social support from family (specifically related to caregiving) than the other groups, as well as a generally pessimistic appraisal of their caregiving situation.

An additional study investigating similar variables was reported by Polich and Gallagher-Thompson (1997). Forty-two female Hispanic caregivers in the greater San Francisco Bay area were interviewed to assess the impact of caregiving on several indices of stress and well-being. They found, as did Kemp and Adams (1996), high levels of self-reported depression, which were best predicted by two variables: dissatisfaction with family support with caregiving, and a perceived negative effect on the caregivers' overall physical health. When level of acculturation was analyzed in the results, it was found that more bicultural caregivers were most depressed when family support was low, whereas more traditional caregivers were not as affected by low family support. Other studies have also found that low acculturation is a buffer against depression when family support is low, whereas high acculturation and low family support (together) are more likely to lead to higher levels of depression. These finding are a reminder that, in this complex area of research, many factors need to be studied in combination, and not just in an isolated manner.

The final study of which we are aware was reported by John and McMillian (1998). They conducted several focus group discussions with Mexican American caregivers in Texas, to learn more about how the concept of caregiver burden (which is so popular and widely used in the Anglo caregiving literature) was viewed and experienced by them. They found that the concept of burden was not palatable to these caregivers, although what they reported would be termed as burdensome by most. To use that term was to go against cultural values that required them not to complain about their difficult situations. What the caregivers in this study did report was situational frustration (developing into genuine anger at times), resentment due to the lack of assistance with caregiving from other family members, and isolation from the outside world. For a family-oriented group like Mexican Americans, these last two experiences were particularly difficult, and were at the basis of requests for interventions like respite programs and day care programs that would increase the quality of care the caregiver could provide, without reliance on other family members. However, financial constraints and other barriers to access (such as language) made this a difficult option to really use.

Taken together, findings from these several studies indicate that distress—particularly depression—can be quite high among Hispanic caregivers, which in turn suggests that the development and utilization of interventions designed to reduce depression could be very helpful to this group. The fact that depression was related to low levels of perceived or actual support from other family members further suggests that interventions designed to increase family support might be helpful as well.

## Cultural Beliefs about Dementia and Implications for Caregiving among Asian Americans

Asian Americans are a highly diverse group, as suggested earlier. Besides diversity in language, cultural norms, religious beliefs and practices, and socio-political history and experiences, there are also great differences in migration patterns to the U.S. This in turn means that first-, second-, or third-generation American-born Asian Americans will differ greatly on the acculturation continuum and thus may hold strikingly disparate beliefs about health and illness in general, and dementia in particular. It is beyond the scope of this chapter to describe these many different cultures (and their beliefs) in detail. The reader is referred to several excellent sources, including: for Chinese Americans: Matocha (1998), for Filipino Americans: Miranda, McBride, and Spangler (1998); for Japanese Americans: Sharts-Hopko (1998); for Korean Americans: Sabet (1998), and for Vietnamese Americans: Nowak (1998). These chapters, in a single, comprehensive, edited book, provide an excellent starting point for obtaining specific information on health beliefs and practices of each group. An additional (but much briefer) monograph on age-related health care issues among Asian and Pacific Islanders is that by Morioka-Douglas and Yeo (1990). However, the direct application of these varying beliefs and practices to the field of dementia and family caregiving has been sparse; only a few studies have been done that specifically address this illness.

In general, it can be said that one of the most common Asian responses to memory problems and associated behavioral problems in elderly relatives is to see these as a normal consequence of growing old. Terms used for dementia in Chinese include ones that translate into English as "stupid and silly" or "less smart"—because of this, many Chinese families do not perceive dementia as an illness requiring attention and intervention (Elliott, Di Minno, Lam, & Tu, 1996). Alternatively, Chinese and other Asian persons very often interpret the signs and symptoms of dementia as indicative of a mental disorder, especially since many demented persons (particularly in the later stages of the disease) experience hallucinations, paranoia, and severe disorientation, which are common in severe mental illness as well. As a result, sometimes dementia is translated using two Chinese characters: one that means "crazy" and the other "catatonic" (Elliott et al., 1996). If that is the perception, a strong negative response will be triggered among the family, which in turn inhibits their help-seeking for a proper diagnosis and treatment. As in the Hispanic culture, *mental illness* among the Chinese and Japanese is extremely stigmatizing, and considered shameful (Elliott et al., 1996). Yet among Japanese Americans, a somewhat less negative view seems to be held, overall, compared to that held by the Chinese. This may be due to the fact that multi-infarct dementia (MID), rather than classic Alzheimer's disease, may be more common among Japanese Americans (Larson & Imai, 1996). MID is often preceded by several strokes, which cause specific, visible types of dysfunction. Also, there may be opportunity for rehabilitation and for some functions to be regained. Finally, since MID is described as having more of a step-wise course, compared to the inexorable downward progression of AD, it may be less difficult for families to understand and to seek appropriate medical help (Tempo & Saito, 1996). On the other hand, most Asian cultures believe that "bad deeds that happen in a family should not be disclosed to outsiders"—this will bring shame to the family. Families with this view (regardless of their ancestry) prefer to hide their demented elder and his or her problems within the immediate family and may not seek help until the disease is very far advanced.

In most Asian cultures, a key value is that of filial piety: taking care of one's family first, particularly one's elders. This value is rooted in beliefs about the importance of the collective over the individual: Asian families value social interaction, interdependency, hierarchical relationships, and empathy, in contrast to most forms of Anglo culture, which value democracy and individuality. These strong family values tend to make caregiving a family affair: rather than one designated primary caregiver, as is common among Anglos, most Asians find that the responsibilities are shared (once the situation is faced honestly). However, there is a certain order within the family for who should assume caregiving responsibilities. Among Chinese Americans, the eldest son and his wife are strongly expected to care for his parents in old age (regardless of whether dementia is present or not). Among Japanese Americans, a similar tradition is upheld, although in both cases (for all practical purposes), the actual tasks of caregiving fall to the female relative (daughter-in-law) while the eldest son may retain decision-making power within the family for how the parents are to be cared for. To ease the burden among the more acculturated, who often have jobs and families of their own, a common practice is to have the demented relative stay with different adult children or other family members at different times of the year. This type of rotation system reduces the burden on any one member, but can make it difficult to access services on a regular basis (Tempo & Saito, 1996). As was noted with Hispanic Americans, intergenerational disagreements can occur when the expectations of the elderly parent for care come in conflict with the values and preferences of their adult children.

One of the few empirical studies undertaken with Chinese American caregivers was reported by Elliott et al. (1996) in which ethnographic data were collected in San Francisco's Chinatown in order to shed some light on this hidden and difficult-to-reach population. Besides the family values noted above, the researchers found that a great deal of importance was ascribed to the Chinese-speaking community there and to being cared for by members of that community, rather than by "outsiders" who represented Western medical practices and research agendas. This underscores the importance of bilingual and/or bicultural health care providers, to gain trust and to be in a better position to negotiate treatment options with key family members. Elliott et al. (1996) also recommends that health care practitioners collaborate actively with Chinese families to devise treatment and care plans that will not cause shame or other difficulties in their community. For example, it is not wise to suggest that it is in any way "dysfunctional" for the daughter-in-law to assume full caregiving responsibilities for a mother-in-law with advanced dementia with no help from that person's three grown daughters who also live in the area. To do so would violate long-standing cultural norms (as noted above), and would only result in the family turning away even more from formal services. We would suggest, however, that when caregiving causes substantial distress, it is necessary to explore culturally accepted strategies to help the caregiver obtain relief and respite.

For Japanese American caregivers, one of the only empirical studies to be found in the literature is that described earlier by Kemp and Adams (1996) in which this group was compared with three other groups of caregivers on several distress indices. Among the Japanese Americans interviewed, it was found that they were generally more pessimistic than the other three groups in terms of their appraisal of caregiving. They used few formal supports and, like the other caregivers studied, scored high on the depression measure used. They also tended to seek more informal support from their family, and reported being generally more satisfied with help from family members than the other groups of caregivers who were interviewed. For the Japanese Americans, their depression was predicted most by an escape or avoidant coping style, which although not common, had a strong negative impact when present. Those who were more acculturated were less pessimistic about caregiving, which, in turn, was associated with less depression, and more satisfaction with the caregiving role. Kemp and Adams (1966) unfortunately did not speculate about the possible causes of the pessimistic orientation.

Taken together, these findings suggest that extra caution is necessary in designing interventions for Asian Americans (as a group), so as not to impinge on the family values and hierarchical nature of most family relationships, as well as not to heighten the family's sense of shame. This further suggests that group oriented interventions (such as support groups where participants are urged to share their personal thoughts and feelings) would probably not be appropriate for most Asian American caregivers—particularly those who are not highly acculturated. On the other hand, family-based inter-

ventions in which the son is encouraged from his position of leader-
ship to create support systems for his wife (who is doing much of
the hands-on work of caregiving) may be worth exploring because
they would respect culturally defined hierarchies, yet have the potential to bring relief where it is most needed.

## Cultural Beliefs about Dementia and Implications for Caregiving among Native Americans/Alaska Natives

Very little is known about dementia and family caregiving in these
groups—partly due to the high prevalence of alcohol-related dementia which tends to shorten the life span and leads to different kinds
of caregiving stress. The interested reader is referred to chapters by
Kramer (1996) and John, Hennessy, Roy, and Salvini (1996) for
more extensive discussion of this topic. However, we will briefly
present some information here that may be relevant to working with
demented individuals and their families.

As with the other ethnic groups discussed in this chapter, the use
of a single term or category neglects the enormous diversity that is
present. For example, Native Americans consist of approximately
500 federally recognized tribes spread out over the entire U.S. However, to simplify the presentation, we will talk about findings that
seem to be in general, across tribes.

The Native American population has a larger percentage of people
under the age of 30 and a smaller percentage over the age of 60,
compared to U.S. Whites. They are much more likely to have incomes
below the poverty line and to be in poor health; in fact, a significant
percentage of those over 60 have the diagnosis of organic brain
syndrome, possibly due to a combination of arteriosclerosis, stroke,
and chronic alcohol abuse (National Indian Council on Aging,
1978). Since other medical problems and depression are also common conditions among Native Americans, it can be very difficult to
diagnose dementing disorders accurately (Neligh & Scully, 1990).

Edwards and Egbert-Edwards (1990) point out that Native American elders may relate to others in new situations by being passive,
so initial contacts with a professional care provider may go rather
slowly and be difficult to conduct, particularly when pointed questions need to be asked (e.g., about memory loss and inability to

function in everyday life) and specific answers are required. As far as intervention goes, many tribes endorse the belief of respect for the natural unfolding of personality; this leads to the concept of noninterference, meaning that individuals are typically allowed to decide how they will behave. For example, Native American adult children may try to convince their ill elderly relative to keep medical appointments, eat a proper diet, and act in sensible ways. However, the ill elder (no matter how severe the dementia) would be allowed to continue making their own decisions (Attneave, 1982).

Similar to other groups we have discussed, Native Americans have a strong sense of community and have great respect for their elders. Those living on reservations tend to rely on the extended family for caregiving; it is not unusual for four generations to live under one roof and to expect to engage in mutual assistance (Edwards & Egbert-Edwards, 1990). Thus, reservation elders may have a distinct advantage over urban elders who must rely more on the formal service system, although there are few nursing homes owned and operated by tribes, and even fewer trained staff in existing nursing homes who can promote Native American culture.

## Summary of This Section

The cultural context within which caregiving occurs includes cultural beliefs, attitudes, and values about health and illness, as well as about family relationships. How caregiving is perceived and executed also depends on many other factors including the caregiver's gender, the nature of their prior relationship, and the family's socioeconomic status, level of education, immigration status, and the like. It goes without saying that a number of factors unique to the care receiver also exert a strong influence on the caregiving process, such as the person's level of cognitive and functional impairment, remaining strengths and weaknesses, behavioral problems, and other health problems which may complicate care. Besides these variables, there are other indicators of stress and vulnerability, and other strengths within the caregiver (e.g., personality structure, spirituality, self-efficacy beliefs) that affect the overall course of caregiving. These are shown in Figure 5.1, which presents the sociocultural context of caregiving, as conceptualized by our research group (Coon, Schulz, Ory, et al., in press).

It is only by carefully studying the relative contribution of all of these factors (singly and in their interaction) that we can truly understand the caregiving process and design interventions that will be culturally appropriate, accessible, and helpful to those in need.

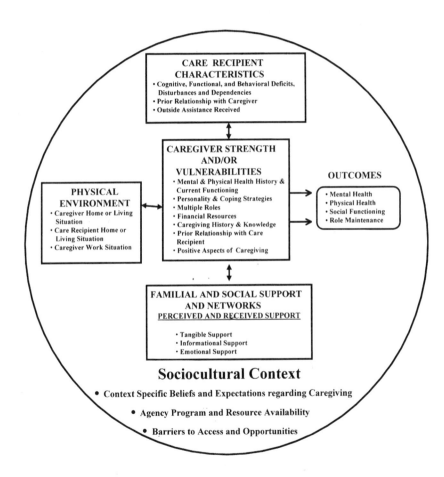

**FIGURE 5.1   Context of caregiving.**

## DESIGN OF CULTURALLY APPROPRIATE AND RELEVANT INTERVENTIONS FOR CAREGIVERS

Even if one plans to follow a well-defined theoretical model (as is depicted in Figure 5.1, for example) there still remain a number of general principles to consider before tackling the task of designing culturally appropriate and sensitive interventions for caregivers of different ethnic and cultural backgrounds. Many of these are explained in greater detail in Bourgeois et al. (1996); they are summarized here. First, interventions must be theoretically derived and based; second, they need to have clearly specifiable and measurable goals; and third, they should be able to be conducted according to specific guidelines or protocols, following specific precautions, and be carried out in an ethical manner. In addition, interventions should be conducted by trained personnel whose work is monitored and who are supervised, if necessary (according to the complexity of the intervention and its "clinical" versus educational or other, less personal, emphasis). Finally, intervention delivery needs to be monitored, so that it can be determined whether or not the intervention is being given as planned. All of these are *general* points that would need to be followed in any intervention research program. Following are some *unique* points that need to be addressed when designing an intervention for a particular cultural/ethnic group:

### Designing Interventions That Are Culturally Sensitive and Appropriate

As we have seen so far in this chapter, this is a lot easier said than done. It should be clear by now that no "one size fits all" when it comes to interventions.

In order to attempt to "tailor" existing interventions, the following questions may be worth considering as the modified intervention is being planned. First, what is the theoretical basis for the intervention? Why is it anticipated that this particular form of treatment will be helpful to this particular racial, ethnic, or cultural group? To answer these questions, one must be thoroughly familiar with the culture, either through one's own knowledge base, or by hiring knowledgeable consultants from the community itself who are interested in the problem you are trying to address—in this case, dementia caregiving. Second, it is generally recommended that pilot work be done at the outset to evaluate it and receive feedback from participants before full-scale implementation, whether the intervention is truly new or is essentially a modification of an existing, successful approach.

If a brand-new intervention is being designed, then work should begin by broadly defining the target population and then seeking both immediate and continued input from the community. The latter can be done in a variety of ways, such as consulting with health and mental health leaders in that community, participating in community-based and community-wide activities relevant to the proposed project (such as health screening fairs, in the case of dementia), and becoming knowledgeable about prior efforts that may have occurred to reach the same target population, and what results they obtained. Next, conducting focus groups is generally recommended. They could be held with care providers and/or possible future participants, in order to learn how the individuals themselves perceive the problem, what help they think they need, and how they would like it delivered. Focus groups have become very popular in the past decade as the field of dementia caregiving has grown. Detailed information about how to organize and run focus groups can be found in such sources as Greenbaum (1998) and Morgan and Krueger (1998). In general, this would be considered the preferred way to begin, particularly when dealing with such sensitive content matter as dementia and its impact on family members. However, researchers do not always have the time or the training to conduct focus groups properly; so, for many clinically oriented researchers in this field, modifications of existing interventions will be the approach taken.

Regardless of whether the intervention is brand-new, or already exists and is being "tailored" or specifically modified for the project or particular ethnic group, it is advisable to consider the following guidelines (based on the authors' experience):

- Recognize that when the intervention itself is not designed by a person whose cultural background matches closely that of the group for whom the intervention is intended, then it is critical to receive abundant input from the community. That input must be sought and cultivated throughout the life of the project, so that the community will perceive this as an outgrowth of their participation in the process. Also, most ethnic elders and their families are distrustful of outsiders and will not participate in programs that do not have a seal of approval from key community leaders (Valle, 1988).

- Recognize that the intervention must be culturally relevant and not dystonic. For example, many Hispanic and African-American elders have close ties to their church, so that interventions that are approved by church officials and perhaps actually conducted on church grounds may be more likely to be acceptable. Spiritual themes can be included, and reference to prayer as a form of coping would be likely to be seen as appropriate and perhaps even welcome (Henderson, Gutierrez-Mayka, Garcia & Boyd, 1993).

- Ensure that all verbal and written instructions regarding the intervention and follow-up measures are salient and relevant to the target population. For example, among Spanish-speaking groups, it is essential that translation, back translation, and committee or consensus translation be performed, and that appropriate adjustments be made for local, idiomatic differences in expression with regard to word usage (Loewenstein, Argüelles, Argüelles & Lin-Fuentes, 1994).

- Commit to the fact that the intervention must use language, behaviors, and content that are viewed as appropriate within the context of the particular group. In order to do this effectively, it is crucial to hire members of the community to which the intervention is targeted, so that they can comment early on about its suitability and likely level of acceptability. For example, Cuban Americans in Miami (some of whom are well-educated and may have a professional background) may find offensive language that was tailored to fit the lower educational (and reading) level of some Mexican American elders. The opposite is also true: Mexican American elders with excellent reading skills may feel that they are being treated in a condescending manner if they are presented with material that is too easy for them to read effectively. Thus, they may not return to take part further in the intervention, even though it was well-designed in other respects (Gallagher-Thompson, Leary, Ossinalde, et al., 1997).

- Do not become discouraged by the fact that for maximal effectiveness, the intervention needs to be conducted by leaders who are from the same (or similar) cultural background as the participants. Rapport is usually built more quickly when this is the case. Despite the costs that are involved (in salary, training time, and the like) to hire indigenous staff, this can be extremely helpful for the success of the project. However, ethnic matching is not a substitute for adequate training in the intervention and how it is to be delivered, which must take place for all staff. For non-English speaking caregivers, language facility is obviously also a key factor. Leaders must be able to communicate in the preferred language of the participants—which often is not English, although the caregiver may be bilingual. In addition, intervention leaders must be comfortable enough with the language and its nuances to be able to conduct sensitive discussions using the proper words (not recommended for beginners; see Gallagher-Thompson et al., 1997). Finally, interventionists need to be able to seek assistance and support from senior staff when the participants bring up problems or issues that are beyond the scope of what the interventionist is trained to handle. This will only happen in an environment of multicultural competence, where mutual respect and an atmosphere of learning prevail.

## Outreach Efforts

Since developing and then implementing intervention programs with caregivers from different cultural backgrounds is so labor-intensive and time-consuming, we believe that it is critical to build in a strong outreach component to the research as well. This will enable potential users of the service to become aware of its existence and to see it as a definite resource, likely to be helpful. We often implicitly assume that caregivers will be eager to participate in such programs because of the inherent stress of caregiving; however, many are reluctant to participate because of an unwillingness to acknowledge in themselves, their family, or their community, that they require support and assistance (Argüelles & Loewenstein, 1998). In order to do effective outreach, it is necessary to determine in advance what the obstacles are to participation (e.g., transportation; sitting costs, for dementia caregivers; competing family obligations; etc.), and spend time problem solving so that these barriers can be addressed and hopefully, overcome (see Arean & Gallagher-Thompson, 1996, for a number of specific recommendations for recruitment and retention of minority elders in intervention-oriented research). Several other recent papers have also addressed this topic. For example, Olin, Pawluczyk, Kauman, et al. (1997) recommend a personal approach to doing community outreach with Hispanic caregivers, in order to increase their familiarity with dementia services and staff. This increases the likelihood that they will use needed services before the patient has reached the end stage of the disease. Argüelles and Loewenstein (1998) describe their modification of the adoption process model developed for marketing research to the field of dementia outreach with the Cuban American population in Miami. They found that by applying this model, they were able to increase recruitment into the REACH project considerably among Cuban American caregivers. Finally, Young, Edevie, Young and Peters (1996) recommend the use of African-American staff to do outreach in that community, making the point that this increases trust and promotes more effective communication. Whatever methods are used to reach the target audience, once they start coming to your center or program, you will need to deliver a good "product" or run the risk of negative publicity, which can ruin future research opportunities. Thus, we see outreach and intervention as going hand-in-hand: successful efforts in both areas are needed in order to improve caregivers' quality of life.

## CULTURAL APPROPRIATENESS OF REACH
## PROJECT INTERVENTIONS

As other chapters in this book have described, the REACH project was designed to be the first large-scale, multisite program to evaluate the effectiveness of various kinds of intervention strategies to improve caregivers' quality of life and reduce subjective distress. The sites chosen and the specific interventions offered at each location are described in detail in Coon et al. (in press) so we will not go into detail here. Our purpose now is to illustrate how several of the interventions being evaluated in the REACH protocols were chosen (or designed) to be culturally sensitive and appropriate for the particular populations of ethnic minority caregivers with whom they are being used. This discussion will highlight three of the six sites that are specifically studying ethnic differences in outcome, and that are enrolling relatively large numbers of caregivers from specific ethnic backgrounds. These are Birmingham, Miami, and Palo Alto. The remaining sites (Boston, Memphis, and Philadelphia) are also enrolling minority caregivers, but the study of ethnic differences in outcome does not appear to be one of their primary research goals.

At Birmingham (which is focusing on African American as well as Anglo caregivers) one of the key intervention conditions is behavioral skill training: teaching caregivers how to mange and modify certain problematic behaviors of their care receiver. At Miami (which is focusing on Cuban Americans as well as Anglo caregivers), one of the major interventions involves the use of in-home family therapy: teaching caregivers how to obtain more assistance and support from family members, as well as teaching skills for conflict resolution. Finally, at Palo Alto (which is focusing on Mexican Americans in addition to Anglo caregivers), a key intervention is the psychoeducational class designed to teach caregivers a set of coping skills for managing their negative emotions, such as depression and frustration. Discussions with principal staff at each of these sites has revealed that while none of these interventions was newly designed for the specific ethnic group targeted, each was significantly modified or tailored for that group. A process was followed before the intervention phase of the study began that included community input early on, substantial pilot testing with feedback, and then further modification of the intervention (e.g., its content, manner of presentation, or use of supplemental materials such as handouts to be read or practiced as homework). These steps were taken in order to increase the likelihood that each particular intervention was culturally appropriate and acceptable.

Selection and training of interventionists at each of the sites has emphasized both cultural diversity and cultural competence. For example, at the Birmingham site, training groups are co-led by White and African-American investigators of equal status. Inclusion of ethnic minority staff can help to address the "cultural mistrust" which can occur among African Americans in dealing with health care and other establishment institutions (Barrett, 1998). Similar practices have been used at the Palo Alto and Miami sites where bilingual and bicultural Hispanic staff are prominent.

In the context of this discussion, it may be noteworthy that these three interventions share an emphasis on active learning: caregivers are taught and encouraged to use a variety of skills designed to empower them and help them take more control over their caregiving situations. This seems consistent with at least some of the material presented earlier, on the culturally bound perceptions of dementia and of caregiving that typify these groups. For example, it was noted that African Americans in general may not view caregiving in as negative or burdensome a light as their Anglo counterparts. But those who enroll in a caregiver intervention study probably are stressed and depressed, and experiencing burden from the role. Once they learn how to manage problem behaviors better in the home environment, these caregivers may report a reduction in their levels of stress, because they have learned how to minimize it.

Similarly, Cuban Americans, with their generally high levels of education and success in the professions, may nevertheless feel depressed and burdened by virtue of the fact that other family members (even those living in close proximity) provide little assistance with caregiving. By participating in an intervention designed to improve communication among family members as well as increasing assertion skills (to ask for help when needed), these caregivers may gain more family assistance and support needed to continue in the role.

Finally, Mexican Americans, who may suffer from low socioeconomic status and related problems, may find it very appealing to enroll in a course for coping with caregiving. The fact that they can master the material and gain more control over the strong negative emotions that are experienced (particularly depression) may empower this group sufficiently so that distress is truly reduced over time.

In short, by building on some of the common cultural values and beliefs of each group, these sites have made a deliberate effort to customize their interventions for the particular groups they are serving. Although no comparative outcome data are available at this time, these sites report generally high rates of recruitment, very low drop-out rates, and high "customer satisfaction" with these particular interventions. Taken together, this suggests that the initial hard work has paid off, and these interventions are culturally appropriate for their participants.

## SUGGESTIONS FOR FUTURE RESEARCH

We wish to conclude this chapter by suggesting areas for fruitful continued research investigation. First and foremost, as we have pointed out, no new culturally specific intervention strategies were designed for the REACH project; this is surely a situation that needs to be addressed in the next generation of caregiver outcome studies. For example, it may be that a completely novel intervention is needed for some of the specific subgroups of Asian-American caregivers. They are not being studied in depth in the REACH project; generally, they do not wish to participate in support groups or other group-oriented programs where it is necessary to share personal information with strangers. Anecdotally, it was reported to several of the authors of this chapter that Japanese-American women who are caregivers might attend a quilting group or a similar kind of activity, where the focus is on making things with one's hands, not on revealing inner feelings and family problems. However, in the course of meeting and working together on such a project, trust builds, and over time, that kind of setting may become conducive to sharing and to gaining support from others in a similar caregiving situation. That really does remain to be seen.

A second recommendation would be to urge future researchers to create actual partnerships with community agencies and other facilities serving the frail elderly. Since so little is really known about dementia in most ethnic communities, it may be that education about similarities and differences among normal aging, memory loss, and dementia, is required in order to raise the level of awareness of entire communities. While this may be time-consuming, it will establish the researcher's presence as someone who is contributing to the community—not just taking what he or she needs and then leaving the community essentially as it was.

A final recommendation is the development of interventions that are truly multigenerational. Most of the current research focuses on the needs and struggles of the primary caregiver, which is a uniquely Anglo approach to the situation. We have pointed out that family is valued over the individual in most ethnic groups; therefore, isn't it time we designed interventions that could conceivably benefit the entire family (particularly those who are living under one roof)? This may pose many logistical and methodological problems, and would be very "messy" research to do, but perhaps it is an idea whose time has come.

## REFERENCES

Aranda, M.P. & Knight, B.G. (1997). The influence of ethnicity and culture on the caregiver stress and coping process: A sociocultural review and analysis. *The Gerontologist, 37*, 342–354.

Arean, P., & Gallagher-Thompson, D. (1996). Issues and recommendations for the recruitment and retention of older ethnic minority adults into clinical research. *Journal of Consulting and Clinical Psychology, 64*, 875–880.

Argüelles, T., & Loewenstein, D. (1997). Research says "Si" to the development of culturally appropriate cognitive assessment tools. *Generations, 21*, 30–31.

Argüelles, T., & Loewenstein, D. (1998, November). Challenges in recruiting families into intervention programs: The Miami experience. In C. Eisdorfer & S. Czaja (Co-chairs), Symposium: *Assisting caregiving families: Challenges and new treatments.* Presented at the annual meeting of the Gerontological Society of America, Philadelphia, PA.

Attneave, C. (1982). American Indians and Alaska Native families: Emigrants in their own homeland. In M. McGoldrick, J.K. Pearce, & J. Giordano (Eds.), *Ethnicity and family therapy.* New York: Guilford Press.

Baker, F. (1996). Issues in assessing dementia in African American elders. In G. Yeo & D. Gallagher-Thompson (Eds.), *Ethnicity and the dementias* (pp. 59–76). Washington, DC: Taylor & Francis.

Ballard, E.L., Nash, F., Raiford, K., & Harrell, L.E. (1993). Recruitment of Black elderly for clinical research studies of dementia: The CERAD experience. *Gerontologist, 33*, 561–565.

Barrett, R.K. (1998). Sociocultural considerations for working with Blacks experiencing loss or grief. In K.J. Doka & J.D. Davidson (Eds.), *Living with grief: Who we are, how we grieve* (pp. 83–96). Washington, DC: Hospice Foundation of America.

Bourgeois, M.S., Schulz, R., & Burgio, L. (1996). Interventions for caregivers of patients with Alzheimer's disease: A review and analysis of content, process, and outcomes. *International Journal of Aging and Human Development, 43*, 35–92.

Buchwald, D., Caralis, P.V., Gany, F., Hardt, E.J., Johnson, T.M., Muecke, M.A., & Putsch, R.W. (1994). Caring for patients in a multicultural society. *Patient Care*, June 15, 1994, 105–120.

Burton, L. (1992). Families and the aged: Issues of complexity and diversity. *Generations, 17*.

Connell, C.M., & Gibson, G.D. (1997). Racial, ethnic, and cultural differences in dementia caregiving: Review and analysis. *The Gerontologist, 37*, 355–364.

Coon, D.W., Schulz, R., Ory, M., & the REACH Study Group (in press). Innovative intervention approaches with Alzheimer's caregivers. In D. Biegel & A. Blum (Eds.), *Innovations in practice, service, and delivery across the lifespan*. New York: Oxford.

Cox, C., & Monk, A. (1993). Black and Hispanic caregivers of dementia victims: Their needs and implications for services. In C.M. Barresi & D.E. Stull (Eds.), *Ethnic elderly and long term care* (pp. 57–67). New York: Springer.

Davidson, A. (1997). *Alzheimer's: A love story*. Secaucus, NJ: Carol Publishing Group.

Edwards, E.G., & Egbert-Edwards, M. (1990). Family care and the Native American elderly. In M.S. Harper (Ed.), *Minority aging: Essential curricula content for selected health professionals and allied health professionals*. HRS DHHS Publication No. P-DV-90-4, pp. 145–164. Washington, DC: U.S. Government Printing Office.

Elliott, K., Di Minno, M., Lam, D., & Tui, A. (1996). Working with Chinese families in the context of dementia. In G. Yeo & D. Gallagher-Thompson (Eds.), *Ethnicity and the dementias* (pp. 89–108). Washington, DC: Taylor & Francis.

Gaines, A.G. (1989). Alzheimer's disease in the context of Black (southern) culture. *Health Matrix, 6*, 4–8.

Gallagher-Thompson, D. (1994). Direct services and interventions for caregivers: A review and critique of extant programs and a look ahead to the future. In M.M. Cantor (Ed.), *Family caregiving: Agenda for the future* (pp. 102–122). San Francisco: American Society on Aging.

Gallagher-Thompson, D., Coon, D., Rivera, P., Powers, D., & Zeiss, A. (1998). Family caregiving: Stress, coping, and intervention. In M. Hersen & V.B. Van Hasselt (Eds.), *Handbook of clinical geropsychology* (pp. 469–493). New York: Plenum Press.

Gallagher-Thompson, D., Leary, M.C., Ossinalde, C., Romero, J.J., Wald, M.J., & Fernandez-Gamarra, E. (1997). Hispanic caregivers of older adults with dementia: Cultural issues in outreach and intervention. *Group: Journal of the Eastern Group Psychotherapy Association, 21*, 211–232.

Gallagher-Thompson, D., Talamantes, M., Ramirez, R., & Valverde, I. (1996). Service delivery issues and recommendations for working with Mexican-American families. In G. Yeo & D. Gallagher-Thompson (Eds.), *Ethnicity and the dementias* (pp. 137–152). Washington, DC: Taylor & Francis.

Gibson, R.C. (1992). Blacks at middle and later life: Resources and coping. *The Annals of the American Academy of Political and Social Science, 464,* 79–90.

Green, J. (1995). *Cultural awareness in the human services* (2nd ed.). Englewood Cliffs, NJ: Prentice-Hall.

Greenbaum, T. L. (1998). *The handbook for focus group research* (2nd ed.). Thousand Oaks, CA: Sage Publications.

Haley, W.E., Han, B., & Henderson, J.N. (1998). Aging and ethnicity: Issues for clinical practice. *Journal of Clinical Psychology in Medical Settings, 5,* 393–409.

Haley, W.E., Roth, D.L., Coleton, M.I., Ford, G.R., West, C.A.C., Collins, R.P., & Isobe, T.L. (1996). Appraisal, coping, and social support as mediators of well-being in Black and White family caregivers of patients with Alzheimer's disease. *Journal of Consulting and Clinical Psychology, 64,* 121–129.

Haley, W., West, W., Wadley, V., White, F., Barrett, J., Ford, G., Harrell, L., & Roth, D. (1995). Psychological, social and health impact of caregiving: A comparison of Black and White dementia caregivers and noncaregivers. *Psychology and Aging, 10,* 540–552.

Henderson, J.N., & Gutierrez-Mayka, M. (1992). Ethnocultural themes in caregiving to Alzheimer's patients in Hispanic families. *Clinical Gerontologist, 11,* 59–74.

Henderson, J.N., Gutierrez-Mayka, M., Garcia, J., & Boyd, S. (1993). A model for Alzheimer's disease support group development in African-American and Hispanic populations. *Gerontologist, 33,* 409–414.

Hinrichsen, G.A., & Ramirez, M. (1992). Black and White dementia caregivers: A comparison of their adaptation, adjustment, and services utilization. *Gerontologist, 32,* 375–381.

John, R., Hennessy, C.H., Roy, L.C., & Salvini, M.L. (1996). Caring for cognitively impaired American Indian elders: Difficult situations, few options. In G. Yeo & D. Gallagher-Thompson (Eds.), *Ethnicity and the dementias* (pp. 187–203). Washington, DC: Taylor & Francis.

John, R., & McMillian, B. (1998). Exploring caregiver burden among Mexican Americans: Cultural prescriptions, family dilemmas. *Journal of Aging and Ethnicity, 1,* 93–111.

Kato, P.M. (1996). On nothing and everything: The relationship between ethnicity and health. In P.M. Kato & T. Mann (Eds.), *Handbook of diversity issues in health psychology* (pp. 287–300). New York: Plenum Press.

Kemp, B., & Adams, B. (1996). *The role of caregiver appraisal, coping method, and social support in the stress of dementia caregivers of four different ethnic groups.* Final Report: Alzheimer's Disease Diagnostic and Treatment Center, Rancho Los Amigos Hospital, Downey, CA.

Kleinman, A., Eisenberg, L., & Good, B. (1978). Clinical lessons from anthropologic and cross-cultural research. *Annals of Internal Medicine, 88,* 251–258.

Kramer, B.J. (1996). Dementia in American Indian populations. In G. Yeo & D. Gallagher-Thompson (Eds.), *Ethnicity and the dementias* (pp. 175–182). Washington, DC: Taylor & Francis.

Lacayo, C.G. (1993). Hispanic elderly: Policy issues in long-term care. In C.M. Barresi & D.E. Stull (Eds.), *Ethnic elderly and long-term care* (pp. 223–234). New York: Springer.

Landrine, H., & Klonoff, E.A. (1992). Culture and health-related schemas: A review and proposal for interdisciplinary integration. *Health Psychology, 11,* 267–276.

Larson, E.B., & Imai, Y. (1996). An overview of dementia and ethnicity with special emphasis on the epidemiology of dementia. In G. Yeo & D. Gallagher-Thompson (Eds.), *Ethnicity and the dementias* (pp. 9–20). Washington, D.C.: Taylor & Francis.

Lawton, M.P., Rajagopal, D., Brody, E., & Kleban, M. (1992). The dynamics of caregiving for a demented elder among Black and White families. *Journal of Gerontology: Social Sciences, 47,* S156–S164.

Lewis, I.D., & Ausberry, M.C. (1996). African-American families: Management of demented elders. In G. Yeo & D. Gallagher-Thompson (Eds.), *Ethnicity and the dementias* (pp. 167–174). Washington, D.C.: Taylor & Francis.

Lockery, S.A. (1991). Caregiving among racial and ethnic minority elders. *Generations, 15,* 58–62.

Loewenstein, D., Argüelles, T., Argüelles, S., & Lin-Fuentes, R. (1994). Potential cultural bias in the neuropsychological assessment of the older adult. *Journal of Clinical and Experimental Neuropsychology, 16,* 623–629.

Mace, N., & Rabins, P. (1991). *The thirty-six hour day* (2nd ed.). Baltimore: Johns Hopkins University Press.

Matocha, L.K. (1998). Chinese Americans. In L.D. Purnell & B.J. Paulanka (Eds.), *Transcultural health care: A culturally competent approach* (pp. 163–188). Philadelphia: F.A. Davis Co.

Mintzer, J.E., Rubert, M.P., Lowenstein, D., Gamez, E., Millor, A., Quinteros, R., Flores, L., Miller, M., Rainerman, A., & Eisdorfer, C. (1992). Daughters caregiving for Hispanic and non-Hispanic Alzheimer patients: Does ethnicity make a difference? *Community Mental Health Journal, 28,* 293–303.

Miranda, B.F., McBride, M.R., & Spangler, Z. (1998). Filipino Americans. In L.D. Purnell & J. Paulanka (Eds.), *Transcultural health care: A culturally competent approach* (pp. 245–272). Philadelphia: F.A. Davis Co.

Morgan, D.L., & Krueger, R.A. (1998). *The focus group kit* (6 volumes). Thousand Oaks, CA: Sage Publications.

Morioka-Douglas, N., & Yeo, G. (1990). *Aging and health: Asian/Pacific Island American elders.* Stanford, CA: Stanford Geriatric Education Center SGEC Working Paper Series #3.

Mui, A. (1992). Caregiver strain among Black and White daughter caregivers: A role theory perspective. *Gerontologist, 32,* 203–212.

National Indian Council on Aging. (1978). *The continuum of life: Health concerns of the Indian elderly.* Final Report on the Second National Indian Conference on Aging.

Neligh, G., & Scully, J. (1990). Differential diagnosis of major mental disorders among American Indian elderly. In M.S. Harper (Ed.), Minority aging: Essential curricula content for selected health and allied health professionals. DHHS Publication No. HRS (P-DV-90-4), pp. 165–178. Washington, DC: U.S. Government Printing Office.

Nowak, T.T. (1998). Vietnamese Americans. In L.D. Purnell & B.J. Paulanka (Eds.), *Transcultural health care: A culturally competent approach* (pp. 449–477).

Olin, J., Pawluczyk, S., Kauman, G.T., Taussig, I.M., Henderson, V.W., & Schneider, L.S. (1997). A comparative analysis of Spanish- and English-speaking Alzheimer's disease patients: Eligibility and interest in clinical drug trials. *Journal of Clinical Geropsychology, 3,* 183–190.

Orona, C.J., & Alkayyali, M. (1992). *Alzheimer's disease, Latino caregivers, and the social construction of moral obligation.* Final report submitted to the Dept. of Health Services, State of CA, from San Jose State University.

Peskind, E.R., & Raskind, M. (1996). Cognitive disorders. In E.W. Busse & D.G. Blazer (Eds.), *Textbook of geriatric psychiatry* (pp. 213–234). Washington, DC: American Psychiatric Press.

Polich, T., & Gallagher-Thompson, D. (1997). Preliminary study investigating psychological distress among female Hispanic caregivers. *Journal of Clinical Geropsychology, 3,* 1–15.

Sanchez, C.D. (1992). Mental health issues: The elderly Hispanic. *Journal of Geriatric Psychiatry, 25,* 60–84.

Schulz, R., O'Brien, A.T., Bookwala, J., & Fleissner, K. (1995). Psychiatric and physical morbidity effects of dementia caregiving: Prevalence, correlates and causes. *Gerontologist, 35,* 771–791.

Segall, M., & Wykle, M. (1988–89). The Black family's experience with dementia. *Journal of Applied Social Sciences, 13,* 170–191.

Sharts-Hopko, N. C. (1998). Japanese Americans. In L. D. Purnell & B. J. Paulanka (Eds.), *Transcultural health care: A culturally competent approach* (on computer disk). Philadelphia: F. A. Davis Co.

Tang, M., Stern, Y., Marder, K., et al. (1998). The APOE-E allele and the risk of Alzheimer disease among African Americans, Whites, and Hispanics. *Journal of the American Medical Association, 279,* 751–755.

Tempo, P.M., & Saito, A. (1996). Techniques of working with Japanese American families. In G. Yeo & D. Gallagher-Thompson (Eds.), *Ethnicity and the dementias* (pp. 109–122). Washington, DC: Taylor & Francis.

Valle, R. (1988). Outreach to ethnic minorities with Alzheimer's disease: The challenge to the community. *Health Matrix, 6,* 13–27.

Valle, R. (1989). Cultural and ethnic issues in Alzheimer's disease family research. In E. Light & B.D. Lebowitz (Eds.), *Alzheimer's disease and family stress: Directions for research* (pp. 122–154). Rockville, MD: National Institute of Mental Health.

Villa, M.L., Cuellar, J., Gamel, N., & Yeo, G. (1993). *Aging and health: Hispanic American elders* (2nd ed.). Stanford, CA: Stanford Geriatric Education Center, SGEC Working Paper Series #5.

Wood, J., & Parham, I. (1990). Coping with perceived burden: Ethnic and cultural issues in Alzheimer's family caregiving. *Journal of Applied Gerontology, 9,* 325–339.

Wykle, M., & Segall, M. (1991). A comparison of Black and White family caregivers' experience with dementia. *Journal of National Black Nurses Association, 5,* 29–41.

Yeo, G. (1996). Background. In G. Yeo & D. Gallagher-Thompson (Eds.), *Ethnicity and the dementias* (pp. 3–8). Washington, DC: Taylor & Francis.

Young, R.F., Edevie, S., Young, J.H., & Peters, J. (1996). Issues of recruitment and retention in Alzheimer's research among African and White Americans. *Journal of Aging and Ethnicity, 1,* 19–25.

# 6

# Measurement Issues in Intervention Research

*Galen E. Switzer, Stephen R. Wisniewski,*
*Steven H. Belle, Robert Burns, Laraine Winter,*
*Larry Thompson, and Richard Schulz*

Although many excellent texts have been written on general principles of instrumentation (e.g., McDowell & Newell, 1996; Nunnally, 1978; Nunnally & Bernstein, 1994; Rosenthal & Rosnow, 1991), few of them provide concise statements concerning the practical application of measurement issues to the selection and development of instruments for new projects. The primary goals of this chapter are to provide a) a guide that includes an organizational structure for making decisions concerning instrument selection, development, and evaluation, b) a practically oriented discussion of the basic issues involved in such decisions, and c) specific examples of measures that are appropriate for use in caregiver intervention research.

Authors of this text are currently engaged in a multi-site project involving intervention research with elderly caregivers (Resources for Enhancing Alzheimer's Caregiver Health; REACH, 1995) and thus, the examples we use here focus primarily on mental and physical health issues. One of the initial steps undertaken by REACH investigators was to form a Measurement Workgroup. This Workgroup was charged with selecting instruments for the project by first identifying key domains to be assessed, identifying suitable measures within each domain, and finally prioritizing measures based on multiple factors such as their appropriateness for the target population, their ability to fulfill the research goals, and their psychometric properties. In addition to these universal considerations in measurement selection, the Workgroup was concerned in particular with measurement goals central to multi-site intervention studies. Because REACH investigators targeted a diverse set of groups but maintained the objective of conducting cross-site comparisons of intervention effectiveness, it was important to select a set of instruments that would characterize potential participants on a number of factors (e.g., socio-demographics, cognitive functioning) for initial screening and for future descriptive purposes. A second set of issues was related to tracking study participants across time. The Workgroup identified instruments that were sensitive to longitudinal changes in caregiver status, and selected or developed instruments that were specific to key transition points that are part of the caregiving role (e.g., bereavement, out of home placement). Thus, instruments assessing a core set of outcomes (e.g., health effects, service utilization, burden, positive aspects of caregiving), and designed to capture the impact of the interventions in a way that allowed for direct comparison of intervention effectiveness, were selected. The Workgroup's final goal was to create measures to assess the integrity and intensity with which interventions were delivered, thus allowing for a more fine-grained analysis of intervention effectiveness. The remainder of this chapter focuses on the type of measurement issues that emerged in the process of selecting, developing, and evaluating instruments for the REACH project, and concludes with a brief overview of instruments appropriate for caregiver intervention research.

The following discussion focuses initially on two broad issues central to decisions about instrumentation; context and psychometrics (see Table 6.1). Context refers to factors exogenous to the assessment tool itself, such as characteristics of individuals to be assessed, the goals of the research endeavor, and constraints on data gathering capabilities. Addressing issues of context is critical because such

---

**TABLE 6.1 Key Contextual Measurement Issues**

Contextual Issues

---

Participant Characteristics
—age
—gender
—education level
—health status
—recent life experiences

Cultural Context
—ethnicity
—cultural traditions and norms

Historical Context
—language
—knowledge base
—beliefs, attitudes, values
—political and historical events

Research Goals
—content of measurement
—specificity of measurement
—comparisons to normative groups

Administration Issues
—feasibility
—format of instrument

---

issues may help guide the selection of instruments and may delineate the generalizability of study results to other groups and settings. Psychometrics refers to the properties of the instrument as it functions within the context. Failure to demonstrate the psychometric properties (e.g., reliability and validity) of instruments in any research endeavor may lead to questions about the meaningfulness of fundamental study findings.

## CONTEXTUAL ISSUES IN THE SELECTION AND/OR DEVELOPMENT OF INSTRUMENTS

### Participant Characteristics

In selecting or developing an instrument, one of the primary considerations should be the characteristics of the study participants (see

Table 6.1 for a summary of key contextual issues). Recent studies have indicated that factors such as the respondent's age, gender, education level, physical and mental health status, and other recent life experiences (e.g., recent pregnancy and delivery, recent bereavement, traumatic life experience) affect responses to items. These factors may lead to under endorsement or over endorsement of items, biases in recalling events, and/or respondent difficulty in interpreting questions. Several measurement issues have been raised in the assessment of physical and psychological functioning among the elderly (Ory, 1988; Ory & Cox, 1994). For example, questionnaires assessing limitations in physical activity in terms of inability to work may make little sense for retired individuals. Stressful life events scales that include questions about the birth of a child and one's job, and fail to include stressful events associated with retirement and growing older, may underestimate life stress among the elderly (Ory, 1988). Age biases can exist even in well established measures such as the Beck Depression Inventory; certain items (e.g., body-image change) are over endorsed by the elderly, producing falsely elevated ratings of depression among older respondents (Talbott, 1989). Other research has shown that many depression instruments may *underestimate* depression in the elderly because older persons tend to deny depressive symptoms, or to attribute them to physical health problems (Maier et al., 1988). The respondent's gender may also affect responses. It has been argued that observed gender differences in depression may be at least partially due to a greater willingness of women to endorse symptoms included in these measures, rather than a true gender difference in depression levels (Miller et al., 1985).

Education level is also important to consider for many types of assessment. Mental status assessment instruments (e.g., The Cognitive Capacity Screening Examination, The Clock Drawing Test, The Short Portable Mental Status Questionnaire, The Mini-Mental State Examination), have been shown to overestimate cognitive impairment among groups with little education and to underestimate impairment among the highly educated (Berkman, 1986; Brayne & Calloway, 1990; Kay et al., 1985; Murden et al., 1991; Uhlmann & Larson, 1991).

Other instruments assessing mental health that include a relatively high proportion of somatic symptom items may be inappropriate for physically ill groups in which such symptoms may reflect medical status rather than emotional distress (Dew, in press; Williams & Richardson, 1993). Reporting of health problems may also be affected by other health-related behaviors such as visiting the hospital; current chronic illness is increasingly underreported as the length of time since the last hospital visit increases (Cannell, Marquis, & Laurent, 1977; Madow, 1973). Finally, it is important to ascertain whether measures of health status or physical functioning are "pitched" to the appropriate level for the population under study. For example, measures of activities of daily living that assess whether a care recipient needs help accomplishing specific tasks (e.g., using the telephone, handling finances) may be inappropriate for severely disabled individuals who have not even attempted to complete those tasks for several years.

## Cultural Context

A second important issue to consider is the cultural appropriateness of the instrument for the study population. Most instruments used in social and behavioral research are based on middle-class, Western European/North American assumptions, values, and norms and thus may not be entirely appropriate for other cultural groups. For example, many of the classic symptoms of schizophrenia as defined by the *Diagnostic and Statistical Manual IV* (DSM; American Psychiatric Association, 1994; e.g., delusions, hallucinations, disorganized speech) are part of the religious ceremonies or daily spiritual experiences of many cultural groups (Eaton, 1980). Conversely, it appears that some mental disorders—for example, "ataques de nervios" among Puerto Ricans—are recognized only among non-European cultures (Guarnaccia, Good, & Kleinman, 1990). Specifically in the area of aging research, it has been noted that race may affect individuals' subjective and objective reports of physical health status, primarily, it is argued because of differing cultural-specific interpretations of meaning of health and disability (Gibson, 1991). Culture-bound assumptions may pervade virtually all mental and physical health instruments. Consequently, it is important to determine whether the instrument has been used successfully with the particular cultural/ ethnic groups included in the sample.

## Historical Context

The effects of historical and political events on measurement issues are rarely discussed, but may be as critical as any of the other contextual issues discussed here, especially for classes of measures that have been used for several years. The basic argument is that societies as a whole experience changes in knowledge, beliefs, attitudes, language, and values that, in turn, may affect how individuals interpret groups of items. Researchers must be aware of, and modify measures to suit the particular social climate within which they are operating. There are several recent examples of responses to changes in historical context. For example, tests of IQ have a long history of revision and updating to accommodate the fact that the knowledge base of society has shifted over time, and that on average, individuals are becoming more educated and adept at answering the types of questions that have been used as indicators of IQ.

Measures of health behaviors also require continual revision as our knowledge about health indicators improves. Until a few years ago, questions about smoking, alcohol consumption, and diet that are currently regarded as central to health assessment, were rarely included in health questionnaires. Thus, the language and other implicit assumptions of a given measure should be part of the initial considerations in instrument selection, especially for instruments that are several years old.

## Research Goals

It may seem obvious to suggest that the goals of a specific research effort should guide instrument selection, but there are multiple considerations in this regard. When assessing global health status, for example, it is critical to determine whether it is most important to measure symptoms (e.g., Were you short of breath?), performance (e.g., Would you have trouble running the length of a football field?), feeling-states (e.g., I feel I am a burden to people.), general quality of life (e.g., In general, how satisfying is your life?), or some combination of these. Health measures vary greatly in their relative emphasis on physical, emotional, and social health, and the extent to which information reported across these domains is based on perceptions and feeling-states, or on symptom frequencies.

A second consideration that is common to most areas of mental and physical health research is whether a general (generic) measure or a specific measure should be used. The relative advantages and disadvantages of generic versus specific measures are currently being discussed prominently in the physical health, psychiatric, and quality of life literatures. Disorder-specific health measures (e.g., Arthritis Impact Measurement Scales; Meenan, 1992) enhance the ability to discover fine-grained distinctions among individuals suffering from the disorder under consideration, but may not be adequate if comparisons of status across individuals with different disorders is central to the research goals.

Finally, decisions about instrumentation may be based on the importance of making comparisons across studies, or with normative samples. If it is desirable to make such normative comparisons, it will be critical to utilize a measure that has been used extensively in other populations, even if it does not address the full range of issues important to the project. It may be possible to supplement existing measures with items that address more specific research goals (see discussion of Modified and Hybrid measures below).

## Administration Issues

Depending on the study instrument, researchers may have several choices about how to gather information from respondents. An initial consideration should be the feasibility of using a particular instrument with the population of interest. Feasibility issues include the burden to potential respondents and the financial cost per subject of gathering the information. Respondents may be reluctant to complete a lengthy interview or survey, both because of the time involved and perceptions that they will be asked to give confidential or sensitive types of information. Groups receiving medical or psychiatric treatment, for example, depending on the nature or severity of their illnesses, may have more difficulty in completing certain types of assessments such as self-administered questionnaires. Reluctance to participate may be addressed with careful explanation of the study procedures and how the data will be used, assurances of anonymity, and with monetary, or other types of incentives offered to participants. Incentives will increase participation rates, but will also increase the cost per participant of gathering data (Dew, 1993; Dillman, 1978). An initial cost consideration is that of the instrument itself; many established measures are copyrighted and the authors may charge a fee each time the instrument is administered or scored. Other important considerations are the cost of the assessment modality and of the person who will administer the assessment. Clinician interviewers necessary for most unstructured diagnostic interviews are most costly, followed by trained lay interviewers and research assistant administered questionnaires/interviews; self-administered questionnaires are the least costly.

In terms of the format of data gathering, in-person interviews are generally the most costly mode of assessment, followed by telephone interviews, and self-administered questionnaires. Although self-report forms may be the least costly to administer, this method is limited by the respondent's ability to read and understand questions, greater potential for non-response bias, and difficulties in presenting complicated question sequences. Telephone interviews may provide a middle ground in terms of cost and quality of information gathered. They also have been shown to yield highly reliable data if the interviewers are carefully trained and supervised (Aneshensel et al., 1982a, 1982b; Aneshensel & Yokopenic, 1985; Fenig et al., 1993; Paulsen et al., 1988; Wells et al., 1988). The use of computers to aid in recording responses to both interviews and self-administered questionnaires has also become more prevalent, and seems to provide a reliable, valid, and highly efficient means of assessing some attributes (e.g., Brugha et al., 1996; Dignon, 1996; Erdman et al., 1992; Kobak et al., 1993; Steer et al., 1994; Thornicroft, 1992; for a review, see Kobak et al., 1996).

## ISSUES IN THE PSYCHOMETRIC EVALUATION OF INSTRUMENTS

In this section, we discuss the general meaning of instrument reliability and validity—the two primary concerns of psychometric evaluation—and methods for examining whether measures meet these minimum psychometric requirements (see Table 6.2 for a summary of key psychometric issues).

## TABLE 6.2 Key Psychometric Measurement Issues

Psychometric Issues

Reliability
—internal-consistency
—multiple measurement consistency
—test-retest
—alternate form
—split-half
—inter-rater

Validity
—content
—criterion
—construct
—factor analytic
—group differences
—within-subject variation across time
—correlations with other measures
—internal consistency
—explication of process

# Reliability

The score or value obtained by an individual on a measure traditionally has been viewed as comprising two components: an underlying "true" score, and error caused by imprecision in measurement (see McDowell and Newell, 1996; Nunnally, 1978 for extended discussions of reliability). Reliability or consistency of a measure refers to the measure's ability to detect the true score rather than measurement error. A perfectly reliable instrument would detect only the true score. The concept of reliability is based on two central considerations: 1) Do items purportedly belonging to a scale actually assess a single construct?, and 2) Do scales measuring a single construct produce consistent estimates of that construct across multiple measurements? The first consideration is usually labeled "internal-consistency reliability" and is most commonly assessed with Cronbach's alpha which provides an estimate of the extent to which items covary, or "hang-together" as a common unit (Cronbach, 1951). Alpha ranges from 0.00–1.00 with higher scores indicating greater internal-consistency of the scale. In general, decisions about whether internal-consistency reliability is high enough depend on the purpose of the analyses. Comparisons between individuals, such as those necessary in case-finding, require high reliability (above .90). Research focused on group comparisons and research in the early stages does not require reliability as high. It has been suggested that a good standard for the latter two situations is a reliability coefficient of .50–.80 (Helmstadter, 1964; Nunnally, 1978; Ware, 1984). Attempting to achieve reliability coefficients above .80 may require considerable time and money, and may lead to redundancy among items in the measure (Boyle, 1985; McDowell & Newell, 1996; Nunnally, 1978).

The second reliability consideration—consistency across multiple measurements—has several variations including test-retest, alternate form, split-half, and intra- and inter-rater reliability and is based on the assumption that many human attributes are relatively stable in the short-term. Thus, reliable instruments should produce consistent estimations of such attributes across multiple measurements administered in relatively close temporal proximity. It should be noted that for intervention or longitudinal research, the optimal measure would produce consistent results in the short-term, but also have high sensitivity to changes that may take place longitudinally and/or during an intervention (Kraemer, 1992). Test-retest reliability, which is probably the most commonly used method of estimating the consistency of a measure, is obtained by reassessing individuals with the same measure at a second time point after the initial measurement. There are some serious limitations in using test-retest methods to estimate reliability, explicated in detail by Nunnally (1978). For example, the selection of the second administration point is critical and is based on the competing goals of minimizing the chance that respondents will remember and attempt to duplicate their responses from the first administration (implying that a longer time interval should be used), and minimizing the chance that any true change in the attribute will have occurred between the two administrations (implying that a shorter time interval is needed). Although judgments about when to administer the retest must be based on the specific instrument under consideration, testing experts suggest that an interval of 2–4 weeks from initial administration may be most appropriate (Nunnally, 1978).

To overcome the liability of respondents' recalling their previous responses inherent in test-retest reliability, alternate form (a second, similar version of the instrument) and split-half methods of establishing reliability were developed. Conceptually, both methods are based on the idea that high correlations between two different versions of a measure—both designed to assess the same construct—is evidence that a construct is being assessed reliably. The split-half method assesses the degree of correlation between two halves of an instrument (often odd versus even items) or between all possible pairs of items administered at a single administration of the instrument. Intra- and inter-rater reliability is similar to these methods, but is appropriate for data involving researchers' judgements (e.g., ratings by interviewers, observational assessments), rather than by respondent self-report. Reliability of assessments conducted by a single rater at different timepoints, or two different raters or judges, is typically evaluated with the Intraclass r for continuous variables and Kappa for dichotomous or ordinal-level variables; high correlations or agreement scores are taken as evidence of measurement reliability.

## Validity

Validity is most often defined as the extent to which an instrument measures what it was intended to measure. This is probably the most appropriate definition for researchers who are selecting or developing instruments for specific purposes. It is important to note, however, that instruments may fail validity criteria for one construct but be valid measures of a different construct (e.g., the Health Opinion Survey, developed to assess mental health may be a better indicator of generalized stress; Butler & Jones, 1979) *or* may be valid indicators of constructs in addition to the one for which they were originally intended (e.g., measures of physical functioning that are also useful as quality of life indicators). In addition, instruments that may be valid in one context (i.e., population, culture, historical period, administration format), may not be valid in another context; validity is always context-specific.

Because validity is context specific, validating a measure must be viewed as a process of accumulating evidence that supports the meaningfulness of the measure rather than a discrete endpoint at which validity is proven (Stewart et al., 1992). Many types of validity have been identified and described, but three broad types of validity are most often cited as central to any validity argument: content, criterion, and construct. Because extended discussions of these types of validity exist elsewhere (e.g., Helmstadter, 1964; McDowell & Newell, 1996; Nunnally, 1978; Stewart et al., 1992), we will define and discuss each type briefly here. Before we do so, however, we should note that *reliability* of an instrument is a necessary, but not sufficient, condition for establishing the validity of an instrument (Nunnally, 1978). In other words, if an instrument is not assessing something consistently, the meaningfulness of the measure is called into question even before validity arguments can be addressed.

Content or face validity concerns the extent to which items in a measure accurately reflect the full breadth of the construct of interest. Nunnally (1978) suggests that if we imagine a sampling universe of all possible items that might identify a construct, content validity is established by demonstrating that a representative set of items has been selected for our measure. Validity of content is usually established by having experts in the field and subjects or patients from the population for whom the instrument would be appropriate, review the instrument and provide critical evaluations of content; there are no formal empirical tests that will verify that content validity has been established. Recently, focus groups and in-depth interviews have gained popularity as methods for gathering content validity information for instruments in the early stages of development. Although evidence of content validity may provide the least powerful validity argument, such evidence is a prerequisite for establishing other types of validity.

Criterion or correlational validity is the extent to which the measure correlates with a "gold standard" of the intended construct. The gold standard (or criterion) can be another accepted measure of the same construct, or in rare cases, observed behavior, characteristic, or attribute that the measure is designed to assess (e.g., self-reported physical functioning validated against observer-ratings of actual physical capabilities). Criterion validity is typically established by examining the correlation of each item and/or the full scale with the criterion score or behavior. Low correlations—either item-criterion or scale-criterion—suggest that particular items, or the scale as a whole, may not measure the intended construct. (Note that this conclusion rests on the assumption that an appropriate criterion has been selected.) Criterion validity can be further divided into concurrent validity—in which the intended construct and criterion are assessed simultaneously—and predictive validity—in which the intended construct is measured first and then used to predict the criterion.

As noted by Helmstadter (1964), construct validity is the most recent addition to ideas about required validity evidence (APA Committee, 1952, 1954; Cronbach & Meehl, 1955), and requires that an instrument be a) viewed as measuring an underlying construct, and b) tested to see whether its hypothesized or theoretical relationships with other variables can be established. Factor analytic techniques are one way of exploring and/or confirming whether a group of items comprises a single unified construct, multiple components of a single construct, or multiple divergent constructs. Factor analysis is useful in determining whether a group of items hypothesized to assess a construct actually do cluster together when they are analyzed with items from other scales, and whether items *within* a measure describe a unified versus a multicomponent construct. Factor analysis should be undertaken in the early stages of examining an instrument to help determine the relationship among items, and to provide evidence of construct validity (Nunnally, 1978). Factor analyses may be confirmatory—if *a priori* hypotheses about which items will load together are specified—or exploratory—if no such hypotheses are made. Structural equation modeling is also increasingly used as a highly sophisticated and flexible means of conducting confirmatory factor analysis (Ullman, 1996)

Cronbach and Meehl (1955) outline five additional ways that construct validity can be established. First, *group differences* may be examined; groups of individuals expected to differ—based on additional characteristics (e.g., ethnicity, gender)—should score differently on the measure. For example, elderly individuals living in the community should score better on a measure of global health than those confined to a nursing home. Second, *within-subject variation* measured across time should indicate minimal changes for trait-like variables and more substantial changes for state-like variables. Thus, measures of major depression should exhibit much less within-subject variation across time than do measures of depressed affect. Third, strong *correlations with other measures* of the same construct (convergent validity), and weak correlations with measures of other constructs (discriminant validity) should be observed. For example, measures of physical functioning (e.g., Functional Status Index, Disability Interview Schedule, Health Assessment Questionnaire) should correlate highly with one another, and less highly with measures of social health and adjustment (e.g., Duke Social Support and Stress Scale, Katz Adjustment Scales). The multitrait-multimethod approach (Campbell & Fiske, 1959) is one framework that can be used to examine such interrelationships among items and scales purported to assess different psychosocial domains. Fourth, the *internal consistency* of an instrument or subscale provides evidence that a single construct is being assessed. Low internal consistency coefficients sometimes found in the early stages of measure development and pilot testing may be evidence that multiple constructs are being assessed. Finally, it is important to conduct a thorough examination and *explication of the assessment process* in which all the steps necessary to answer a certain item are analyzed to eliminate alternate hypotheses about observed patterns of responses (e.g., response set, social desirability).

## ISSUES IN SELECTING, DEVELOPING, AND EVALUATING FOUR CLASSES OF INSTRUMENTS

Instruments used in most research efforts can be divided into four broad categories based on the extent to which the full instrument, or items within the instrument, have been used in other research and have well established psychometric properties. The following section is organized around these four categories which we have labeled a) established measures, b) modified measures, c) hybrid measures, and d) new measures (see Figure 6.1). Established measures are those that have been used in more than one research setting and have exhibited good reliability and validity in each of these settings; published measures that do not meet these criteria should be treated as new measures. Modified measures are those that have been modified in some way (e.g., shortened, altered response categories) to fit the research goals. Hybrid measures combine items from more than one source to assess a single construct. New measures

# Established Psychometric Properties?

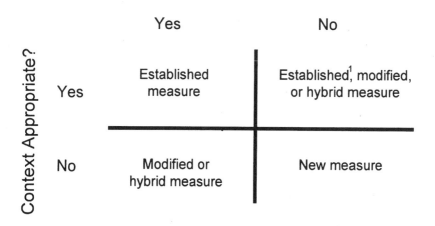

FIGURE 6.1    **Basic template for measure selection.**
[1]Here, "established" refers only to the fact that the measure is appropriate for the context; psychometric properties of the instrument must still be evaluated carefully.

are those that are newly developed with a specific research goal in mind.

Two questions should guide the search for an appropriate study measure: 1) Do appropriate established measures exist? If so, the issues in the Established measures section below should guide instrument selection. 2) Do measures that are nearly appropriate for the study goals exist? If so, a modified or hybrid measure should be considered. If no appropriate or nearly appropriate measures exist, creation of a new measure may be justified.

## Established Measures

As noted at the outset of this discussion, the two primary considerations in evaluating whether or not an existing measure is suitable for a particular research endeavor are contextual and psychometric.

These two sets of issues are linked in the sense that using an inappropriate measure for a given context (e.g., unclear wording, gender biased) often lead to psychometric liabilities such as poor reliability or validity. Thus, the first consideration should be whether an established measure meets the contextual considerations we have outlined. If there are characteristics of the population to be studied (e.g., age, culture, historical period) or the administration format that are significantly different from those that were used to establish the psychometric properties of the instrument, pilot tests should be conducted to establish the psychometrics of the instrument in the new population.

An excellent example of efforts to establish the psychometric properties of and the potential pitfalls that are inherent in such efforts, involve the 20-item Center for Epidemiological Studies Depression Scale (CES-D; Radloff, 1977). The CES-D has been widely used to assess general depressive symptomatology or distress as a combination of affective, somatic, and interpersonal symptoms. Initial evaluations of the instrument conducted among English-speaking, middle class, Anglo individuals of various ages yielded evidence of good reliability and validity (Hertzog et al., 1990). However, subsequent studies of CES-D characteristics among diverse ethnic groups including American Indians (Manson et al., 1990) and Hispanics (Guarnaccia, Angel, & Worobey, 1989), *and* comparisons of men and women (Guarnaccia et al., 1989; Stommel et al., 1993), suggest that the factor structure and/or the operation of individual items differed across ethnic groups and by gender. Such differences in the characteristics of a measure when it is applied to new populations have serious implications for construct validity, and have been addressed by researchers in a variety of ways. For example, it may be possible to identify a different measure of the construct—in this case a different measure of distress—that operates similarly across the population groups of interest. Alternatively, items that are biased may be eliminated or altered—Stommel et al. (1993) used a 15-item version of the CES-D to reduce gender bias—and the newly discovered factor structure may be used in the analyses—alternative CES-D factors have been used in analyses involving minority populations (e.g., Guarnaccia et al., 1989). If a decision is made to proceed with a measure despite differences in psychometric characteristics, extreme caution should be used in the interpretation of intergroup comparisons even though the ability to examine such comparisons may be one of the primary advantages of utilizing an established measure.

Evidence of criterion-related validity, if available, should also be evaluated carefully. For example, Roberts et al. (1990) found that although CES-D scores were highly associated with diagnosed depression (as assessed by the Diagnostic Interview Schedule) in Anglo and English-speaking Mexican-American populations, there was poor agreement between the CES-D and diagnosed depression in Spanish-speaking Mexican-Americans. Although questions about the appropriateness of the criterion (in this case the DSM) should always be considered seriously, intergroup differences between the measure and the criterion should also raise validity concerns.

After an established measure is selected and used in a research effort, evaluating its psychometric properties in the current research effort is still critical, but may entail a less rigorous process than for the other types of measures discussed in the following sections. At a minimum, initial psychometric analyses should include an evaluation of the internal consistency of the measure, as well as analyses designed to verify the factor structure (e.g., confirmatory factor analysis) of measures comprising more than one subcomponent. In the case of the CES-D, for example, the four-factor structure should be verified, and overall and subscale internal consistency values should be computed and reported. The extent of new validation work necessary for an established measure depends on the type of validation that already exists for the scale, and the similarity of the sample of interest to those with which validity was originally established. A conservative approach would suggest that, at minimum, some evidence of construct validity is necessary. Findings such as the evidence of the unstable factor structure of the CES-D across some research settings suggest that assuming validity may not always be warranted. If novel intergroup comparisons are part of the research goals (e.g., gender or ethnic group comparisons), it is important to conduct the psychometric analyses described here *within* each group of interest. Divergent factor structures or internal consistency coefficients imply that the measure is not equivalent across groups and thus, that main effect differences among groups should be interpreted with caution.

## Modified Measures

Perhaps the first issue in modifying an established measure should be to explicate a detailed rationale for the alterations to be made. Shortening a measure substantially, changing the response categories, or altering the item stems may have serious psychometric consequences for the scale. Comparisons with studies employing the original version of the scale may not be valid. In other words, depending on the extent of the modifications, a modified measure may be only moderately superior to a newly created measure in terms of the ability to rely on previously reported psychometric work. The primary advantages of modifying a measure over developing a new measure are that there are some assurances that this set of items has operated as an indicator of a unified construct in the past, and that clarity of item wording and content has been demonstrated.

Justifications for modifying a measure are not limited to, but may include, that a) the original measure is too long for the current research purpose, b) the original response categories are not expected to produce sufficient variation, c) the original response categories are too broad or inclusive, and d) the original item wording is unclear or not relevant to the current population. In presenting findings based on a modified measure, it is important to describe the original measure, outline the steps that were taken to alter the measure, and discuss any anticipated differences in the performance of the modified measure.

Many published examples are available of measures that have been modified in some way after the original psychometric work was conducted. In fact, the majority of instruments undergo adaptations or modifications in the development process or for specific research purposes that make them substantially different from the original measure. One of the most common modifications is to reduce the number of items in a measure in order to reduce respondent burden. The 20-item Short Form Health Survey assessing six health-related domains provides an excellent example of the process of selecting and evaluating items from longer health surveys (Stewart et al., 1988; Ware et al., 1992). When there were criticisms that the 20-item version was too limited in scope, a 36-item, 8-domain version of the

Short Form was developed and evaluated (Ware et al., 1993; Ware & Sherbourne, 1992). Finally, in response to calls for an abbreviated instrument, a 12-item, 2-domain version of the instrument was developed and evaluated (Ware et al., 1996). Each step in the refinement of the instrument was fully reported, and psychometric evaluations were described (Jenkinson et al., 1997; Ware et al., 1996).

Modifications to the Revised Memory and Behavior Problems Checklist (RMBPC; Teri et al., 1992) as part of our own research with elderly caregivers (REACH, 1995) provides another example of this process. The original measure included twenty-four items designed to assess the extent to which persons with cognitive impairments had recently experienced depressive affect, disruptive behavior, or memory-related problems. Because our research is primarily concerned with *caregivers* of persons with Alzheimer's disease or related dementias, we were interested not only in the behaviors themselves, but also in the caregiver burden associated with such behaviors. Response categories to the items were thus modified from Likert-type to dichotomous categories (behavior present or absent), and subquestions asking how much the caregiver was bothered or upset by the behavior were added. We are still able to construct a scale that provides an estimate of the frequency of memory and problem behaviors, and in addition have assessed the construct of caregiver burden associated with each problem. We should note that our modification of the response categories means that our estimates will not be directly comparable to the original version.

Substantial psychometric work is needed to assess the reliability and validity of modified measures. Depending on the extent of the modifications, the full range of reliability tests may need to be conducted. In addition, at least some validity work is necessary. Content validity and evaluation of internal factor structure may be especially important for measures that are reduced in length from their original versions to ensure that the same number, and full breadth of, the original constructs are represented. Conversely, evaluating construct validity to determine whether the measure seems to support anticipated theoretical relationships may be more of a concern when there are additions to, or modifications in, item wording (e.g., RMBPC).

## Hybrid Measures

Hybrid measures—created by combining items from more than one established scale, or by combining items from an established scale with newly created items—are one step further removed from their original psychometric properties than are measures that have been modified. When existing scales do not adequately cover all the issues of interest, or have questionable psychometric properties, creating a composite measure from more than one scale or developing new items to supplement a scale may be justified.

As with the modified measures, the rationale for creating a hybrid measure should be developed with the foreknowledge that previous psychometric work with these items may no longer be valid. In presenting work involving a hybrid measure, it is important to provide the following information: a) description of the original measure(s), b) inadequacies in existing measures that led to the creation of a hybrid measure, c) steps in selecting or creating items, d) modifications that were made to item stems or response categories, and e) how the hybrid measure is expected to function differently from existing measures (e.g., It will assess the same construct but with better psychometric properties, or will assess a broader construct.).

An example from our research with caregivers of individuals with Alzheimer's disease or dementia is the Caregiver Health and Health Behaviors Form (REACH, 1995). Because no single existing measure assessed the full range of health and health-related behaviors important to our caregiver cohort, we drew items from several measures to examine specific aspects of health that might be particularly affected by the caregiving role. For example, items concerning perceived physical health and stress-related health symptoms were selected from the SF-36 (Ware et al., 1993; Ware & Sherbourne, 1992), comorbidity items were selected from the AHEAD study (Asset and Health Dynamics Among the Oldest Old; Health Retirement Study, 1993), and health behavior items were selected from the Nutrition Screening Initiative (NSI; Posner et al., 1993).

The psychometric work necessary for evaluating hybrid measures may equal that required for any category of measure discussed here. Advantages of utilizing items that come from well established measures include the fact that most items have been evaluated for clarity, and the fact that tentative comparisons of responses to individual items as assessed in previous studies may be possible. Disadvantages include the fact that slight modifications to item stems or response categories are almost always necessary to enhance the flow of the items, and, response categories of items from different scales are seldom similar. Dissimilar response categories that are retained in the hybrid measure may be confusing to respondents and necessitate the transformation of item distributions. For example, the response format of health behavior items discussed above is dichotomous while that of the stress-related symptoms is a three-point scale, making item transformations necessary prior to computing the scale.

Because hybrid measures present items in a novel combination, often with some alterations in wording, heavy emphasis should be given to preliminary analyses in order to evaluate whether the items belong together in a scale. Item distributions, and inter-item and item-scale correlations should be carefully examined. In addition, given that the factor structure of this particular set of items will not have been previously evaluated, factor analysis should play a prominent role in the early analyses. At this stage, the results of the factor analysis can be used to make judgements about which items to retain or eliminate and about how (and if) subscales will be computed. After all of these various changes, psychometric analyses of the resulting measure should be comprehensive.

At a minimum, more than one technique for establishing the reliability of the hybrid measure should be utilized. As noted above, content validity concerns may have already been addressed in the creation of the hybrid measure and, in fact, may have been the primary justification for creating the measure in the first place. However, construct validity—and, if possible, criterion validity—should be evaluated.

## New Measures

The creation of a new measure should be undertaken only as a last resort, after a rigorous search for existing measures of the construct of interest has been conducted. The willingness of researchers to create new measures has led to an explosion of published instruments assessing similar constructs (e.g., more than 500 assessing depression, more than 3,000 assessing general or specific health status), many with virtually no reported psychometric properties (Health and Psychosocial Instrumentation database; HaPI-CD; BMDS, 1997).

However, there are emerging research questions for which no appropriate instruments may exist, for example, physician attitudes about palliative care, acceptance of new forms of organ and tissue donation, and issues surrounding aging and caregiving. In other circumstances, although relevant instruments may exist, they may have poor psychometric properties that would be difficult to correct (e.g., questionable construct validity). In these situations, the creation of a new measure may be justified. Advantages of creating a new measure include the fact that researchers can a) conduct focus groups and reviews by experts to ensure that the content of the measure is specific to their research goals, b) control item wording and response categories, and c) establish the length of the measure at the outset. Disadvantages include a) the intensive psychometric work that is critical to conduct *prior* to analyzing (or even collecting) the data in terms of central study hypotheses, b) the possibility that a new measure may fail some critical reliability or validity criterion, and c) the inability to compare results with any other previous research. (The first two disadvantages may be less important if the primary purpose of the research is to create the measure.)

In the process of developing and/or reporting on a newly created measure, comprehensive justifications for developing the measure— including a description of why the measure was necessary and the unavailability of appropriate established instruments—should be provided. The steps followed in generating ideas about specific items and the constructs they identify should be explained in detail. Ideally, a large pool of potential items should be generated on the basis of focus groups or expert opinion, pilot tested, reevaluated, and reduced to form some final draft of the measure. As part of the process of identifying a construct and creating the measure, the purpose of the measure (i.e., proposed theoretical relationships) should also be clearly described. After data using the measure are collected, researchers should extensively evaluate the measure's reliability and validity.

For new measures especially, it is important to discuss how the instrument could be further refined for application to future research questions. For example, items that may be altered or deleted should be identified, indications for additional psychometric work should be discussed, appropriateness of the measure for groups outside the normative sample should be addressed, and implications for the development of additional complementary items or scales should be described.

The value of any research effort rests to a high degree on the foundation of appropriate measurement. What constitutes "appropriateness" is a complex issue that has generated individual reports, full volumes, and entire journals devoted to the problem of ensuring that the assessment tools we use produce accurate information. The initial goal of this chapter was to reinforce the seriousness of measurement issues and to provide a basic template to guide nonexperts in the selection, development, and evaluation of study instruments. Because verification of the psychometric properties of an instrument—even those that are well-established—is context-specific and must be reestablished to some degree for every research effort, it is critical for all researchers to have a basic understanding of measurement issues. We now move to a more specific discussion of established measurement tools available for caregiver research.

## CAREGIVER ASSESSMENT IN ALZHEIMER DISEASE RESEARCH

The following discussion provides a brief summary of existing measurement approaches for assessing a variety of factors among caregivers of persons with Alzheimer disease and related disorders (ADRD). We address seven major measurement domains that are prevalent in the caregiving literature: health effects, caregiver characteristics and contextual measures, service utilization, burden, positive aspects of caregiving, quality of care provided, and measures related to normative caregiver transitions such as institutionalization and death of the care recipient. The measures described in each of the following sections have been used widely and have proven psychometric properties.

### Health Effects of ADRD Caregiving

Schulz and Williamson (1997) recently reported the results of a review focused on health effects of ADRD caregiving in studies published since 1990 to identify the range of outcome variables used. As summarized in Tables 6.3 and 6.4, health effects are most often conceptualized as comprising psychiatric and physical domains. Indicators of psychiatric morbidity (Table 6.1) can be further divided into four types of measures. Although individual self-report items assessing global ratings of mental health are often used, the majority of studies reviewed used standardized self-report measures such as the CES-D. The advantage of self-report measures of mental health is that they are often short, can be easily administered, and provide a good indication of an individual's mental health state along the dimension being assessed. Their primary disadvantage according

**TABLE 6.3 Examples of Mental Health Indicators Used in Caregiving Research**

I.   Individual self-report items
     Global mental health ratings

II.  Self-report scales
     Beck Depression Inventory (BDI)
     Bradburn Affect Balance Scale (BABS)
     Center for Epidemiological Studies Depression Scale (CES-D)
     Depression Adjective Checklist
     General Health Questionnaire (GHQ)
     Geriatric Depression Scale (GDS)
     Hopkins Symptom Checklist (SCL-90 or SCL-58)
     Profile of Mood States (POMS)
     State-Trait Anxiety Inventory (STAI)
     Zung Depression Scale

III. Diagnostic interviews
     Diagnostic Interview Schedule (DIS)
     Hamilton Depression Rating Scale (HDRS)
     Psychiatric Epidemiological Research Interview (PERI)
     Research Diagnostic Criteria (RDC)
     Schedule for Affective Disorders and Schizophrenia (SADS)
     Short Psychiatric Evaluation Schedule (SPES)
     Structured Interview for DSM-III-R (SCID)

IV.  Psychotropic drug use
     Self-report
     Direct transcription

**TABLE 6.4 Examples of Physical Health Indicators Used in Caregiving Research**

I.  Individual self-report items
    Global physical health ratings
    Impact on health
    Number of heath problems or illnesses

II. Symptom checklists or scales
    Caregiver Health Scale
    Cohen-Hoberman Inventory of Physical Symptoms
    Cornell Medical Health Index
    Duke-UNC Health Profile
    Health Review
    Louisville Health Scale
    Physical Health Section of OARS
    Physical Symptoms Index
    Rosencranz Health Inventory

III. Service use
     Hospitalizations
     Physician visits
     Aggregate use of health services
     Drug utilization

IV. Health-related behaviors
    Alcohol consumption
    Smoking behavior
    Sleep
    Eating behavior/nutrition

V.  Clinical assays/assessments
    Immune function
    Wound healing
    Heart rate
    Blood pressure
    ICD-9 Diagnoses
    Medication use

to some researchers is their failure to provide an actual diagnosis of disorder.

Thus, several recent studies (e.g., Schulz et al., 1995, 1997) have used structured diagnostic interviews (Table 6.1, III.) to provide diagnoses of depressive and anxiety disorders as defined by the

*Diagnostic and Statistical Manual* (American Psychiatric Association, 1994). In contrast to self-report measures, the major disadvantages of structured diagnostic instruments is that they often require a lengthy interview conducted by a highly trained interviewer, making them relatively costly to use. A final indicator of psychiatric morbidity frequently reported in the literature is psychotropic drug use. Methods for collecting drug utilization information range from simple self-reporting to the direct transcription from medication containers of all drugs taken by the respondent. The latter method generally is believed to be a more reliable indicator of drug use. Overall, studies of caregiver mental health show a consistent pattern of increased depressive and anxiety symptomatology as compared to age- and gender-based norms.

Measures of physical health outcomes (Table 6.4) are assessed using a broad range of indicators including: self-report items such as global physical health ratings, symptom checklists or scales such as the Duke-UNC Health Profile and the Rosencranz Health Inventory, service utilization, such as physician visits and hospitalizations, health-related behaviors such as alcohol consumption and sleep patterns, and clinical assays and assessments such as immune function and blood pressure. In contrast to the consistent caregiver-related effects found on indicators of psychiatric morbidity, the effects of caregiving on physical health are less clear. Although caregivers tend to rate themselves as slightly less healthy and to report more symptoms than noncaregivers, they are not necessarily more likely to report more chronic conditions or illness episodes. An important emerging area of caregiving health outcomes in research focuses on changes in subclinical disease such as hypertension, pulmonary function, blood chemistries, and cardiac arrhythmias as indicators of health effects. The demands of caregiving may not precipitate an illness event per se, but rather may aggravate existing vulnerabilities. Thus, attempts should be made to assess whether illness results from existing conditions being exacerbated or represents new conditions unrelated to prior medical history or risk factors.

## Caregiver Characteristics and Caregiving Context Measures

In addition to providing a variety of health-related outcome measures from which to choose, the literature on ADRD caregiving also provides insight about the patient and caregiver characteristics that may be associated with health outcomes. Factors consistently linked to negative health outcomes include: lower socioeconomic status, being married to the patient, low levels of social support, low levels of self-esteem and mastery, and poor prior relationship with the patient. Patient problem behaviors consistently are predictive of negative outcomes, and level of patient cognitive function has been found to correlate positively with physical health outcomes of the caregiver (Schulz et al., 1995). In addition to standard sociodemographic data about both caregivers and care recipients, Schulz and Williamson (1997) recommend that researchers gather data on the relationship of caregiver to patient, living arrangements, family structure, role responsibilities of the caregiver, history and duration of caregiving, and other stressful life events that may affect caregiving outcomes. A good source for the measurement of these constructs is the National Institute on Aging/National Institute for Nursing Research spon-sored Alzheimer disease intervention REACH project, and surveys such as the Health and Retirement Study (HRS), and the Asset and Health Dynamics Among the Oldest Old (AHEAD).

## Caregiver Burden

Virtually all caregiving studies include standardized measures of the subjective and/or objective burden experienced by caregivers. This construct usually is defined as the "physical, psychological, or emo-tional, social and financial problems that can be experienced by family members caring for impaired older adults" (George & Gwyther, 1986, p. 253). Although caregiver burden measures are widely used, questions have been raised recently regarding their psychometric properties. It has been noted, for example, that al-though reliability data typically are reported for these measures, few researchers address issues of validity or sensitivity to change (Deimling, 1994; Vitaliano et al., 1991). Some of the more recently developed burden measures (e.g., Vitaliano et al., 1991) are designed to address the psychometric shortcomings of previously published scales.

It is also important to recognize that caregiver assessments of the functional, cognitive, and behavioral status of the care recipient are likely to be influenced by the dispositional characteristics of the caregiver (Bookwala & Schulz, 1997). Existing literature generally supports the conclusion that caregivers are likely to overestimate the disability of the person they care for (Magaziner et al., 1988) and that the magnitude of bias is related systematically to the personality attributes of the caregiver, such as the level of neuroticism and mastery. Caregivers who are high on neuroticism or mastery tend to rate the care recipient more negatively than individuals who are low on these dispositional attributes.

## Positive Aspects of Caregiving

As a counterpoint to the negative aspects of caregiving emphasized in the majority of the literature, positive aspects of caregiving has received increasing attention in recent years. It may be that the many stresses associated with caregiving may be counteracted by the positive aspects of caregiving, and thus, maintain the quality of life for these individuals. Representative items on instruments assessing positive aspects include indicators of the extent to which caregiving has made the caregiver feel more useful, feel needed, feel good about him/herself, learn new skills, and give more meaning to life. A scale developed by the Caregiver Health Effects Study (CHES; Schulz et al., 1997) has high internal validity and good fit based on confirmatory factor analysis. These analyses yield two subscales representing caregiver self-esteem and meaning in life that are distinct, but correlated fairly highly. Future studies should endeavor to systematically assess the positive aspects of caregiving.

## Quality of Informal Care

Because caregiving often is based on behaviors learned during a lifetime and on affectional bonds between two individuals, it is assumed that the care delivered generally is of high quality. However, empirical evidence evaluating this assumption is very limited. Moreover, the available literature focuses primarily on the negative end of the quality continuum—abuse, neglect, and exploitation (Table

6.5 lists five categories of poor quality elder care.). Federal agencies such as Health and Human Services and caregiver researchers alike have noted that there is insufficient information about the quality of informal care provided to the elderly (Schulz & Williamson, 1997).

Given the lack of empirical research in this area, it should not be surprising that assessment methods are in the early stages of development. Available measurement strategies focus on what constitutes poor care rather than defining high quality care. At the broadest conceptual level, poor care is defined as any act by a caregiver that harms, or has the potential to harm, the care recipient physically, psychologically, or financially. Many states have statutes and accompanying reporting forms which represent a measurement strategy of sorts, although in practice they are applied only rarely. Other

**TABLE 6.5 Examples of Physical Health Indicators Used in Caregiving Research**

I.  Physical abuse
    Restraints (e.g., tying to bed or chair)
    Forcing food/medications
    Withholding food/medications
    Hitting/slapping
    Shaking
    Pinching
    Excess sedation

II. Psychological abuse
    Screaming/yelling
    Threats to institutionalize
    Threats of physical force
    Locking in a room
    Moving to other location without consent

III. Physical neglect
    Failure to provide food, utilities, safe living environment,
    medical care, adequate supervision

IV. Psychological neglect
    Failure to provide affection or a cheerful living environment,
    include in family and holiday celebrations, etc.

V.  Exploitation
    Theft of resources
    Misuse of resources

important sources for measurement of quality of elder care are found in the works of Steinmetz (1988), Godkin et al. (1989), Fulmer (1991), and Pillemer and colleagues (Pillemer & Finkelhor, 1989; Pillemer & Suitor, 1992).

According to Schulz and Williamson (1997), a comprehensive multidimensional assessment of quality of care would include: 1) physical abuse, 2) psychological abuse, 3) physical neglect, 4) psychological neglect, and 5) financial exploitation. Representative indicators of each category are listed in Table 6.5. Self-report measures of physical and psychological abuse including many of the indicators listed in the first two headings of Table 6.5 have been developed by Straus (1979) and Steinmetz (1988). Physical and psychological neglect scales have been developed by Quinn and Tomita (1986) and Williamson and Miller (Unpublished manuscript, University of Georgia, 1996) respectively. Self-report instruments may not be adequate for gathering information about poor care given that caregivers may tend to underreport incidents which may incriminate them, and care recipients may be unable to provide accurate reports because of cognitive deficits, fear, and/or the sense of obligation associated with receiving care. One alternative to self-reporting is to use an observation checklist including information on overt signs of abuse or neglect such as bruises or bleeding.

The measurement of abuse, neglect and exploitation clearly is in need of further development. Promising strategies for the future might include the validation of caregiver self-report through care recipient interviews, secondary caregivers, or other proxies, or through the examination of archival records.

## Service Utilization

Service utilization often is viewed as either a mediator or an outcome of the caregiving experience in descriptive studies of caregiving. Many intervention studies treat service use as the major independent variable because the provision of a specific service such as respite care constitutes the primary intervention. Researchers interested in assessing the stress-related effects of caregiving frequently assess service use as a potential buffer of negative health outcomes (e.g., Biegel et al., 1993). Investigators focused on policy issues related to caregiving typically view service use as an outcome when addressing questions of substitution or determinants of institutionalization. Many instruments are available to assess the types, frequency, and usefulness of services available to caregivers. These measures have strong face validity but have questionable reliability when they are based exclusively on the self-report of the caregiver. In general, the self-report data collected from caregivers should be supplemented with utilization data collected from medical and social service records and/or other informants.

## Caregiving Transitions

It is probable that one of the important future directions for caregiving research will include a focus on the impact of transitions involving the institutionalization or death of the care recipient. It will therefore be valuable to employ specific measures that capture aspects of these transitions and unique outcomes associated with these transitions, particularly in the case of bereavement. Aneshensel et al. (1995) has identified measures that serve as good starting points assessment of transitional stressors associated with institutionalization and adaptation to institutionalization.

The existing empirical literature on bereavement effects in a caregiving context suggest several conclusions. Overall, the preponderance of findings suggest that caregivers experience relatively little difficulty in the long term (1 year or more) in adjusting to the loss of the recipient. There is some evidence for short-term negative effects associated with bereavement, but also evidence for positive outcomes, including feelings of relief and improved quality of life. The measurement of bereavement outcomes in a caregiving context have included global well-being (George & Gwyther, 1984), depression (Bodner & Kielcolt-Glaser, 1994; Collins et al., 1994; McHorney & Mor, 1988; Norris & Murrell, 1987), family and personal strain (Bass et al., 1991), and reported social and emotional difficulties (Collins et al., 1993; Bass et al., 1991). Greater uniformity in the conceptualization of stressors and physical and psychiatric outcomes are needed to advance this research area. In addition, it is also recommended that measures be developed to assess circumstances surrounding the death, specific bereavement-related outcomes, and complicated grief (Prigerson et al., 1995; Schulz & Williamson, 1997).

In sum, the existing literature provides valuable guidance in the selection of health-related measures for caregivers. Measures should be chosen based on the specific question being asked, the contextual issues discussed at the beginning of this paper, and the psychometric properties of the available instruments. Although it is usually advisable to select an instrument that is well established, there may be situations—especially in the emerging area of caregiver research—that require the modification or development of an instrument. Such situations should be approached deliberately, and with a clear idea of the types of psychometric evidence that will be necessary to deem the instrument reliable and valid.

## REFERENCES

American Psychiatric Association. (1994). *Diagnostic and statistical manual of mental disorders*, 4th ed, revised. Washington, DC: American Psychiatric Association.

American Psychological Association Committee on Psychological Tests. (1952). Technical recommendations for psychological tests and diagnostic techniques: Preliminary proposal. *American Psychologist, 7*, 461–476.

American Psychological Association Committee on Psychological Tests. (1954). Technical recommendations for psychological tests and diagnostic techniques: Preliminary proposal. *Psychological Bulletin Supplement, 51*, 1–38.

Aneshensel, C.S., Frerichs, R.R., Clark, V.A., & Yokopenic, P.A. (1982a). Measuring depression in the community. *Public Opinion Quarterly, 46*, 110–121.

Aneshensel, C.S., Frerichs, R.R., Clark, V.A., & Yokopenic, P.A. (1982b). Telephone versus in person surveys of community health status. *American Journal of Public Health, 72*(9), 1017–1021.

Aneshensel, C.S., Pearlin, L.I., Mullan, J.T., Zarit, S.H., & Whitlatch, C.J. (1995). *Profiles in caregiving*. New York: Academic Press.

Aneshensel, C.S., & Yokopenic, P.A. (1985). Tests for the comparability of a causal model of depression under two condition of interviewing. *Journal of Personality and Social Psychology, 49*(5), 1337–1348.

AHEAD: Asset and Health Dynamics among the Oldest Old. (1993). Health Retirement Study, Institute for Social Research and the National Institute on Aging.

Bass, D.M., Bowman, K., & Noelker, L.S. (1991). The influence of caregiving and bereavement support on adjusting to an older relative's death. *Gerontologist, 31*, 32–42.

Behavioral Measurement Database Services. (1997). HaPI-Health and Psychosocial Instruments, Pittsburgh, PA.

Berkman, L.F (1986). The association between educational attainment and mental status examinations: Of etiologic significance for senile dementias or not? *Journal of Chronic Disorders, 39*, 171–174.

Biegel, D.E., Bass, D.M., Schulz, R., & Morycz, R. (1993). Predictors of in-home and out-of-home service use by family caregivers of Alzheimer's disease patients. *Journal of Aging and Health, 5*, 419–438.

Bodner, J.C., & Kielcolt-Glaser, J.K. (1994). Caregiver depression after bereavement: Chronic stress isn't over when it's over. *Psychology of Aging, 9*, 372–380.

Bookwala, J., & Schulz, R. (1997). Contagion among elderly couples. *Psychology of Aging, 11*, 582–591.

Boyle, G.J. (1985). Self-report measures of depression: Some psychometric considerations. *British Journal of Clinical Psychology, 24*, 45–59.

Brayne, C., & Calloway, P. (1990). The association of education and socioeconomic status with the Mini-Mental State examination and the clinical diagnosis of dementia in elderly people. *Age Ageing, 19*, 91–96.

Brugha, T.S., Kaul, A., Dignon, A., Teather, D., & Wills, K.M. (1996). Present state examination by microcomputer: Objectives and experience of preliminary steps. *International Journal of Methods in Psychiatric Research, 6*(3), 143–151.

Butler, M.C., & Jones, A.P. (1979). The Health Opinion Survey reconsidered: Dimensionality, reliability, and validity. *Journal of Clinical Psychology, 35*, 554–559.

Campbell, D.T., & Fiske, D.W. (1959). Convergent and discriminant validation by the multitrait-multimethod matrix. *Psychological Bulletin, 56*, 81–105.

Cannell, C.F., Marquis, K.H., & Laurent, A. (1977). A summary of studies of interviewing methodology. *Vital Health Statistics, 2*, 1–78.

Collins, C., Liken, M., King, S., & Kokinakis, C. (1993). Loss and grief among family caregivers of relatives with dementia. *Qualitative Health Research, 3*, 236–253.

Collins, C., Stommel, M., & Wang, S. (1994). Caregiving transitions: Changes in depression among family caregivers of relatives with dementia. *Nursing Research, 43*, 220–225.

Cronbach, L.J. (1951). Coefficient alpha and the internal structure of tests. *Psychometrika, 16*, 297–334.

Cronback, L.J., & Meehl, P.E. (1955). Construct validity in psychological tests. *Psychological Bulletin, 52,* 281–302.

Deimling, G.T. (1994). Caregiver functioning. In M.P. Lawton & J.A. Teresi (Eds.), *Annual Review of gerontology and geriatrics. Vol. 14, Focus on assessment techniques.* New York: Springer.

Dew, M.A. (in press). Psychiatric disorder in the context of physical illness. In B.P. Dohrenwend (Ed.), *Adversity, stress and psychopathology.* Washington, DC: American Psychiatric Press.

Dew, M.A. (1993). Assessment and prevention of expectancy effects in community mental health studies. In *Interpersonal expectations: Theory, research, and application* (Edited by Blanck, P.D.). Cambridge University Press: New York.

Dignon, A.M. (1996). Acceptability of a computer administered psychiatric interview. *Computers in Human Behavior, 12*(2), 177–191.

Dillman, D.A. (1978). *Mail and telephone surveys: The Total Design Method.* New York: John Wiley & Sons.

Eaton, W.W. (1980). *The sociology of mental disorders.* New York: Praeger Publishers.

Erdman, H.P., Klein, M.H., Greist, J.H., Skare, S.S., et al. (1992). A comparison of two computer-administered versions of the NIMH Diagnostic Interview Schedule. *Journal of Psychiatric Research, 26*(1), 85–95.

Fenig, S., Levav, I., Kohn, R., & Yelin, N. (1993). Telephone vs. face-to-face interviewing in a community psychiatric survey. *American Journal of Public Health, 83*(6), 896–898.

Fulmer, T. (1991). Elder mistreatment: Progress in community detection and intervention. *Family and Community Health, 14,* 26–34.

George, L.K., & Gwyther, L.P. (1986). A multidimensional examination of family caregivers of demented adults. *Gerontologist, 24,* 253–259.

Gibson, R.C. (1991). Race and the self-reported health of elderly persons. *Journal of Gerontology, 46,* 235–242.

Godkin, M.A., Wolf, R.S., & Pillemer, K.A. (1989). A case-comparison analysis of elder abuse and neglect. *International Journal of Aging and Human Development, 28,* 207–225.

Guarnaccia, P.J., Angel, R., & Lowe Worobey, J. (1989). The factor structure of the CES-D in the Hispanic Health and Nutrition Examination Survey: The influences of ethnicity, gender, and language. *Social Science and Medicine, 29*(1), 85–94.

Guarnaccia, P.J., Good, B.J., & Kleinman, A. (1990). A critical review of epidemiological studies of Puerto Rican mental health. *American Journal of Psychiatry, 147*(11), 1449–1456.

Helmstadter, G.C. (1964). *Principles of psychological measurement.* New York: Appleton-Centruy-Crofts.

Hertzog, C., Van Alstine, J., Usala, P.D., Hultsch, D.F., & Dixon, R. (1990). Measurement properties of the Center for Epidemiological Studies Depression Scale (CES-D) in older populations. *Psychological Assessment: A Journal of Consulting and Clinical Psychology, 2*(1), 64–72.

Jenkinson, C., Layte, R., Jenkinson, D., Lawrence, K., Petersen, S., Paice, C., & Stradling, J. (1997). A shorter form health survey: Can the SF-12 replicate results from the SF-36 in longitudinal studies? *Journal of Public Health Medicine, 19,* 179–186.

Kay, D.W.K., Henderson, A.S., Scott, R., et al. (1985). Dementia and depression among the elderly living in the Hobart community: The effect of the diagnostic criteria on the prevalence rates. *Psychological Medicine, 15,* 771–788.

Kobak K.A., Greist J.H., Jefferson J.W., & Katzelnick, D.J. (1996). Computer administered clinical rating scales: A review. *Psychopharmacology, 127*(4), 291–301.

Kobak, K.A., Reynolds, W.M., & Greist, J.H. (1993). Development and validation of a computer-administered version of the Hamilton Rating Scale. *Psychological Assessment, 5*(4), 487–492.

Kraemer, H.C. (1992). Coping strategies in psychiatric clinical research. In A.E. Kazdin (Ed.), *Methodological Issues and Strategies in Clinical Research.* Washington, DC: American Psychological Association.

Madow, W.G. (1973). Net differences in interview data on chronic conditions and information derived from medical records. *Vital Health Statistics, 2,* 1–58.

Magaziner, J., Simonsick, E., Kashner, M., & Hebel, J.R. (1988). Patient-proxy response comparability on measures of patient health and functional status. *Journal of Clinical Epidemiology, 41,* 1065–1074.

Maier, W., Philip, M., Heuser, I., et al. (1988). Improving depression severity assessment: I. Reliability, internal validity and sensitivity to change of three observer depression scales. *Journal of Psychiatric Research, 22,* 3–12.

Manson, S.M., Ackerson, L.M., Wiegman, D.R., Baron, A.E., & Fleminig, C.M. (1990). Depressive symptoms among American Indian adolescents: Psychometric characteristics of the Center for Epidemiologic Studies Depression Scales (CES-D). *Psychological Assessment: A Journal of Consulting and Clinical Psychology, 2*(3), 231–237.

McHorney, C.A., & Mor, V. (1988). Predictors of bereavement depression and its health services consequences. *Medical Care, 26,* 882–893.

McDowell, I., & Newell, C. (1996). *Measuring health: A guide to rating scales and questionnaires, 2nd ed.* New York: Oxford University Press.

Meenan, R.F., Mason, J.H., Anderson, J.J., et al. (1992). AIMS2: The content and properties of a revised and expanded Arthritis Impact Measurement Scales health status questionnaire. *Arthritis and Rheumatology, 35,* 1–10.

Miller, I.W., Bishop, S., Norman, W.H., et al. (1985). The Modified Hamilton Rating Scale for Depression: Reliability and validity. *Psychiatry Research, 14,* 131–142.

Murden, R.A., McRae, T.D., Kaner, S., et al. (1991). Mini-Mental State Exam scores vary with education in blacks and whiles. *Journal of the American Geriatrics Society, 39,* 149–155.

Norris, F.H., & Murrell, S.A. (1987). Older adult family stress and adaptation before and after bereavement. *Journal of Gerontology, 42,* 606–612.

Nunnally, J.C. (Ed.). (1978). *Psychometric Theory, 2nd ed.* New York: McGraw-Hill.

Nunnally, J.C., & Bernstein, I.H. (1994). *Psychometric Theory, 3rd ed.* New York: McGraw-Hill.

Ory, M. (1988). Considerations in the development of age-sensitive indicators for assessing health promotion. *Health Promotion, 3*(2), 139–150.

Ory, M., & Cox, D.M. (1994). Forging ahead: Linking health and behavior to improve quality of life in older people. *Social Indicators Research, 33,* 89–120.

Paulsen, A.S., Crowe, R.R., Noyes, R., & Pfohl, B. (1988). Reliability of the telephone interview in diagnosing anxiety disorders. *Archives of General Psychiatry, 45*(1), 62–63.

Pillemer, K., & Finkelhor, D. (1989). Causes of elder abuse: Caregiver stress versus problems with relatives. *American Journal of Orthopsychiatry, 59,* 179–187.

Pillemer, K., & Sitor, J.J. (1992). Violence and violent feelings: What causes them among family caregivers? *Journal of Gerontology, 47,* 165–172.

Posner, B.M., Jette, A.M., Smith, K.W., & Miller, D.R. (1993). Nutrition and health risks in the elderly: The nutrition screening initiative. *American Journal of Public Health, 83,* 944–945.

Prigerson, H.G., Maciejewski, P.K., Reynolds, C.F., et al. (1995). The inventory of complicated grief: A scale to measure maladaptive symptoms of loss. *Psychiatric Research, 59,* 65–79.

Quinn, M.J., & Tomita, S.K. (1986). *Elder abuse and neglect: Causes, diagnosis, and intervention strategies.* New York: Springer.

Radloff, L.S. (1977). The CES-D Scale: A self-report depression scale for research in the general population. *Applied Psychological Measurement, 1,* 385–401.

REACH: Resources for Enhancing Alzheimer's Caregiver Health. (1995–2000). National Institute on Aging and National Institute of Nursing Research.

Roberts, R., Rhoades, H.M., & Vernon, S.W. (1990). Using the CES-D Scale to screen for depression and anxiety: Effects of language and ethnic status. *Psychiatry Research, 31,* 69–83.

Rosenthal, R., & Rosnow, R.L. (1991). *Essential of Behavioral Research: Methods and Data Analysis, 2nd ed.* New York: McGraw-Hill, Inc.

Schulz, R., O'Brien, A.T., Bookwala, J., & Fliessner, K. (1995). Psychiatric and physical morbidity effects of Alzheimer's disease caregiving: Prevalence, correlates, and causes. *Gerontologist, 35,* 771–791.

Schulz, R., Newsom, J.T., Mittelmark, M., Burton, L., Hirsh, C., & Jackson, S. (1997). Health effects of caregiving: The Caregiver Health Effects Study. *Annals of Behavioral Medicine, 19,* 110–116.

Schulz, R., & Williamson, G. (1997). The measurement of caregiver outcomes in Alzheimer disease research. *Alzheimer Disease and Associated Disorders, 11*(6), 117–124.

Steinmetz, S.K. (1988). *Duty bound: Elder abuse and family care.* Newbury Park, CA: Sage.

Steer, R.A., Rissmiller, D.J., Ranieri, W.F., & Beck, A.T. (1994). Use of the computer administered Beck Depression Inventory and Hopelessness Scale with psychiatric inpatients. *Computers in Human Behavior, 10*(2), 223–229.

Stewart, A.L., Hays, R.D., & Ware, J.E. Jr. (1988). The MOS Short-Form General Health Survey: Reliability and validity in a patient population. *Medical Care, 26,* 724–735.

Stommel, M., Given, B.A., Given, C.W., Kalaian, H.A., Schulz, R., & McCorkle, R. (1993). Gender bias in the Measurement Properties of the Center for Epidemiologic Studies Depression Scale (CES-D). *Psychiatry Research, 49,* 239–250.

Straus, M. (1979). Measuring intrafamily conflict and violence: The Conflict Tactic (CT) scales. *Journal of Marriage and Family, 1,* 75–88.

Talbott, M.M. (1989). Age bias in the Beck Depression Inventory: A proposed modification for use with older women. *Clinical Gerontologist, 9,* 23–35.

Teri, L., Truax, P., Logsdon, R., Uomoto, J., Zarit. S., & Vitaliano, P.P. (1992). Assessment of behavioral problems in dimentia: The Revised Memory and Behavior Problems Checklist. *Psychology and Aging, 7*(4), 622–631.

Thornicroft, G. (1992). Computerised mental health assessments. In G. Thornicroft, C.R. Brewin, & J. Wing (Eds.) *Measuring mental needs* (pp. 258–272). London, England: University of London.

Uhlmann, R.F., & Larson, E.B. (1991). Effect of educations the Mini-Mental State Examination as a screening test for dementia. *Journal of the American Geriatric Society, 39,* 876–880.

Ullman, J.B. (1996). Structural equation modeling. In B.G. Tabachnick & L.S. Fidell, *Using multivariate statistics 3rd ed.* (pp. 709–811). Harper Collins College Publishers.

Vitaliano, P.P., Russo, F., Young, H.M., Teri, L., & Maiuro, R.D. (1991). Predictors of burden in spouse caregivers of individuals with Alzheimer's disease. *Psychology of Aging, 6,* 392–402.

Ware, J.E. (1984). The General Health Rating Index. In N.K. Wenger, M.E. Mattson, C.D. Furberg, & J. Elinson (Eds.), *Assessment of quality of life in clinical trials of cardiovascular therapies* (pp. 184–188). New York: Le Jacq.

Ware, J.E. Jr., Kosinski, M., & Keller, S.D. (1996). A 12-item Short-Form Health Survey: Construction of scales and preliminary tests of reliability and validity. *Medical Care, 34,* 220–233.

Ware, J.E. Jr., & Sherbourne, C.D. (1992). The MOS 36-item Short-Form Health Survey (SF-36). I. Conceptual framework and item selection. *Medical Care, 30,* 473–483.

Ware, J.E. Jr., Sherbourne, C.D., & Davies, A.R. (1992). Developing and testing the MOS 20-item Short-Form Health Survey: A general population application. In A.L. Stewart & J.E. Ware Jr., (Eds.), *Measuring functioning and well-being: The medical outcomes study approach* (pp. 277–290). Durham, NC: Duke University Press.

Ware, J.E. Jr., Snow, K.K., Kosinski, M., et al. (1993). *SF-36 Health Survey: Manual and interpretation guide.* Boston, MA: The Health Institute, New England Medical Center.

Wells, K.B., Burnam, M.A., Leake, B., & Robins, L.N. (1988). Agreement between face-to-face and telephone-administered versions of the depression section of the NIMH Diagnostic Interview Schedule. *Journal of Psychiatric Research, 22*(3), 207–220.

Williams, A.C., & Richardson, P.H. (1993). What does the BDI measure in chronic pain? *Pain, 55,* 259–266.

Williamson, X., & Miller, X. (1996). Inadequate care of impaired elderly family members. *Unpublished Manuscript,* University of Georgia.

# 7

## Identifying Mechanisms of Action: Why and How Does Intervention Work?

*Laura N. Gitlin, Mary Corcoran,*
*Jennifer Martindale-Adams, Charlotte Malone,*
*Alan Stevens, and Laraine Winter*

### INTRODUCTION

An important new direction in clinical trial research with AD family caregivers is the systematic documentation and evaluation of intervention processes. This approach to caregiver intervention research is critical for several compelling reasons. First, whereas a range of service programs for AD family caregivers has been tested (see chapter 2), our understanding of why and how interventions work is limited. Second, previous reports have found variable results among intervention studies (Bourgois, Schulz, & Burgio, 1996; Knight, Lutzky, & Macofsky-Urban, 1993). Some research has also shown that family caregivers tend to underutilize available formal services (Gill, Hinrichsen, & diGiuseppe, 1998; Hamilton, 1996). Finally, a lack of accepted and standard methods for documenting intervention characteristics and processes has made it difficult to generalize study findings and implement interventions in different service settings (Bala, Austin, Ewigman, Borwn, & Mitchell, 1995). These limitations have intensified the importance of identifying specific intervention features and caregiver characteristics that are associated with treatment outcomes. An understanding of intervention processes may suggest new approaches to support family members. Moreover, it may enhance knowledge of which strategies work best and for whom and at which caregiving stage interventions are most beneficial.

Of particular importance to the study of intervention processes is identifying the underlying *mechanism(s) of action* of an intervention. Mechanism of action refers to the theoretical and empirical accounting of why and how a particular change in a caregiver or care recipient occurs as a consequence of participating in an intervention. A mechanism of action seeks to elucidate underlying associations or pathways through which desired changes in behavior, cognition, or affect are achieved through intervention. Mechanisms also delineate how change proceeds, the particular conditions under which an intervention achieves beneficial results, and why a change may occur for certain groups of participants and not others.

Caregiver intervention studies are implicitly grounded in a particular understanding of how a behavioral or cognitive change may take place or the mechanism of action. Unfortunately, to date, few clinical trials with AD family caregivers have included adequate design features and measures to adequately explain the underlying mechanisms for the effect of an intervention. Thus, little is presently known about the psychological, social, and physiological mechanisms that predispose caregivers to achieve or not achieve positive outcomes from interventions. To advance this area of research, clinical trials must consider mechanisms as a specific research query and include the evaluation of intervention effects as specific design and measurement goals.

Mechanisms have traditionally been examined in the biological and pharmocologic sciences. However, identifying mechanisms of behavioral change may require a different approach due to the complexity and multifactorial nature of caregiver interventions. This chapter provides an overview of the mechanisms of action concept and its application to the study of interventions for AD family caregivers. First, the significance of the study of mechanisms of action is discussed. Next, we identify three recent developments in research that may advance this form of inquiry. Following this, we delineate and discuss two interrelated considerations in examining mechanisms as shown in Table 7.1. Foremost in the study of mechanisms is the requirement to pose relevant theoretical frameworks which underpin the intervention and from which to generate specific hypotheses and testable causal pathways. In this chapter we discuss select theoretical frameworks to illustrate different causal pathways through which interventions may work. Another important consideration in the study of mechanisms is clearly specifying the structural elements and processes of delivering an intervention. Accordingly, we identify key dimensions of caregiver interventions such as dose, intensity, methods of delivery, and discuss approaches to their measurement. These dimensions describe the conditions of treatment and how change may proceed. It may be that only one dimension or a combination of factors produce an intervention effect. Thus, in this chapter, we suggest that the study of mechanisms of caregiver interventions requires the integration of a theoretical model with the measurement of its treatment components. To illustrate each of these points, we draw on the experiences of the REACH study group.

## SIGNIFICANCE OF MECHANISMS OF ACTION

The concept, *mechanism of action*, is relatively new to social and behavioral clinical trial research, and virtually absent in the study of caregiver interventions. By contrast, identifying mechanisms of action

**TABLE 7.1 Components to the Study of Mechanisms of Action**

| 1.  Why intervention works | 2.  How intervention works |
|---|---|
| • Theory to explain caregiver change<br>• Theory to explain care recipient change<br>• Causal pathways (direct, mediation, moderation) | • Structural elements<br>• Entity and targeted domains<br>• Fidelity components<br>—Delivery<br>—Receipt<br>—Enactment |

has been a fundamental aspect of inquiry in the physiologic basis of aging. For instance, specifying the mechanisms by which aging occurs at the cellular level remains a primary focus of biologic research and is central to the understanding of age-related disease processes and physical frailty (Morrison, Katz, Parmelee, Boyce, & Ten Have, 1998).

The significance of understanding mechanisms of action is best illustrated by clinical trial research in pharmacology. The centrality of this concept to this field is reflected in the more than 3,234 citations found in a Medline database search conducted from 1990 to April, 1998. Searches on this topic in Psychlit, Health Star, and CINHAL databases yielded similar results with all citations referring to pharmacological studies. Mechanisms of action in pharmacology include two components: (1) identifying the physiologic or biologic actions that occur, and (2) specifying the drug regimen such as the strength of dose, time of dose, and form of dose (e.g., liquid, tablet). Thus, identifying mechanisms, or how a particular drug activates physiologic or biologic change, is critical in that it informs dosing decisions and the conditions for its administration. Examining mechanisms of action in caregiver intervention studies include parallel components: (1) identifying relevant theoretical models, and (2) specifying the treatment dosage such as the number of contacts or type of contacts (e.g., face-to-face, telephone, computer).

It is important to recognize that identifying mechanisms of action represents an ongoing research process in which knowledge is gained incrementally through repeated research endeavors. The ongoing efforts of scientists to discern the effects of cholinergic agents on memory functioning in dementia patients illustrates this knowledge-building process. At present, cholinergic agents are considered one of the most promising pharmacological treatments for cognitive impairment. In research on the first generation of cholinergic agents, the proposed mechanism of action was described as the "cholinergic hypothesis." This hypothesis suggested an association between cognitive decline and cholinergic cell loss in areas of the brain. Currently, with the second generation of cholinergic agents, investigators are suggesting that cognitive symptoms improve through synaptic effects. Still other researchers are suggesting that these agents provide neuroprotective effects through activating nicotinic receptors (Schneider, 1996). Thus, the mechanisms by which these agents function have not been fully disclosed and competing hypotheses continue to be tested.

## RESEARCH DEVELOPMENTS TO ADVANCE THE STUDY OF MECHANISMS

Several recent developments in social science and behavioral research significantly advance the study of the mechanisms of action in caregiver interventions. First, well-developed theories and models of behavior change have been proposed and tested in other fields. These theories and models provide useful frameworks for developing hypotheses and identifying specific factors and pathways by which caregiver interventions may function.

Another factor facilitating the study of mechanisms is a growing literature on methodological issues in clinical trial research (Egan, Snyder, & Burns, 1992; Spilker, 1996; Teri & Logsdon, 1996; Weissert & Hedrick, 1994). This literature has identified specific factors that may confound treatment effects and which must be controlled or tested in clinical trials. For example, research on psychotherapeutic interventions has shown that therapist attributes may influence the treatment process and its outcomes (Crits-Christoph & Mintz, 1991; O'Leary & Borkovec, 1978). Studies suggest that information about the characteristics of those who provide intervention should be collected. Statistical analyses can be performed to examine differences in outcomes between interventionists and the relationship between therapist factors and treatment outcomes.

Recent advances in statistical modeling techniques also permit a more focused examination of mechanisms. Mechanisms of action are conceptually linked to the statistical ideas of mediation and moderation. The distinction between mediators and moderators has been carefully explicated in the experimental psychology literature, most notably by Baron and Kenney (1986). Mediation refers to the generative mechanism through which an independent variable influences an outcome. A mediator is a third variable that affects the relation between an independent or predictor variable and a dependent variable or outcome.

A variable functions as a mediator to the extent that it accounts for the relationship between a predictor and an outcome. Mediation is especially important in the context of intervention research since variables identified as such may be likely candidates for the foci of interventions, assuming, of course, that the identified factors are amenable to change. For instance, if psychosocial resources such as self-efficacy and social support emerge as mediators of well-being, interventions may be designed to enhance these resources.

In contrast, a moderator considers the subgroups of a particular independent variable to determine which group or level leads to maximal effectiveness in a designated dependent variable. Examples of typical moderating variables in caregiving research include gender, ethnicity, and spousal relationships. Independent variables may have differential effects on intervention outcomes as a function of these variables. While direct, mediation, and moderation models have been used to predict change in caregiver well-being in prospective studies (Haley, Roth, Coleton, Ford, West, Collins, & Isobe, 1996), these models have not been applied to intervention research but may be useful for describing mechanisms of action.

Unquestionably, providing care to a family member with dementia represents a complex activity that potentially may have multiple consequences for caregiver health and well-being. Consequently, interventions for caregivers are generally multifaceted and are designed to effect multiple caregiver and care recipient outcomes, such as behaviors, cognition, and emotional responses. Thus, a given intervention may have more than one mechanism through which it operates. A combination of theoretical frameworks may be necessary to explain the role and impact of various intervention components. Likewise, statistical modeling techniques will be required to account for mechanisms by which change is evinced in the different domains that are targeted by an intervention.

## UNDERSTANDING WHY CHANGE OCCURS

One of the first set of tasks in the study of mechanisms is articulating a relevant theoretical framework or the underpinning of an intervention, developing appropriate hypotheses, and testing a causal pathway by which change in the targeted area may occur. For this effort, a vast array of theories from related fields of inquiry are available. Here we highlight select theories that may be particularly useful to the study of why interventions do or do not work with AD family caregivers.

## Stress Process Models

Stress process models have been used extensively in prospective studies to examine the mechanisms by which psychosocial factors influence caregiver well-being (Goode, Haley, Roth, & Ford, 1998; Schulz, Visintainer, & Williamson, 1990; Schulz, O'Brien, Bookwala, & Fleissner, 1995). Briefly stated, this vast body of research has shown that psychosocial resources such as caregiver appraisals, coping responses, and level of social support mediate the effect of caregiving stressors on caregiver well-being. As described in detail in chapter 2, a broad stress-process health model is used by the REACH study group as a basis for understanding the outcomes and underlying mechanisms of its diverse interventions. The model is useful in this context because it accounts for the environment, physical health, and psychosocial influences on caregiver well-being. Also, the model considers the impact of various interventions on each of these factors. For example, an intervention may provide education to enhance a caregiver's understanding of and ability to cope with the demands of caregiving. Alternately, an intervention may be directed at changing the caregiver's physical and social environment to reduce the impact of problem behaviors. Thus, the model provides the framework for testing caregiver interventions and elucidating the specific pathways by which burden is reduced or other behavioral and cognitive changes occur.

## Motivational Theories

Motivation is an important concept in the study of mechanisms of interventions that involve behavioral change. Motivation refers to the notion that human activity is grounded in or stems from goals. Goals orient people to particular interpretations of events, organize behavior, and guide actions which result in the pursuit of desired outcomes (Gollwitzer & Bargh, 1996). There are numerous theories of motivation, but each attempts to link cognitive processes to actual behaviors.

As applied to caregiving, these theories suggest that caregivers have implicit ideas about best care practices with dementia patients (e.g., keep routines normal and unchanged). As suggested in Figure 7.1, a theory of best care may lead to the formation of specific goals, and subsequently, to behavioral actions that caregivers wish to accomplish (e.g., bathe family member daily as he used to do). However, as the disease progresses, goals may become difficult to achieve. Caregivers may become motivated to learn new strategies that will enable them to either achieve their implicit or stated goals or to reframe these goals. One mechanism suggested by motivational theory is that tailoring an intervention to individual goals, as opposed to using a structured group intervention, may elicit desired outcomes by tapping into the specific goals and personal motivational frameworks of caregiver participants.

Caregiver theory of best care  ⇒  Formation of specific caregiving goals  ⇒  Actions

**FIGURE 7.1   Application of motivational theory to caregiving.**

## Behavior Change Theories

Behavior change theories provide a framework for understanding mechanisms of changing lifestyle-type behaviors (Meillier, Lund, & Kok, 1997). The transtheoretical model of behavioral change, developed by Prochaska and colleagues (Prochaska & DiClemente, 1983; Prochaska, Redding, & Evers, 1997) may be helpful in understanding mechanisms of action of caregiver interventions. The transtheoretical model views behavior change as occurring incrementally, through a series of well-defined stages. These stages may be used to classify individuals so that intervention approaches can be tailored to a specific level of readiness for modifying actions. Levels of readiness also may be used to explain why some intervention participants achieve behavior gains while others do not. The stages of readiness have been used extensively to examine the effects of varied interventions that are designed to alter health-related behaviors such as tobacco use and weight loss.

With regard to caregiving, the acquisition of new skills that allow a caregiver to manage daily care problems requires a sequence of behavioral changes. A caregiver may need to have a certain level of readiness before being able to modify or change what may be long-standing care routines. In this way, readiness for behavior change may mediate caregiver outcomes. This behavior staging framework is currently used by the Memphis and Philadelphia REACH study sites to understand which caregiver participants may benefit most from intervention. Memphis REACH modified Prochaska's four basic stages of change to fit the caregiving situation. This is illustrated in Figure 7.2. At each of the two sites, interventionists classify caregivers according to four levels of readiness to accept intervention strategies. By cross-tabulating readiness data with components of treatment implementation such as dose and intensity rates, investigators hope to discern patterns of treatment effects. Additionally, the moderating

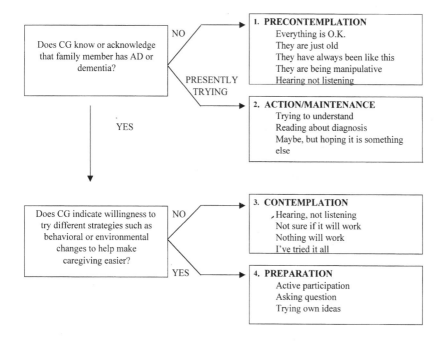

**FIGURE 7.2   Readiness form.**

role of factors, such as gender and ethnicity, can be evaluated. For example, analyses will be conducted to determine if gender moderates treatment effects at each stage of readiness. This theory offers a useful framework from which to refine our understanding of mechanisms of action and how interventions operate for different ethnic and gender groups.

## Personal Control Theory

Another useful framework for the study of mechanisms is the construct of self-efficacy. Bandura (1997) has suggested that self-efficacy beliefs influence the initiation of actions, and therefore, serve as important mediators of behavior in different domains of daily life. A substantial body of research supports this theory and indicates that strong self-efficacy beliefs are related to positive health outcomes and the adaptation of health promoting behaviors (McAvay, Seeman, & Rodin, 1996). Caregiver studies also have shown that strong self-efficacy beliefs and a personal sense of control are important psychological resources that have a negative relationship with depression (Intrieri & Rapp, 1994; Miller, Campbell, Farran, Kaufman, & Davis, 1995).

Schulz, Heckhausen, and O'Brien (1994) have applied the concept of personal control to the study of disability. These researchers have advanced a theory of personal control which suggests that as people are threatened with loss in their ability to control daily life outcomes, they seek adaptive strategies to compensate for this threat. If adaptive strategies cannot be used or do not adequately compensate for the threat of loss of control, then the result may be heightened anxiety and depression.

Applied to caregiving, personal control theory suggests caregivers may be motivated to learn and use new care techniques in order to maintain direct personal control over important life domains. The successful use of strategies to manage new problems may provide caregivers with a sense of mastery or self-efficacy. Theoretically, enhanced feelings of self-efficacy will, in turn, result in less caregiver depression, upset and burden. As shown in Figure 7.3, personal control theory offers a testable pathway as to the mechanism by

Caregiver motivated to maintain control

⇓

Caregiver adapts new care strategies

⇓

Care strategies are effective solutions to new problems

⇓

Caregiver feels sense of self-efficacy

⇓

Caregiver burden is reduced

**FIGURE 7.3**    Application of personal control theory to caregiving.

which caregivers may benefit from an intervention involving skills training or behavioral management techniques.

Table 7.2 summarizes these and other theoretical approaches that may be useful in explaining the mechanisms through which different caregiver interventions result in reduced burden, just one of the potential outcomes of a caregiver intervention.

## IDENTIFYING STRUCTURAL AND PROCESS DIMENSIONS OF INTERVENTIONS

Another component in the study of mechanisms of action (see Table 7.1) is determining the way in which change occurs. This involves identifying the structural dimensions of an intervention and the process of its implementation. Examining structural and process

**TABLE 7.2  Common Caregiver Interventions, Possible
Theoretical Frameworks and Hypothetical Mechanisms of Action
to Explain Reduced Burden**

| Intervention | Theoretical framework | Implied mechanism of action |
|---|---|---|
| Family therapy | Social exchange theory/equity theory | Individuals use exchanges to maximize rewards and minimize costs. Reciprocation of exchanges need to be perceived as equal or fair to maintain stable family relationships and caregiver well-being. Caregivers benefit from family therapy because it equalizes exchanges and enhances social support. Increased social support that is perceived as beneficial reduces burden. |
| Individualized skills training | Motivational theories | Personal goals provide a framework for initiating behaviors. Caregivers become motivated to adapt new skills and change behaviors to address self-identified goals of caregiving. Attainment of personal goals to achieve desired outcomes leads to reduction of burden. |
| Behavior management techniques | Self-efficacy/ personal control theory | Individuals need to control daily life events to maintain positive affect and well-being. When faced with loss of control, caregivers are motivated to adapt new care strategies that enhance their control and improve self-efficacy. Improved self-efficacy leads to reduced burden. |
| Home environmental modifications | Competence-environmental press framework | Competence-environmental press framework emphasizes a just right fit between the individual and environment to optimize behavior. This suggests that a change in the environment to decrease its press will enhance abilities of the dementia patient to carry out tasks and reduce excess behaviors associated with the disease. Maintenance of function and control of difficult behaviors reduces objective caregiver burden. |

elements allows researchers to discern the optimal conditions under which an intervention is effective. For instance, some evidence suggests that psychoeducational counseling enhances psychological resources and feelings of self-efficacy among caregivers (Mittleman, Ferris, Shulman, Steinberg, Ambinder, Mackell, & Cohen, 1995). However, it is unclear which delivery format (standard group or individualized session) and for which group of caregivers this intervention is most beneficial (Brodaty, Gresham, & Luscombe, 1997). Describing, manipulating, and testing conditions of delivery enable researchers to determine how changes in behavior, cognition, and/ or affect occur. Developing an understanding of the basic elements of an intervention is necessary before service efficiency and effectiveness can be maximized (Basler, 1995).

## Structural Dimensions of Interventions

To categorize the structural dimensions of interventions, REACH has developed two matrices from which to map and compare interventions (see chapter 2 for a complete description of the conceptual underpinning of this approach and definitions of the components of the matrices).

*Attributes of Service Delivery.* Briefly, one matrix characterizes 19 attributes of service delivery. Examples of these attributes include the frequency and duration of contacts, location of intervention (e.g., home versus clinic), and whether delivery is standardized (e.g., group-end goals), tailored (e.g., individualized goals), or involves others (e.g., care recipient, other family members). These dimensions represent the pragmatics of implementing an intervention, but are rarely described comprehensively in caregiver intervention studies. Nevertheless, these attributes may either hinder or enhance the enactment of treatment strategies by caregivers, and thus, are important to understanding mechanisms of action.

For example, each REACH intervention introduces behavior management strategies in some form to improve caregiver skills. However, the method of delivery and the care setting in which strategies are introduced vary across sites. Memphis REACH implements its interventions in a primary care setting; Palo Alto provides interventions in clinical settings, and Miami, Philadelphia, and Birmingham implement interventions in caregiver homes. REACH will be able to examine whether an attribute such as the setting of service delivery enhances or hinders caregiver acceptance and use of new skills. Investigators also will be able to discern the extent to which the setting of service delivery is a condition of an intervention that either enhances or hinders its effectiveness.

*Domains Targeted for Change.* The second matrix developed by REACH characterizes interventions in terms of two domains or aspects that an intervention targets for change. The first aspect concerns the primary entity that an intervention targets. Although the caregiver is the point of implementation of an intervention, the content of the intervention may target issues that are related to either caregivers, care recipient behaviors, and/or to the social (e.g., family, social supports) and/or physical environment (use of objects). Each intervention may be directed at any one or a combination of these three primary entities.

The second aspect of the matrix concerns the primary domain within each entity that is the focus or content of the intervention. Four domains have been identified. The intervention may seek to (1) build knowledge, (2) address cognitions, (3) change behaviors, or (4) improve affect. Again, any one intervention may target multiple areas. In summary, the primary entity and the domain of interventions represent two orthogonal dimensions which result in a 3 (entity) by 4 (domain) or 12 component matrix by which all caregiver interventions can be mapped (see chapter 2 to examine the matrix). For instance, a common intervention is to enhance caregiver understanding of the disease process using education materials. In this case, the primary entity that is the target of intervention is the care recipient and the disease process, and the primary domain or content is knowledge-building. Another common intervention is to enhance a caregiver's sense of mastery and well-being through support group programs. In this case, the primary entity that is the target of the intervention is the caregiver, and the domain or content of the intervention is cognitions. Thus, the mechanisms underlying a change in knowledge level via an education-based intervention may differ from the mechanisms underlying a change in cognitive processes that occur in a support group intervention.

This point is illustrated by a recent intervention study of women with breast cancer. This study compared an education-based intervention to a peer discussion group (Helgeson, Cohen, Schulz, & Yasko, in press) and evaluated mechanisms for the interventions' effects. Clear benefits were derived only in the education group and participants in the peer group demonstrated negative psychological outcomes. The primary mechanism by which patients benefitted from the education intervention centered on self-image. The authors showed that the educational materials normalized the experience of having breast cancer. In contrast, women in the peer group demonstrated negative effects because they increased their rate of negative downward comparisons. That is, they experienced greater anxiety by interacting with women who were worse off.

To further illustrate the utility of this approach, consider the three interventions that are being tested at Memphis REACH. Each intervention builds on the other so that there are incremental increases in duration, dose, and intensity from one group to the next. The most basic intervention is the Information and Referral group which has the lowest levels of duration, dose, and intensity. This intervention provides information about the disease process and referral to local resources for family caregivers. Thus, the intervention targets the domain of knowledge-building for two entities, the caregiver and care recipient. This is considered a minimal treatment group. Conversely, the Memphis Behavioral Care intervention provides information. Additionally, it introduces caregivers to behavior management techniques, presents coping strategies, and ways of modifying the social and physical environment. The intervention targets three entities: caregiver, care recipient, and the social/physical environment. The content of the intervention is directed at three domains improving knowledge building, behaviors, and affect. The third intervention, the Memphis Enhanced Care group, has the highest levels of duration, dose, and intensity. This intervention provides information about and referral to local resources, introduces and has caregivers practice behavior management techniques, presents coping strategies, and provides suggestions for modifying the social and physical environment. It not only targets the caregiver's and care recipient's cognition-knowledge, the care recipient's behavior and affect, but also the caregiver's cognition-skills, behavior, and affect. As in the second intervention group, this level of intervention also targets the caregiver's cognition-knowledge of the social and physical environment. Each of these interventions occur on-site at a primary care physician's office and involves repeated contacts with caregivers over two years.

The intervention tested by Philadelphia REACH provides a different set of contrasts along the 3 by 4 matrix. The Philadelphia intervention involves home visits during which multifaceted strategies are introduced to address specific caregiver-identified difficulties in managing dementia. Strategies include knowledge building about the progression of the disease, management techniques such as task breakdown and effective communication, and modifying the social and physical environment, including the use of adaptive equipment. The intervention is individualized and specific strategies are tailored to fit the particular concerns that are identified by the caregiver, the characteristics of the physical and social environment, and the level of function of the care recipient. Therefore, the intervention is directed at three primary entities: the caregiver, care recipient, and social/physical environment. The domains that are targeted include knowledge building and behavior change.

The two REACH matrices provide a categorical approach from which to analyze and contrast interventions along key elements of delivery and the specific target areas. For each cell of the matrix (e.g., care recipient by behavior), a different mechanism of action may be posed. REACH investigators will be able to use hierarchical analytic models to investigate the relationship between components of various interventions and treatment outcomes. Also, with this approach, REACH will be able to derive expanded measures for comparing and contrasting interventions. For example, dose, duration, and intensity measures (e.g., frequency and duration of contacts, and number of strategies introduced) can be combined with other dimensions such as method of contact, environmental setting, and/or the number of domains and entities that the intervention targets.

## Process Dimensions of Interventions

To understand process dimensions of interventions, it is helpful to apply the concept of treatment fidelity. Typically, treatment fidelity refers to a set of measures that document treatment implementation. Measures serve two purposes. The first purpose is to examine the extent to which independent variables are manipulated (Moncher & Prinz, 1991). That is, fidelity assessments enable investigators to systematically analyze the relationship between process and treatment outcomes. The second purpose of fidelity assessment is to monitor the actions of interventionists to ensure consistency and adherence to study protocols. Since measures of treatment fidelity provide invaluable detail of content and procedures, the data informs the mechanisms by which the intervention achieves its effectiveness. Thus, treatment fidelity measures serve the dual purposes of determining the relationship between degree of implementation and treatment effects and monitoring the integrity and consistency of intervention implementation.

Lichstein, Riedel, and Grieve (1994) have recommended the systematic evaluation of three elements of treatment fidelity: treatment delivery, receipt, and enactment. These researchers also have recommended a number of strategies to enhance and measure each element. Although strategies must be customized to specific interventions, those developed by the REACH study group and summarized in Table 7.3, exemplify this approach.

Lichstein, Riedel, and Grieve (1994) describe treatment delivery as the degree to which an interventionist presents the treatment to participants as intended. Treatment delivery addresses basic questions such as whether interventionists are adequately trained and render the intervention consistently and accurately. Obviously, if an intervention is not delivered in the intended manner, it is not possible to interpret findings. A number of factors potentially threaten the ability to deliver an intervention according to protocol and thereby impede the mechanisms that lead to direct actions. These threats include, but are not limited to, the following conditions: a) the intervention is long-term, b) there are multiple components to its implementation, c) multiple experimental groups are being tested simultaneously, d) more than one interventionist is involved, and e) there is attrition of interventionists. Common strategies to enhance treatment delivery include development and use of a treatment manual, systematic training and a certification process for interventionists, and developing a mechanism for ongoing monitoring and feedback.

**TABLE 7.3  Treatment Fidelity Enhancement Strategies and Measures**

| Fidelity component | Enhancement strategies | Measures |
|---|---|---|
| Delivery | • Manual guidance<br>• Standard scripts<br>• Protocol monitoring<br>• Training interventionists | • Intended/actual dose<br>• Intended/actual intensity<br>• Characteristics of interventionists |
| Receipt | • Client-centered approach<br>• Active therapeutic techniques (role play)<br>• Use of visual-auditory aids | • Number and type of intervention strategies introduced<br>• Record of who (CG or therapist) suggests strategy<br>• Number and type of techniques used (role play, demonstration, video, etc.)<br>• Knowledge gains |
| Enactment | • Provide opportunities to practice strategies<br>• Provide intervention over long time frame | • Number and type of strategies in use (observation and self-report)<br>• Reasons for nonuse/abandonment<br>• Caregiver report of effectiveness of each strategy |

Treatment receipt refers to the extent to which study participants receive the treatment as intended. Potential threats to receipt include use of only one teaching method, a lack of sufficient opportunity to practice new strategies, and communication difficulties or cultural differences between interventionist and study participant (e.g., use of technical or medical terms, differences in value systems). Common strategies to enhance treatment receipt include the use of multiple active therapeutic techniques (e.g., role play, demonstration), use of multimedia (e.g., video, written materials), and an approach that is either client-centered or collaborative.

Treatment enactment refers to the extent to which study participants actually enact or apply the knowledge and skills learned in treatment. If participants do not use the knowledge and skills transmitted in intervention, then little benefit will likely be derived. Enactment then is an important component of treatment fidelity and represents a measure of intervention utilization.

## MEASUREMENT CONSIDERATIONS

Thus far we have defined fidelity components and discussed methods to strengthen the mechanisms of delivery, receipt, and enactment of an intervention. The measurement of each of these components also is an important aspect in studying mechanisms of action. In developing measures of delivery, receipt, and enactment, several methodological issues must be considered. These are listed in Table 7.4.

To date, an accepted and standard set of measures to assess the components of treatment fidelity has not been developed. Consequently, investigators must develop their own assessments and test their psychometric properties. One recommended strategy to accomplish this task is to triangulate data by combining different data types and sources from which information is gathered. For example, to examine the receipt and enactment of intervention strategies, a rating scale can be devised by the investigator and completed by the interventionist, caregiver, another family member, and/or an independent, objective evaluator. Also, data can be collected using a range of methodologies including videotape or audiotape of inter-

---

### TABLE 7.4 Measurement Considerations

- Source of ratings:

  —Caregiver
  —Observation
  —Audio/videotape
  —Interventionist

- Inter-rater reliability
- Validity
- Level of measurement
- Type of expected change:

  —Change from absence to presence of a particular behavior
  —Change from low to high occurrence of a particular behavior

---

vention sessions, fieldnotes/progress notes written by intervention-ists at each caregiver contact, caregiver narratives and personal journals, and/or behavioral logs that track the occurrence of tar-geted problem areas. These documents can then be coded and analyzed for evidence of delivery, receipt, and enactment. The data can also be triangulated to obtain validity or convergence of emerg-ing themes and other findings.

The specific measures developed by the REACH study group and summarized in Table 7.3 illustrate the use of a range of effective strategies. To examine treatment delivery across study sites, REACH uses a standard form to document the dose, intensity, and other elements of delivery. This form records several aspects of each care-giver contact including its length, the setting, the presence of others, and who initiated contact. Summary scores can be derived to describe dose and intensity rates, variation in delivery settings, and the num-ber of occasions in which others are involved in any one particular intervention. Another important measure of delivery assesses the personal characteristics of interventionists. REACH uses a simple demographic form that is completed for each interventionist at each site. Attributes such as race, age, years of experience, and gender will be examined in relation to treatment outcomes.

To measure treatment receipt, a variety of measures are being used by REACH sites. For example, some sites have developed forms that are completed by interventionists at each contact. These forms record detailed information such as the specific recommendation or strategy provided to a caregiver and at which contact the recom-mendation is offered, who initiates the strategy (e.g., caregiver, inter-ventionist, both or other), and whether the strategy is attempted and ultimately enacted. These data will yield frequency distributions as to the number and type of recommended strategies offered for each caregiver problem area, the number and type of strategies that caregivers themselves derive during intervention, and the number and type of strategies successfully used.

Several REACH sites also measure caregiver knowledge to deter-mine level of treatment receipt. Varied methodologies are used including audiotaping intervention contacts, having an objective evaluator randomly observe the interventionist and study participant, and, in two sites, using computer technology to record the number of times caregivers access the technology.

Finally, to measure treatment enactment, REACH sites have developed specific approaches tailored to the contours of their individual interventions. Direct observation of whether a caregiver uses recommended intervention techniques is perhaps the most reliable method for evaluating enactment. However, this approach may not always be feasible and may be augmented by self-report. Several REACH sites collect information from caregivers about the frequency with which they use each recommended strategy, reasons for abandoning a strategy or its nonuse, the length of time a particular strategy is used, and the perceived effectiveness of the strategy in addressing a problem area.

## SUMMARY

Mechanisms of action have been inadequately addressed in AD family caregiver intervention research. To date, we can only speculate about the particular pathways through which behavioral, cognitive, or emotional changes occur in caregivers and/or care recipients as a consequence of intervention participation. In this chapter we have argued that future studies must not only test treatment effectiveness, but must also systematically identify the mechanisms through which interventions achieve or fail to achieve desired outcomes among diverse caregiving groups. To advance this new direction in caregiver research, a more rigorous approach to theory formulation and measurement of treatment implementation is necessary.

Recent progress in theory development, clinical trial methodology, and statistical techniques may contribute to advancing the study of mechanisms. Specifically, stress process models, motivational theories, and behavior change models are being used to predict a range of health-related behaviors, and may be particularly helpful in articulating the pathways through which treatment effects are achieved in caregiver interventions. Furthermore, to expand our understanding of mechanisms, intervention studies must include the systematic assessment of treatment processes as a measurement goal. To this end, the REACH study group has developed an effective categorization scheme for comparing interventions along 19 service delivery components and have devised a 3 by 4 matrix that summarizes the primary entities and domains that reflect the specific target areas of interventions. These matrices are useful in deriving summary scores and creating delivery indices from which to examine which elements contribute to and strengthen mechanisms of action. Additionally, the tripartite concept of treatment fidelity facilitates a methodical evaluation of treatment components from which to disentangle process from outcomes and discern the optimal conditions for delivering interventions.

Knowledge about why and how families derive benefit from formal intervention has immense clinical and theoretical import. The search for explanations as to why and how interventions work promises to yield significant knowledge about regulatory systems that guide caregiving activity and the conditions under which desired behavioral, cognitive, and/or affective change occurs. From such knowledge, interventions can be more effectively developed to meet the multiple needs of caregivers at each stage of caregiving and as the disease progresses.

## REFERENCES

Bala, E.A., Austin, S.M., Ewigman, B.G., Borwn, G.D., & Mitchell, J.A. (1995). Methods of randomized controlled clinical trials in health services research. *Medical Care, 33,* 687–699.

Bandura, A. (1997). *Self-efficacy: The exercise of control.* New York: W.H. Freeman & Co.

Baron, R.M., & Kenney, D.A. (1986). The moderator-mediator variable distinction in social psychological research: Conceptual, strategic, and statistical considerations. *Journal of Personality and Social Psychology, 51,* 1173–1182.

Basler, H. (1995). Patient education with reference to the process of behavioral change. *Patient Education and Counseling, 26,* 93–98.

Brodaty, H., Gresham, M., & Luscombe, G. (1997). The Prince Henry Hospital dementia caregiver's training program. *International Journal of Geriatric Psychiatry, 12,* 183–192.

Bourgois, M.S., Schulz, R., & Burgio, L. (1996). Interventions for caregivers of patients with Alzheimer's Disease: A review and analysis of content, process, and outcomes. *International Journal of Aging and Human Development, 43,* 35–91.

Crits-Christoph, P., & Mintz, J. (1991). Implications of therapist effects for the design and analysis of comparative studies of psychotherapies. *Journal of Consulting and Clinical Psychology, 59,* 20–26.

Egan, E.C., Snyder, M., & Burns, K.R. (1992). Intervention studies in nursing: Is the effect due to the independent variable? *Nursing Outlook, 40,* 187–190.

Gill, C.E., Hinrichsen, G.A., & DiGiuseppe, R. (1998). Factors associated with formal service use by family members of patients with dementia. *The Journal of Applied Gerontology, 17,* 38–52.

Gollwitzer, P.M., & Bargh, J.A. (1996). *The Psychology of Action: Linking Cognition and Motivation to Behavior.* New York: The Guilford Press.

Goode, K.T., Haley, W.E., Roth, D.L., & Ford, G.R. (1998). Predicting longitudinal changes in caregiver physical and mental health: A stress process model. *Health Psychology, 17,* 190–198.

Haley, W.E., Roth, D.L., Coleton, M.I., Ford, G.R., West, C.A.C., Collins, R.P., & Isobe, T.L. (1996). Appraisal, coping, and social support as mediators of well-being in black and white family caregivers of patients with Alzheimer's Disease. *Journal of Consulting and Clinical Psychology, 64,* 121–129.

Hamilton, E.M. (1996). Factors associated with family caregivers' choice not to use services. *American Journal of Alzheimer's Disease, 11,* 29–38.

Helgeson, V.S., Cohen, S., Schulz, R., & Yasko, J. (in press). Group support interventions for people with cancer: Benefits and hazards. *Annals of Psychiatry.*

Intrieri, R.C., & Rapp, S.R. (1994). Self-control skillfulness and caregiver burden among help-seeking elders. *Journal of Gerontology: Psychological Sciences, 49,* P19–P23.

Knight, B.G., Lutzky, S.M., & Macofsky-Urban, F. (1993). A meta-analytic review of interventions for caregiver distress: Recommendations for future research. *The Gerontologist, 33,* 240–248.

Lichstein, K.L., Riedel, B.W., & Grieve, R. (1994). Fair tests of clinical trials: A treatment implementation model. *Advances in Behavioral Research Therapy, 16,* 1–29.

McAvay, G.J., Seeman, T.E., & Rodin, J. (1996). A longitudinal study of change in domain-specific self-efficacy among older adults. *Journal of Gerontology: Psychological Sciences, 51B,* P243–253.

Meillier, L.K., Lund, A.B., & Kok, G. (1997). Cues to action in the process of changing lifestyle. *Patient Education and Counseling, 30,* 37–51.

Miller, B., Campbell, R.T., Farran, C.J., Kaufman, J.E., & Davis, L. (1995). Race, control, mastery, and caregiver distress. *Journal of Gerontology: Social Sciences, 50B,* S374–382.

Moncher, F.J., & Prinz, R.J. (1991). Treatment fidelity in outcome studies. *Clinical Psychology Review, 11,* 247–266.

Morrison, M.F., Katz, I.R., Parmelee, P., Boyce, A.A., & TenHave, T. (1998). Dehydroepiandrosterone Sulfate (DHEA-S) and Psychiatric and Laboratory Measure of Frailty in a Residential Care Population. *The American Journal of Geriatric Psychiatry, 6,* 277–284.

O'Leary, K.D., & Borkovec, T.D. (1978). Conceptual, methodological, and ethical problems of placebo groups in psychotherapy research. *American Psychologist,* September, 821–830.

Prochaska, J.O., & DiClemente, C.C. (1983). Stages and processes of self-change in smoking: Toward an integrative model of change. *Journal of Consulting and Clinical Psychology, 5,* 390–395.

Prochaska, J.O., Redding, C.A., & Evers, K.E. (1997). The transtheoretical model and stages of change. In K. Glanz, F.M. Lewis, & B.K. Rimer (Eds.), *Health behavior and health education: Theory, research, and practice.* San Francisco: Jossey-Bass.

Schneider, L.S. (1996). New therapeutic approaches to Alzheimer's Disease. *Journal of Clinical Psychiatry, 57*(Suppl. 14), 30–36.

Schulz, R., Heckhausen, J., & O'Brien, A.T. (1994). Control and the disablement process in the elderly. *Journal of Social Behavior and Personality, 9,* 139–152.

Schulz, R., Visintainer, P., & Williamson, G.M. (1990). Psychiatric and physical morbidity effects of caregiving. *Journal of Gerontology: Psychological Sciences, 45,* P181–191.

Schulz, R., O'Brien, A.T., Bookwala, J., & Fleissner, K. (1995). Psychiatric and physical morbidity effects of dementia caregiving: Prevalence, correlates, and causes. *The Gerontologist, 35,* 771–791.

Spilker, B. (1996). *Guide to clinical trials.* Philadelphia: Lippincott-Raven.

Teri, L., & Logsdon, R.G. (1996). Methodologic issues regarding outcome measures for clinical drug trials of psychiatric complications in dementia. *Journal of Geriatric Psychiatry and Neurology, 8,* S1–S17.

Weissert, W.G., & Hedrick, S.C. (1994). Lessons learned from research on effects of community-based long-term care. *Journal of the American Geriatric Society, 42,* 348–353.

# 8

## From Intervention Studies to Public Policy: Translating Research into Practice

*Diane Feeney Mahoney, Robert Burns,*
*and Brooke Harrow*

### OVERVIEW

In the research arena, we can no longer be satisfied with conducting research and reporting scholarly findings. Rather, the scientific community, funding agencies, and the public increasingly expect researchers to report their findings in a manner that informs public policymakers' initiatives. Although researchers universally report the direct outcomes from their intervention studies, policy implications and outcomes are not necessarily discussed. In this chapter our intentions are to provide a background on the rationale for addressing policy issues in caregiving studies, to describe common cost analysis methodologies used in policy analyses, and to integrate examples that illustrate the linkage between research findings and public policy.

# POLICY BY DESIGN

Ideally, studies should be designed with policy implications in mind. In the classic words of Harold Lasswell (1936) public policies determine "who gets what, when, [and] how." The logic of policy deliberation defines the problem to be addressed, the participants involved, the ways the policy will affect them, its intended effects on society, and specifies the social and political values that the policy promotes (Fischer, 1995). While retrofitting research policy implications after study completion is not impossible, research findings may be limited when key policy relevant variables have been omitted. More robust and relevant findings can be achieved when policy implications are integrated into the research planning stage.

As discussed in chapter 2, although numerous studies have been conducted on caregiving issues, not all of these studies meet rigorous research standards. Since the relevance of research-derived policy implications is a recent development, studies that include research-driven policy implications comprise a smaller subset in the literature. One direction for future caregiving studies is to address policy-relevant data in research. A key question researchers need to consider is whether findings from a caregiving intervention research should become public policy? To answer this question, researchers must clearly understand the framework of policy analysis and contemporary caregiving policy issues.

In general, policy studies examine the organization, finance, and delivery of care and related services from the economic framework of supply and demand. The supply side considers the economic resources available to support the demand for services by a population. In chapter 1, the financial costs associated with caregiving were reviewed. That discussion reinforces the prevailing view understanding that caregiving services consume significant economic resources. The review also noted that demographers are projecting a growth in demand by the frail geriatric population most in need of services during a period when the pool of available family caregivers is expected to decline. The tension between the forces of supply and demand underpin policy analysis and form the basis for the concept of competing interests which is discussed later in our section on policy political analysis.

## Access

Issues of access to, quality, and appropriateness of services have traditionally been of interest to policy makers. During the early 1990s, public awareness and concerns arose from the realization that 37 million Americans did not have health insurance. With rising unemployment rates and fear of an economic recession, people became aware of the link between employment and insurance coverage (Young & Cohen, 1991). Later, as workers became re-employed, many still were unable to regain full insurance coverage because of the reduced benefits associated with part-time employment or insurance denial due to preexisting illness. A constituency of the uninsured and the underinsured was formed that gained policymaker's attention (Monheit, 1994).

Concurrently, business interest groups petitioned policymakers to reduce the escalating costs of health care that threatened their ability to remain competitive in the world marketplace while sustaining worker's health care benefits. Eventually, health care reform and cost containment became a major theme for President Clinton's first administration. The process and issues involved in the health care reform effort has made an intriguing policy case study and the interested reader is referred to Ginzberg and Ostow (1994) for their analysis.

Reform was doomed when policymakers and the stakeholders failed to reach consensus on a single plan for health care reform. Increasing pressures on the federal budget, public skepticism about a government-run health care program, and in-fighting among special interest groups derailed the momentum for health care reform. Whether macro (large scale) or micro (small scale) policy initiatives are proposed, the adoption of policy research findings is subject to the interplay of sociopolitical factors. The resulting fragmentation in coverage for long-term care services and a lack of access to and coverage for chronic care needs such as dementia caregiving (U.S. Office of Technology Assessment, 1987) remain as consequences of failed health care reform. Ironically, cost containment reforms have aggressively continued with the introduction of managed competition, capitated payments, and risk sharing initiatives. However, these cost reforms have raised questions about the quality of, access to health care, and the appropriateness of service delivery (Born &

Geckler, 1998; Brody & Bonham, 1997; Brook, 1997; Epstein, 1997; Fraser, 1997; Thurber, 1997).

In response to the growing concern of the public and its policymakers over quality issues, in March of 1997, President Clinton appointed an Advisory Commission on Consumer Protection and Quality in the Health Care Industry (Advisory Commission, 1997). The Agency for Health Care Policy and Research (AHCPR), a government agency whose mission is to improve health care quality through research and education, supported several research studies that began to investigate the impact of managed care on quality and the cost of care (Health Affairs, 1997). Analysts have suggested that solutions to long-term care issues may be found in partnerships between government insurance programs, private insurance policies, innovative forms of elder housing that integrate social and health care programs (Rivlin, Wiener, Hanley, & Spence, 1988). Caregiving studies are needed that scientifically assess the effects of health care reform as well as program innovations on service access, quality, and appropriateness of care.

## Disenfranchised Groups

Being portrayed as a group in need of assistance can be advantageous. Policymakers often promote policies that favor addressing underserved and disadvantaged populations, and researchers may consider highlighting their findings that have relevance for a disenfranchised group. Thoughtful consideration should be given to the policy implications. For example, older adults have held the status of an underserved population for many years. Social Security policies effectively addressed widespread poverty associated with older age at the turn of the century (Kingston & Schultz, 1996). Health care policymakers fostered support for programs to improve access to geriatric health care services through better insurance coverage. By the 1980s, an image of the "Greedy Geezer" arose. Fairlie (1989) portrayed older adults as selfishly consuming social resources to the detriment of other needy groups, specifically children's services. Callahan (1987, 1990) suggested that a disproportionate share of limited health care resources are spent on extending elderly lives without attention to the quality of life. He proposed rationing health care. Colorado's Governor Lamm viewed the elderly as an economic burden that compromised society's resources and the younger generation's future (Lamm, 1985). Although many gerontologists critique the accuracy of the Geezer image and argue that generational interdependence is a better policy framework (Binstock & Kahana, 1988; Kingson, Hirshorn, & Cornman, 1986; Bass & Caro, 1996), the need to do so demonstrates that the risk of successful policy initiatives is losing support when one group is perceived as advantaged relative to other population groups. Strategically, advocates agree that the Social Security and Medicare programs benefit older adults. They argue, however, that older people would be sorely disadvantaged without this government assistance given their considerable health care issues and that unmet needs remain, especially in long-term care (Bass, Kutzat, & Torres-Gil, 1990; Feder, 1990; National Committee to Preserve Social Security, 1996; Quadagno, 1996). The irony is that a major policy success can create a paradox with the loss of the disadvantaged status and preferential policy initiatives.

## Effectiveness, Efficiency, and Equity

When making determinations about the best course of action, public policy makers carefully consider effectiveness, efficiency, and equity (Eastaugh, 1987). Effectiveness assesses whether or not a project attained its intended goals or generated publicly recognized benefits. Efficiency is measured by the degree to which benefits outweigh resource costs. Equity assesses who benefits from a study; whether the program benefits many people or only a few with specialized needs.

From a research perspective relevant issues to be considered might be whether a new program or policy recommendation meets the target objectives more efficiently than alternative options, whether costs and benefits of the program/policy will be equitably distributed, and whether the program/policy has social relevance and societal value. Caregiver interventions that test new programs designed to change reimbursement policy should anticipate evaluations based on effectiveness, efficiency, and equity. Programs that consume scarce resources but remain underutilized by caregivers are inefficient. Program policy evaluations should examine the reasons for a potential subject's refusal to participate as well as participant's utilization characteristics and disenrollment trends for issues related to effectiveness, efficiency, and equity. For example, health services researchers have critiqued the effectiveness of common clinical treatment approaches and found that many that were assumed to be therapeutic were not effective (U.S. Preventive Services Task Force, 1996). Researchers should anticipate that caregiving interventions will be subjected to similar scrutiny for their effectiveness, efficiency, and equity.

## POLICY POLITICAL ANALYSIS

Policy analysis addresses the tensions between desirable goals and limited resources amid social and political forces. These forces can radically overturn policy directions (Mechanic, 1986), yet the reasons for such shifts are obscure.

Pessimists suggest that policy decisions emerge from an interplay of facts and ideals mediated by politics and therefore give little consideration to the public interest or wisdom. Conversely, optimists believe that social improvements based on compromise, mutual accommodation, and reliable information can emerge under such circumstances (Ricci, 1993). The Medicare catastrophic legislation passed in 1988 and repealed in 1989 illustrates how political forces influenced policy changes. Although the major intent of this legislation was to cover catastrophic medical care costs, a provision of the bill expanded Medicare coverage for 80 hours of home care per year. This provision was designed to give respite to primary informal caregivers after the deductible was met. Beneficiaries soon realized that significant payment increases would be levied on all participants for these benefits. In addition, projections indicated less than 20 percent of beneficiaries would meet the substantial deductible and be eligible for benefits. Public discontent escalated leading to rapid repeal of the legislation. Retrospective analyses showed that the preferences of the key stakeholders, the Medicare beneficiaries, had not been adequately considered, a critical error in determining the feasibility of program implementation.

## Stakeholders

Who are the stakeholders in caregiving research? They are the parties influencing or being influenced by the acceptance or rejection of a policy proposal. Generally in the field of caregiving research a constellation of entities have been identified as the key stakeholders: providers, insurers, payors, consumers of the care, and family members. The more organized and mobilized a group becomes, the more likely they will receive policymakers' attention.

Typically when special interest groups are discussed, thoughts turn to lobbyists and agents of business and industry. However, the health care field has counterparts in organizations such as the American Medical Association (AMA) and the American Hospital Association (AHA). Organized labor, though present, is less influential in the health and social welfare fields than in business. Think tanks, which multiplied rapidly in the 1970s and 1980s, also might be categorized as special interest groups whose purpose is to analyze and discuss policy relevant topics with governmental officials, the media, interest groups, sponsors, and the public (Ricci, 1993). According to Kingdon (1995, p. 47), "the lower the partisanship, ideological cast, and campaign visibility of the issues in a policy domain, the greater the importance of interest groups."

Public interest groups, comprised of consumers and advocates, have arisen to counterbalance efforts of business, labor, and professional interest groups. Two major advocacy groups concerned with caregiving are the Alzheimer's Association and the American Association of Retired Persons (AARP). The following comparison illustrates the differences in approaches taken by these groups to advocate for their constituencies. To form a larger constituency in need of legislated programs for long-term care, Lombardo (1991), a member of the National Board of Directors for the Alzheimer's Association, advocates combining the estimated 4 million Americans with Alzheimer's disease with the two million non-Alzheimer's cognitively impaired Americans. She cites similarities in needs among the two groups and among their caregivers and notes that some programs have been able to successfully combine care for "developmentally disabled and physically handicapped [persons] with dementia patients." She also acknowledges that "At the same time, the dementia specialized day care and in-home respite care programs [also] have been very well received" (Lombardo, 1991, p. 9). Her statements demonstrate the strategic positioning of the Alzheimer's advocate, hoping to merge different interest groups to form a larger political constituency for the greater good, while supporting the uniqueness of a subgroup's needs when sociopolitical forces indicate benefits are possible for that special interest group.

AARP has over 28 million members and it is the nation's largest advocacy organization for people age 50 plus. The group identifies advocacy, education, and community service as its organizational objectives although it also provides insurance coverage, a mail order pharmacy, and travel services. The advocacy branch of AARP does not position itself by diagnostic disease labels such as Alzheimer's disease but by broader issues such as caregiving for older adults. AARP positions itself as representing both the givers and receivers of care. Recently they cosponsored, along with the National Alliance for Caregiving, a national survey of family caregivers (discussed in chapter 1), that produced a clear portrayal of the magnitude of this constituency group and their important caregiving contributions. Legislatively, AARP supports expansion of services for all caregivers and provides numerous publications and programs to educate caregivers and their families. Kingdon summarizes the influence of interest groups by noting "The work of the interest groups vary according to their missions. Some of it is positive, promoting new courses of government action [based upon their preferred alternatives]; other activity is negative, seeking to block changes in public policy . . . that would reduce their benefits or prerogatives" (Kingdon, 1995, p. 49).

What should researchers share with these stakeholders and interest groups to encourage their support of your recommendations? According to Majchrzak (1984), stakeholders want to know the organizational structure needed for implementing your program or policy, the total resources needed for implementation, the policy mechanisms needed to encourage implementation, possible intended and unintended policy effects, and the anticipated outcomes if your program or recommendation is not implemented. For example, a caregiving intervention is tested using highly skilled professionals yet implementation is recommended in a setting where these professionals do not practice, then this organizational constraint will likely undermine an agency stakeholder's support. Another example might involve a finding that a highly intensive support program such as one-on-one in-home counseling several times a week over a year long period of time significantly improves caregiver well-being. While this intervention may receive support from caregivers, their families, and counselors, other competing interest groups with concerns about the cost and availability of labor resources needed to implement such a program may oppose it. Still others may be concerned about opportunity costs, which are the costs of doing something else with the same resources. In a fixed resource environment, adoption of a new program often is at the expense of an existing program. Researchers should anticipate opposition from stakeholders in the current program.

Being aware of stakeholders' concerns during the research design phase can allow for modifications to address these concerns. For example, instead of using a specialized professional, perhaps a staff member from the agency targeted to adopt this program could be taught how to do the intervention. Alternatively, the program could be tested with the highly specialized professional in one phase and a second research phase could assess results using agency staff members. Ideally, researchers should confer with stakeholders and address identified issues of oppositions during each phase of the study, as noted in chapter 4.

## Proponent and Opponent Views of Family Caregiver Compensation

As described in chapter 1, family and friends provide the most caregiving help to the frail elderly and are the key stakeholders when proposals for compensation of informal caregiving are discussed (Simon-Rusinowitz, Mahoney, & Benjamin, 1998). From a policy perspective, further research is needed to clarify the values that inform the circumstances under which caregiving is considered a family responsibility rather than a public responsibility (Kingson et al., 1986). The critical question remains—How should public and private caregiving responsibilities be divided?

Proponents of policies to offer benefits to family caregivers argue that without the unpaid homecare of family caregivers, public expenditures would be several times greater than current costs. Evidence of widespread substitution effects, that is withdrawal of family support when paid services are introduced, has not occurred (Tennstedt, Crawford, & McKinlay, 1993). Proponents argue that strengthening family caregiving through tax credits and or direct payment for services would ultimately save financial resources by reducing the utilization of formal paid services and costly institutionalization (Linsk, Keigher, & Osterbusch, 1988). The demographic imperative of the baby boomer generation makes this discussion very relevant. More families will be faced with caring for older relatives at a time when fewer family caregivers will be available due to women's entry into the workforce, declining numbers of children, and breaking of family ties due to relocation and divorce (Baines, Evans, & Neysmith, 1991). Feminist scholars favor policies for caregiver compensation to promote gender justice. They argue that society's dependence on women to provide the majority of unpaid caregiving places those who cannot work, or must leave employment to meet caregiving demands at a disadvantage economically (Osterbusch, Keigher, Miller, & Linsk, 1987).

Opponents to family caregiver compensation are concerned about equity issues. Given the large number of family caregivers, offering equitable benefits would be expensive and might result in compensation to minimally involved family members without increasing their caregiving responsibilities. Moreover, the most common recommendation has been to offer benefits in the form of tax credits. However, this compensatory approach disproportionately benefits more affluent families who are more likely able to afford to purchase the support they need. Another suggested alternative has been to model family compensation after entitlement programs that require financial means testing and have eligibility qualification. From an efficiency viewpoint, this solution would add cumbersome bureaucratic components that likely would hinder targeting assistance to primary caregivers in need. Without definitive ways to measure caregiver burden and the cost of caregiving, how can parity in compensating caregivers be judged by social value? Other opponents raise ethical issues suggesting that families are morally obligated to provide care and society should not have to pay them to meet their family responsibilities. And, one test program reported financial fraud from some family members who reported services that were not delivered in order to collect payments (Blaser, 1998). Further analysis of family compensation is beyond the scope of this chapter. For additional information, readers are referred to Linsk, Keigher, England, and Simon-Rusinowitz (1995) for their in-depth analysis of state-administered family compensation programs tested under Medicaid waivers. In summary, these researchers recommend the need for studies that are directed at determining the cost savings and excesses associated with family caregiving, "using different models of compensation, efficiency, and administrative arrangements" (p. 90). The next section will identify relevant data resources for researchers interested in conducting caregiver compensation and other policy-related caregiving studies.

## Data Sources for Policy-Related Secondary and Meta-Analyses

Numerous federally sponsored data sets on policy-relevant caregiving research are available. An inventory of these sources was compiled in the mid-80s at the request of congress (U.S. Congress, Senate 1986) when over 25 national databases were identified. The National Medical Expenditure Surveys (NMES), the Survey of Income and Program Participation (SIPP), and the National Nursing Home Survey (NNHS) have been prime sources for present day cost of care and service utilization studies. For example, findings from the Institutional Population component of the 1987 NMES provided the first national estimate that 7.6% of 22,064 nursing facilities had special units for Alzheimer's residents. The report further identified the characteristics of these facilities and the trend toward specialty programs (Leon, Potter, & Cunningham, 1990).

The 1982, 1984, and 1989 National Long Term Care Survey (NLTCS) of chronically disabled elders living in institutions and the community is another relevant caregiving database. This longitudinal series contains the "characteristics of all spouses and children of a large, nationally representative sample of disabled elders. It also documents the care each caregiver gives. This survey differs from earlier ones in that it is nationally representative and covers all spouses and children including those who do not give care" (Stone & Kemper, 1989, p. 489).

The National Claims History File (NCHF) contains Medicare beneficiary diagnostic data, health care utilization data, and provider costs. The Medicare Current Beneficiary Survey (MCBS), is a nationally representative sample of the Medicare population, provides Medicare utilization, and expenditure data linked to health status and function. The nursing home Minimum Data Set version 2.0 (MDS 2.0) provides resident level health and functional ability data and it is available nationwide. The Outcome and Assessment Statistical Information System (OASIS) has been developed for electronic report submission by home health agencies and is moving toward adoption. Additionally, a separate Minimum Data Set Home Care Version (MDS HC) has been adopted by the Medicaid program in several states. As electronic reporting expands to provide linkage capabilities across systems (while maintaining beneficiary confidentiality), policy-related studies that integrate issues of access, health status, health care utilization, and expenditure data will become more feasible.

National data sets do have limitations, such as difficulty linking files due to administrative, legal, subject confidentiality, and technical issues (Gilford, 1988). For example, to obtain data about the approximately six million Medicare and Medicaid dually eligible beneficiaries requires statewide linking capabilities currently available in only 12 states. Data in the State Medicaid Research Files (SMRF) are limited to claims information sent to HCFA by the 30 participating states and do not contain information on managed care programs or demonstration projects under Medicaid waivers. To promote more policy- and cost-related studies, the Health Care Financing Administration is currently sponsoring an initiative to assist researchers in managing the administrative and technical issues related to using and linking their files (Research Data Assistance Center (ResDAC), personal communication P. Homyak, March 13, 1998. HCFA Contract #500-96-0023/02).


## Policy Resources for Caregiving Issues Available on the Internet

Besides the traditional avenues of research inquiry, the Internet offers ready access to a variety of policy-relevant sites. A selected listing of these pertinent sites follows:

- Administration on Aging (AOA). http://www.aoa.dhhs.gov. Geriatric information for patients and practitioners, including treatment, policy issues, and links to other related resources is available at this site.
- Advisory Commission on Consumer Protection and Quality in the Health Care Industry. http://www.hcqualitycommission. gov. At this site, the commission posts copies of their reports and records the progress of their activities.
- Agency for Health Care Policy and Research (AHCPR). http:// www.nlm.nih.gov/HSTAT/AHCPR/desired guideline. This site provides full text versions of the agency sponsored clinical practice guidelines and the consumer versions.
- Alzheimer's Association. http://www.alz.org. This is the site at the national public advocacy organization for Alzheimer's Disease. The site provides a public policy section that lists the current advocacy activities including legislative initiatives at the state and federal levels.
- Alzheimer's Disease Education and Referral (ADEAR). http:// www.alzheimers.org. A service of the National Institute on Aging (NIA), this site provides information on Alzheimer's research being conducted through federally supported studies, consumer publications, and annual progress reports on Alzheimer's disease research.
- American Association of Retired Persons (AARP). http:// www.aarp.org/wwstand/caregiv.html. This site lists their numerous publications, programs, and resources available to assist older adults and their caregivers. For a fee, users can access AGELine, a database for aging-related information.
- Gerontological Society of America (GSA). http://www.geron. org. This site provides links to publications sponsored by the society and their legislative and policy updates.
- Health Care Financing Administration (HCFA). http:// www.hcfa.gov. As the U.S. governmental agency overseeing the Medicare program, this site provides information and utilization statistics for Medicare and Medicaid programs. State and federal data on long-term care services, Medicare and Medicaid managed care, as well as links to policy-related sites are available at this site.

- Healthfinder. http:// www.healthfinder.gov. This is a government portal website that provides access to consumer health information produced by federal and state governments and their partners. The site provides online documents, publications, databases, and technical medical information.
- National Committee for Quality Assurance (NCQA). http:// www.ncqa.org. A private, nonprofit organization that assesses and reports on the quality of managed care plans maintains this site. It offers a list of accredited HMOs and accreditation reports.
- National Institute on Aging (NIA). http://www.nih.gov/nia/ This site operated by a division of the National Institutes of Health, offers a Health Information section with publications that include the topic of Alzheimer's disease.
- NCOA National Council on the Aging, Inc. http:// www.ncoa.org. This site is maintained by a private nonprofit association of professional caregivers, educators, program administrators, and practitioners in the aging field. The association favors consumer-directed long-term care service models such as giving caregivers (of Americans with disabilities regardless of age) cash grants to purchase desired services.
- Social Security Medicare coverage. http://www.ssa.gov. This site offers the latest information on the Social Security application process, covered benefits, exclusions, and related policies.

## Making Policy Recommendations

Programs designed to address policy concerns are more likely to receive policymakers' attention and influence their actions. Recommendations that entail radical or major reforms, however, rarely are implemented. Although Medicare and Medicaid were initiated during President Johnson's Great Society era, their implementation resulted from a unique combination of bipartisan support, a favorable political and economic climate, and a highly visible large-scale constituency. A policy window of opportunity was created when forces converged to make the agenda of the Great Society, popular and appealing to diverse interest groups. When an issue "catches on" and receives astute stewardship, such as what Johnson provided to navigate the field of opposing forces, a major reform is possible. Thus, poignant vignettes from caregiving research, shared with a mobilized advocacy/special interest group, at a time when the subject is of great public interest, could "catch on" and directly influence a change in programmatic policy given a policy window of opportunity.

More typically, small-scale incremental reforms or marginal policy adjustments are made that result in gradual change (Lindblom, 1977). As the Robert Wood Johnson Foundation's State Initiatives in Health Care Reform program reported (1997), the states serve well as policy laboratories because they provide a manageable scale for testing health policy reforms. The Foundation's experience at the state level, however, informed them that justification cannot overcome public misgivings about instituting major attempts to over-haul the existing system and that incremental reform is more politically achievable. Thus, practical research suggestions should mesh well with the prevailing tendency toward incremental implementation. Rather than suggesting total coverage of supportive caregiving services under Medicare, fixed dollar benefits or hours of service limits may be accepted more readily. If researchers identify caregiver preferences and calculate the cost of benefits gained in terms of the reduction in caregiver stress or burden levels, then findings are translated into policy-relevant data.

Researchers must be wary, however, of making recommendations based upon simplistic models in which economic benefits outweigh resource costs. In caregiving situations, the benefits in productivity experienced by family caregivers due to an intervention substantially increase the benefit-cost ratio of interventions targeted to the chronically ill (Ross-Degan, Soumerai, Avorn, Bohn, Bright, & Aledort, 1995). For example, when a grandparent cares for his or her grandchildren, the average number of hours per week spent in child care giving is 14. The economic value of this care to the country has been estimated to range between $17 billion to $29 billion per year (Bass & Caro, 1996). Similarly, if a respite program allows a caregiver to provide previously unreported childcare services, the financial value of this additional productivity should be considered in the economic analysis.

# COST ANALYSIS

## The Role of Cost Analysis in Intervention Studies

Publicly funded intervention studies need to go beyond answering the question "Does it work?" and begin to answer "If it works, should we do it?" Observational caregiving studies can add to the body of knowledge and provide input into the development of caregiving interventions. However, caregiving intervention studies should implicitly, if not explicitly, provide information needed to make decisions on future implementation. Cost analysis is therefore a necessary component of these studies.

Cost analyses always have been a part of public policy decision making. It is not surprising that the implementation of policies and programs often are the result of political rather than economic decisions. Nevertheless, the cost of a potential program usually is estimated either to assist in the decision to implement a program or to gain support for the program after the decision has been made to implement it. Cost-effectiveness analysis and cost-benefit analysis, two types of cost analyses, are not new methodologies but recently have gained a larger role in policy decisions. Answering the question "Should we do it?" now requires not only cost data but also cost-effectiveness data.

The importance of cost-effectiveness analysis (CEA) is illustrated by the attention the U.S. Public Health Service (PHS) devotes to it. For example, not only is cost-effectiveness analysis considered a necessary component of research grants submitted to the National Institute of Health (NIH), but in 1993 the PHS also convened The Panel on Cost-Effectiveness in Health and Medicine (the Panel) which produced a book outlining their recommendations on methods for standardizing CEA in policy analyses (Gold, Siegel, Russell, & Weinstein, 1996).

## Types of Cost Analysis

The general term cost-effectiveness analysis (CEA) often is used to refer to cost analyses that describe cost per outcome of different interventions and also cost-benefit analysis (CBA) which puts a monetary value on both the intervention and the outcome. However, the results of a CBA often are perceived as more easily interpreted because the results are presented in terms of net benefits: i.e., how many dollars the intervention saved. CBA usually is chosen when the intervention being studied is expected to save dollars in medical costs. When efficiency is the only relevant goal, CBA may be used to look for the largest net benefits. However, CBA is difficult, if not impossible, to perform when the outcomes evaluated are improvements in psychological, social, behavioral, or health status measures.

CEA evaluates interventions or programs in terms of either their costs per unit of intermediate outcome, such as decrease in blood cholesterol level, or a final outcome such as years of life saved (Hurley, 1990; Mandelblatt et al., 1996). The cost per unit of outcome may be perceived as the "price" of an intervention. Using this price, decisions can be made on which programs would achieve the greatest benefits for a given dollar expenditure. Alternatively, if a certain level of outcome is desired, this price can be used to determine which program achieves a desired benefit at the lowest cost. However, it is not sufficient to use this "price" to answer the policy question, "How cost-effective is this intervention?" The cost-effectiveness of an intervention can only be established by comparing it to an alternative strategy designed to achieve the same outcome or by clearly defined cost-effectiveness criteria (Siegel, Weinstein, & Torrance, 1996). CEA calculates incremental costs and effectiveness to determine a cost-effectiveness ratio. This ratio is incremental costs (the difference in costs between an intervention and the alternative of interest) divided by the difference in outcomes of the two alternative options.

When CEA is used to evaluate a health or medical intervention, frequently the outcome is measured in terms of years of life saved or quality-adjusted years of life saved. This calculation, however, requires the incorporation of subjective patient preferences regarding years of life, healthy or sick (Hurley, 1990; Mandelblatt et al., 1997; Neumann & Johannesson, 1994). This type of CEA was once called "cost-utility" analysis. Using "years of life saved" or "quality-adjusted life year (QALY) saved" in CEA facilitates comparison of programs with different goals that may be competing for the same pool of health care resources. For example, the number of QALYs saved per dollar in a program designed to reduce cholesterol can be readily compared with QALYs saved from a cancer prevention program. However, the use of years of life saved or QALYs saved often requires estimates of morbidity and mortality from sources outside the intervention, and may thereby complicate CEA analysis. Further, the use of QALYs may be less appropriate when an intervention is not expected to have an effect on health status or life expectancy; i.e., an intervention designed to reduce caregiver burden.

Cost-of-illness analysis is performed to inform policy. This type of analysis may be part of a CEA or can stand alone. For example, a cost-effectiveness analysis of a new drug to prevent acute myocardial infarctions (AMI) might include a cost-of-illness analysis for AMIs in estimates of the cost of not taking the drug. Or, described below, a study that estimates the cost of caregiving for disabled or cognitively impaired elders can inform policies on public support for community based care (Harrow, Tennstedt, & McKinlay, 1995).

## Cost Perspective: Societal or Program

In any cost analysis the perspective of the analysis must be decided upon and made explicitly prior to any cost measurement activities. This is especially important when making cost-effectiveness comparisons since interventions may appear more or less cost-effective depending on the cost inclusion criteria of the CEA. There are broadly two perspectives, the societal perspective and the program perspective. The societal perspective seeks to find the total costs of an intervention regardless of who incurs the cost (Petitti, 1994). This perspective allows researchers to approximate true economic costs rather than accounting costs. Opportunity costs of resources, that is the cost of the next best alternative use, are included in this perspective, regardless of whether or not financial outlays are incurred. For example, if volunteers were used in an intervention, the dollar value of their time would be included in a cost analysis performed from a societal perspective. One problem using a societal perspective in cost analyses is that the hospital, government, or third-party payers make policy decisions rather than allowing society to make those decisions (Hurley, 1990). These institutional decision makers may be unconcerned about any costs that are not directly incurred by them. In contrast, the program perspective is concerned only with the immediate cost of an intervention and its outcome. The only costs considered are the actual outlays encountered in administering the intervention. Volunteer time would not be considered as a resource cost from the program perspective. Similarly, any intervention-induced savings in medical costs outside the program would not be considered when calculating the cost of the intervention (Petitti, 1994). The choice of which perspective to use depends on the purpose of the analysis. A CEA that compares two interventions may choose either perspective, as long as the same perspective is selected for both interventions. A cost analysis done for program planning purposes may be more appropriate from the program perspective.

## Methodology

Obtaining data on costs can be the most difficult part of cost analysis (Petitti, 1994). When planning the collection of costs, four rules should be followed. First, the greatest amount of attention should be placed on those categories of cost that account for the highest proportion of total cost. For example, for interventions that are very labor-intensive, it may be necessary to carefully measure all labor time with a system such as work logs to measure hours. Focusing the greatest attention on the highest share of costs reduces the potential measurement error. Second, careful recordkeeping practices should be implemented at the beginning of the intervention to avoid loss of cost information. This further avoids the problem of disentangling costs of the intervention from evaluation costs. These recordkeeping procedures should be practical and require minimal effort to assure accuracy and completeness. Third, collection of cost data should be in units (i.e., number of hours) as well as dollars to maximize the generalizability of the information. Recording the number of units allows for flexibility when deciding upon future application of the intervention. The more specific the information available, the more useful the results are from the intervention. Finally, the cost of the intervention should be kept separate from the evaluation or research study. This may be difficult if the same staff administers the intervention and evaluates the effects.

Take a full inventory of all potential costs before beginning the intervention also may be helpful. Weinstein and Fineberg (1980) provide a useful categorization of four types of cost: direct cost, overhead, induced costs, and indirect costs. Direct costs include equipment, labor, materials, and any incentive payments. Overhead encompasses the rent or building depreciation, space preparation, maintenance, utilities, support services, and other administrative services. Induced costs are limited to medical treatments (e.g., physician visits or laboratory tests) added or avoided. Indirect costs include lost wages and productivity. The choice of which category depends upon the perspective of the analysis. For example, if a CEA were to be done from the program perspective, the indirect cost category would not be necessary since this category includes measures of cost relevant only to a societal perspective. For each cost category, costs must be further detailed to include every resource use that would not have existed without the intervention. For example, under direct cost, the labor would include the wages for the staff performing the intervention such as therapists leading the caregiver support groups. It is important to not ignore costs for inputs without market prices (Guyatt et al., 1986). Therefore, if using volunteers in a community intervention, the costs of their time should be considered so that the estimated costs of reproducing the intervention, without the benefit of unpaid volunteers, would be accurate.

Cost-effectiveness ratios can be calculated once the final outcomes of an intervention are known and all costs have been collected. These ratios can reflect either average cost or incremental cost. Average cost-effectiveness ratios reflect the cost per benefit of a particular strategy independent of alternate strategies (Detsky & Naglie, 1990). Incremental cost-effectiveness ratios reveal the cost per unit of outcome of switching from one strategy to another. The numerator and denominator of the ratio represent differences between the alternative interventions. The numerator is the cost of the intervention minus the cost of the alternative, while the denominator is the effect of the intervention minus the effect of the alternative (Detsky & Naglie, 1990; Mandelblatt et al., 1996; Weinstein & Stason, 1977). With cost-benefit analysis, a comparable ratio is not typically calculated. Instead, net benefits are calculated by subtracting the costs of an intervention from the monetized benefits (which could represent avoided costs).

## The Role of Cost Analysis in Caregiving Research and Policy

Of the many evaluation studies of caregiver interventions, (e.g., Brodaty, 1994; Brennan, Moore, & Smyth, 1995; Clark & Rakowski, 1983; Collins, Given, & Given, 1994; Farran & Keane-Hagerty, 1994; Gallagher, 1985; Gallagher, Lovett, & Zeiss, 1989; Haley & Pardo, 1989; Haley, Brown, & Levine, 1987; Lawton, Brody, & Saperstein, 1989; Lombardo & Aronson, 1995; Mittelman, Ferris, Steinberg, Shulman, Mackell, Ambinder, & Cohen, 1993; Ripich, 1994; Robinson & Yates, 1994; Toseland & Rossiter, 1989; Toseland & Smith, 1990; Toseland, Labrecque, Goebel, & Whitney, 1992; Toseland, Rossiter, & Labrecque, 1989; Toseland, Rossiter, Peak, & Smith, 1990; Zarit & Zarit, 1982; Zarit, 1991; Zarit, Anthony, & Boutselis, 1987; Zarit, Orr, & Zarit, 1985), few have included a cost analysis (Brodaty & Peters, 1991; Drummond et al., 1991; Oktay & Volland, 1990; Weinberger et al., 1993). Several possible reasons have been suggested for the lack of cost analyses in the caregiving intervention literature. Lombardo and Aronson (1995) in their overview of caregiving research, argue that caregiving research is still in the early stages of development and suffers from a lack of good definitions of cost-effectiveness. Second, Altman (1986) has contended evaluators of interventions often give cost analysis a lower priority than examining overall endpoint effects. Difficulty in measuring costs also has been noted. When evaluators do perform cost analysis, it is often done ex poste. However, Rossi and Freeman (1993) point out in their book *Evaluation Research,* that the information routinely available from an evaluation may prove insufficient for a retrospective cost analysis.

Relative to the number of cost analyses of caregiver interventions performed, there has been a greater number of studies analyzing the cost of caregiving. A number of studies have attempted to quantify the total costs of caring for older persons with Alzheimer's Disease or other dementia, including the costs of both formal services provided by agencies as well as the informal care provided by family and friends (Ernst & Hay, 1994; Hay & Ernst, 1987; Hu, Huang, & Cartwright, 1986; Max, Webber, & Fox, 1995; Rice et al., 1993; Weinberger et al., 1993). In 1985, Hu et al. (1986) estimated annual caregiving costs at $11,735. Hay and Ernst (1987) made similar estimates of $8,939 for informal services and $1,774 for formal home care. More recent cost estimates suggest annual informal caregiving costs for persons with Alzheimer's Disease to range between $34,000 (Max et al., 1995; Rice et al., 1993) and $36,000 (Weinberger et. al., 1993) while formal home care costs range between $2,900 (Weinberger et al., 1993) and $9,600 (Rice et al., 1993). Harrow, Tennstedt, and McKinlay (1995) have estimated the economic costs of community care in an elder population disabled by limitations in activities of daily living to be $9,600, including both informal care and formal services. These estimates of community based care can inform policy by identifying the quantity, types, and costs of formal services that would be needed if the provision of informal care diminishes (Harrow, Tennstedt, & McKinlay, 1995).

## TRANSLATING RESEARCH INTO HEALTH CARE DELIVERY REFORM AND/OR PUBLIC POLICY

As noted earlier, the relationship between research and policy is complex and often confusing. Numerous obstacles may be encountered in moving from a research finding to an implemented policy; and, unfortunately, there is no precise formula for this translation. Davis and Howden-Chapman (1996, p. 868) note "A theoretical orientation that is open to the possibilities for sociopolitical change and methodological precepts that are appropriate to the analysis of systemic and structural questions are obviously essential preconditions for the conduct of policy-relevant research. Equally important, however, is the need to embed research within a conceptual framework that will facilitate its ready translation into policy."

Thus, as mentioned previously, the translation process actually begins early in the research phase with selection of an appropriate theoretical orientation, methodology, and conceptual framework. To further the translation process of converting research into policy or health care delivery reform, however, requires three major additional steps. The first step is the accumulation of sufficient evidence to support the effectiveness of interventions for a targeted illness or health care problem. This body of evidence may encompass an array of research approaches ranging from epidemiologic research to complex interventions and clinical trials. It would have to be an extraordinary situation for a single study to lead to a policy decision or change in health care delivery. What is necessary is an accumulation of studies clearly supporting the effectiveness of the proposed interventions.

The second major step entails a cost-effectiveness or cost-benefit analysis of the intervention. The analytic approaches to assessing cost in health care interventions have been discussed thoroughly in the preceding paragraphs. In translating research to health care delivery reform or public policy, the objective of cost analysis, of course, is to demonstrate that the proposed intervention, in addition to conferring a health benefit, demonstrates a cost benefit when compared to alternative strategies of treatment. This step has become particularly relevant in today's atmosphere of cost containment and managed care.

The final major step is for the intervention to receive external validation from a consensus group. The consensus group may represent a professional group or organization such as the Gerontological Society of America, a government organization such as the National Institutes of Health, or a component agency, an insurer, or a health plan. The consensus panel or their endorsing statement can help shape and influence policy through the development of a standard of care and potentially a reimbursed intervention.

Given this model, the translation process can be enhanced in several ways; and, ideally, the translation process should be tailored to the individual research strategy. For example, with the REACH research project, a theoretical framework was first developed that encapsulated the fundamentals of behavioral intervention in caregiving. Next, the pragmatics of implementing the proposed range of interventions were carefully scrutinized, incorporating a degree of flexibility that permitted each site to tailor intervention strategies to meet the needs of individual sites. The next step was to develop and/or modify measurement instruments to adequately and accurately assess the interventions and their outcomes, including cost-effectiveness. Thus, as the REACH project demonstrates, during each phase of research design, emphasis should be placed on the feasibility of translating a successful research project into an effective health care reform strategy.

Moving from the realm of research to the application of research as health care reform or public policy often depends to some degree on the nature of the research itself and on the type of health care change being contemplated. For example, when research is funded by an agency or organization that later may elect to apply the research results, translating research into health care reform or public policy may be more easily initiated by that agency than by an agency or organization outside the research setting (Davis & Howden-Chapman, 1996). Though this situation potentially may raise ethical questions or issues about conflicts of interest, the translation process is, nevertheless, simplified. Similarly, research that targets a carefully defined subpopulation of individuals may be more easily translated into health care reform or public policy than one aimed at a less homogeneous patient population.

In today's research climate, media exposure also can adversely or favorably influence the translation process. Grassroots efforts by patient advocacy and support groups often enlist the support of the media to advance their demands for health care changes as demonstrated by the recent changes in the availability of drug "cocktail" treatments for AIDS patients. Conversely, one need look no further than the abortion issue to see the influence media exposure can have when activists rally media support. In this age of dynamic telecommunications innovations, the concept of media exposure now must embrace the computer Internet and Worldwide Web systems, satellite communications, and audiovisual programs. Access to information age technologies can play a significant role in translating research findings into health care delivery and public policy.

Just as advocacy can change the tone and focus of policy decisions, other intangible factors also can influence the conversion of research into health policy. Certain health care conditions, because of their prevalence or cost of care, will be much more visible and therefore more influential in generating policy change. Furthermore, conditions that currently are costly to treat may effect policy change if new interventions are implemented that produce significant cost savings.

Once analyzed and reported, research can and does serve as a springboard for initiating health care change, public policy reform, or both. This translation process may operate at several levels. For example, most researchers conclude their research reports with recommendations or suggestions for further use of their findings, whether for actual application or the need for additional research. Although their influence is indirect, these suggestions and recommendations can effect the translation of research into policy simply by instigating a change in approach for later studies. In some instances, however, specific research projects have blossomed into applied health care policies or reform that are assimilated into mainstream care. As noted earlier, the assimilation process most often takes place at an incremental pace, yet the translation of research to policy is evident. Several examples are discussed below.

Influenza infection subjects older adults to considerable morbidity and increased risk of mortality. Epidemiologic data has demonstrated significant risk of death and utilization of hospital days during influenza infections. However, clinical trials of influenza vaccination have shown a reduction in both morbidity and mortality from influenza. Cost benefit analyses have reported direct savings of $117 per person vaccinated with a total savings of nearly $5 million (Nichol, Margolis, Wuorenmna, & von Sternberg, 1994). All professional medical and public health groups now endorse and advocate yearly influenza vaccination. In addition, after research data indicated a consensus of approval for the vaccine, Medicaid and Medicare policies were changed to include influenza vaccination as a covered benefit. Reimbursement for the vaccination likely provided additional motivation for participation. Influenza vaccination thus may serve as a prototypical clinical intervention that has successfully been translated from research findings to policy for health care delivery.

Screening mammography provides an example of the challenges encountered in translating research findings into health care policy. Although mammography often is viewed as an integral part of early detection of breast cancer, several issues surrounding the translation of breast cancer research to health care policy remain controversial. To date, there is no consensus on the age at which women should receive baseline mammography, the frequency of mammography for various age groups, or guidelines for alteration in the routine schedules based on clinical variables. The confusion and controversy is fueled, in part, by conflicting research data which do not consistently implicate one strategy or approach over others in these issues. Furthermore, Waller and Batt (1995, p. 829) note that an additional issue receiving attention in both the U.S. and Canada is the demand by breast cancer patient advocates for "greater participation in decision making with respect to research." Finally, a recent consensus conference summary was overturned with a conflicting decision, which fundamentally alters the difficult, but logical process from research to policy (Fletcher, 1997). Thus, though research findings have shown that mammography is an effective screening tool, the translation of those findings into health care delivery has resulted in variable implementation and reimbursement for the procedure with an uncertain impact on both health care outcomes and costs.

As with breast cancer screening, prostate cancer screening continues to be shrouded in controversy. Despite decades of research, no consensus has been reached about screening in general. The primary obstacle may be the uncertainty regarding treatment and outcomes of prostate cancer. Although there are effective treatments, translating those treatments into effective clinical outcomes; i.e., decreased mortality, is not clear. Thus, with an uncertainty regarding treatment, the issues surrounding screening such as which populations to screen, how often to screen, and how to actually screen for prostate cancer are made more uncertain. Because of these gaps in knowledge, to date there are no consensus statements regarding guidelines for screening. Furthermore, because of these limitations, Medicare does not pay for prostate cancer screening.

As these examples have illustrated, translating research into public policy or health care delivery reform can be a complicated, protracted task. However, the task can be eased with well-designed studies that incorporate sound theoretical approaches and stringent methodologies within a conceptual framework that fosters commensurable analyses.

Besides strengthening the scientific approach to research, what else can be done to ease the process of translating research findings into health care delivery reform and/or public policy? Recently, Glasgow (1996, p. 1166) observed that "research and policy/advocacy activities" coexist on fields that are "separate but equal." Though his comment was directed toward the field of diabetes care, it could readily apply to research and policy in general. Perhaps more thoroughly integrating research and policy, not just in research design, but conceptually in our ideology would enhance their utility and foster a meshing of these complementary activities.

One effective way to further the union of research and policy is to encourage an interdisciplinary approach to research and to require interdisciplinary training for all research team members. This strategy can accommodate lay persons as well as scientists. As Waller and Batt (1995) suggest, the notion that physicians and scientists are the only individuals capable of making contributions to research policy decisions is outdated.

Another method of narrowing the gap between research and policy lies in dissemination of research findings. No longer should researchers be content with limited distribution of research results. We all have a stake in the research findings and the policy implications of research. Finally, we must all accept the fact that there are limitations to what constitutes health care and the resources available to pay for it. Through a broader understanding of the science of a specific area, coupled with realistic expectations of resources to provide those services, we can begin to shape a rational health care strategy that matches the potential of science to the realities of our resources. At that intersection, then we can begin to meaningfully effect the health status of the population (Blumstein, 1997).

## REFERENCES

Advisory Commission on Consumer Protection and Quality in the Health Care Industry. (1997). http://www.hcqualitycommission.gov.

Baines, C.T., Evans, P.M., & Neysmith, S.M. (1991). Caring: Its impact on the lives of women. In C.T. Baines, P.M. Evans, & S.M. Neysmith (Eds.). *Women's caring: Feminist perspectives on social welfare* (pp. 11–35). Toronto: McClelland & Stewart.

Bass, S., Kutza, E., & Torres-Gil, F.M. (1990). *Diversity in aging: Challenges facing planners and policymakers in the 1990's.* Glenview, IL: Scott, Foresman and Company.

Bass, S., & Caro, F. (1996, Spring). The economic value of grandparent assistance. *Generations*, 29–33.

Binstock, R.H., & Kahana, J. (1988). An essay on setting limits: Medical goals in an aging society. *Gerontologist, 28*, 424–426.

Blaser, C.J. (1998). The case against paid family caregivers: Ethical and practical issues. *Generations, 22*(3), 65–69.

Blumstein, J. F. (1997). The Oregon experiment: The role of cost-benefit analysis in the allocation of Medicaid funds. *Social Science and Medicine, 45*, 545–554.

Born, P., & Geckler, C. (1998). HMO quality and financial performance: Is there a connection? *Journal of Health Care Finance, 24*(2), 65–77.

Brennan, P.F., Moore, S.M., & Smyth, K.A. (1995). The effects of a special computer network on caregivers of persons with Alzheimer's disease. *Nursing Research, 44*(3), 166–172.

Brodaty, H., & Peters, K.E. (1991). Cost effectiveness of a training program for dementia carers. *Int Psychogeriatr, 3*(1), 11–22.

Brodaty, H. Can interventions with family caregivers make a difference to them and to people with dementia? Presented at the Fourth International Conference on Alzheimer's Disease and Related Disorders, Minneapolis, MN (4th ICADRD-MN'94); July 29, 1994, and abstracted in *Neurobiol Aging* August 1994; 15(Suppl I): S3.

Brody, H., & Bonham, V.L. (1997, Oct 13). Gag rules and trade secrets in managed care contracts. Ethical and legal concerns. *Archives of Internal Medicine, 157*(18), 2037–2043.

Brook, R.H. (1997, Nov 19). Managed care is not the problem, quality is. *Journal of the American Medical Association, 278*(19), 1612–1614.

Callahan, D. (1987). *Setting limits.* New York: Simon and Schuster.

Callahan, D. (1990). *What kind of life.* New York: Simon and Schuster.

Clark, N.M., & Rakowski, W. (1983). Family caregivers of older adults: Improving helping skills. *Gerontologist, 23*, 637–642.

Collins, C.E., Given, B.A., & Given, C.W. (1994). Interventions with family caregivers of persons with Alzheimer's Disease. *Nursing Clinics of North America, 29*(1), 195–207.

Davis, P., & Howden-Chapman, P. (1996). Translating research findings into health policy. *Social Science & Medicine, 43*, 865–872.

Detsky, A.S., & Naglie, I.G. (1990). A Clinician's Guide to Cost-Effectiveness Analysis. *Annals of Internal Medicine, 113*(2), 147–154.

Drummond, M.F., Mohide, E.A., Tew, M., Streiner, D.L., Pringle, D.M., & Gilbert, J.R. (1991). Economic evaluation of a support program for caregivers of demented elderly. *Int J Technol Assess Health Care, 7*(2), 209–219.

Eastaugh, S.R. (1987). *Financing Health Care, Economic efficiency and equity.* Dover, MA: Auburn House Publishing Company.

Epstein, A.M. (1997, Nov 19). Medicaid managed care and high quality. Can we have both? *Journal of the American Medical Association, 278*(19), 1617–1621.

Ernst, R.L., & Hay, J.W. (1994). The U.S. economic and social costs of Alzheimer's disease revisited. *Am J Public Health, 84*(8), 1261–1264.

Fairlie, H. (1989, March 28). Talking about my generation. *New Republic,* 19–22.

Farran, C.J., & Keane-Hagerty, E. (1994). Interventions for caregivers of persons with dementia: Educational support groups and Alzheimer's association support groups. *Applied Nursing Research, 7*(3), 112–117.

Feder, J. (1990). Health care of the disadvantaged: The elderly. *Journal of Health Politics, Policy and Law, 15*(2), 259–269.

Fischer, F. (1995). *Evaluating public policy.* Chicago: Newlson-Hall Publishers.

Fletcher, S.W. (1997). Whither scientific deliberation in health policy recommendations? *The New England Journal of Medicine, 336*, 1180–1183.

Fraser, I. (1997). Access to health care. In T.J. Litman & L.S. Robins (Eds.), *Health politics and policy* (pp. 288–305). Boston: Delmar Publishers.

Gallagher, D., Lovett, S., & Zeiss, A. (1989). Intervention with caregivers of frail elderly persons. In M.G. Ory & K. Bond (Eds.), *Aging and health care: Social science and policy perspectives.* New York: Routledge.

Gallagher, D. (1985). Intervention strategies to assist caregivers of frail elders: Current research status and future research directions. In M.P. Lawton & G. Maddox (Eds.), *Annual Review of Gerontology and Geriatrics. Vol. 5.* New York: Springer.

Gilford, D.M. (1988). *The Aging Population in the Twenty-first Century, Statistics for Health Policy.* Washington, DC: National Academy Press.

Ginzberg, E., & Ostow, M. (1994). *The road to reform the future of health care.* New York: The Free Press, Macmillan, Inc.

Glasgow, R.E. (1996). Are research and policy advocacy two separate worlds? *Diabetes Care, 1*, 1165–1166.

Gold, M.R., Siegel, J.E., Russell, L.B., & Weinstein, M.C. (Eds.). (1996). *Cost-Effectiveness in Health and Medicine: Report of the Panel on Cost-Effectiveness in Health and Medicine.* New York: Oxford University Press.

Guyatt, G., Drummond, M., Feeny, D., Tugwell, P., Stoddart, G., Haynes, R.B., Bennett, K., & Labelle, R. (1986). Guidelines for the clinical and economic evaluation of health care technologies. *Social Science and Medicine, 22*(4), 393–408.

Haley, W.E., & Pardo, K.M. (1989). Relationship of severity of dementia to caregiving stressors. *Psychol Aging, 4*(4), 389–392.

Haley, W.E., Brown, S.L., & Levine, E.G. (1987). Experimental evaluation of the effectiveness of group intervention for dementia caregivers. *Gerontologist, 27*(3), 376–382.

Harrow, B.S., Tennstedt, S.L., & McKinlay, J.B. (1995). How costly is it to care for disabled elders in a community setting? *Gerontologist, 35*(6), 803–813.

Hay, J.W., & Ernst, R.L. (1987). The economic costs of Alzheimer's disease. *Am J Public Health, 77*(9), 1169–1175.

Health Affairs. (1997). Special issue on the impact of managed care on quality. *Health Affairs, 16*(6).

Hu, T.W., Huang, L.F., & Cartwright, W.S. (1986). Evaluation of the costs of caring for the senile demented elderly: A pilot study. *Gerontologist, 26*(2), 158–163.

Hurley, S. (1990). A review of cost-effectiveness analyses. *The Medical Journal of Australia, 153*(Suppl.), S20–S23.

Kingdon, J.W. (1995). *Agendas, Alternatives, and Public Policies.* 2nd ed. New York: HarperCollins College Publishers.

Kingson, E.R., Hirshorn, B.A., & Cornman, J.M. (1986). *Ties That Bind, The interdependence of generations.* Washington, DC: Seven Locks Press.

Kingston, E., & Schultz, J. (1996). *Social Security in the Twenty-first Century.* Cary, NC: Oxford University Press.

Lamm, R. (1985). *Mega-Traumas, America at the Year 2000.* Boston: Houghton Mifflin.

Lasswell, H. (1936). *Who Gets What, When, How.* New York: McGraw-Hill.

Lawton, Powell, M., Brody, E., & Saperstein, A. (1989). A controlled study of respite service for caregivers of Alzheimer's patients. *Gerontologist, 29*(1), 8–16.

Leon, J., Potter, D., & Cunningham, P. (1990). *Current and projected availability of special nursing home programs for Alzheimer's disease patients.* (DHHS Publication No. (PHS) 90-3463. National Medical Expenditure Survey Data summary 1, Agency for Health Care Policy and Research. Rockville, MD: Public Health Service.

Lindblom, C.E. (1977). *Politics and markets.* New York: Basic Books Inc.

Linsk, N.L., Keigher, S.M., & Osterbusch, S.E. (1988). States' policies regarding paid family caregiving. *Gerontologist, 28,* 204–212.

Linsk, N.L., Keigher, S.M., England, S.E., & Simon-Rusinowitz, L. (1995). Compensation of family care for the elderly. In R. Kane & J.D. Penrod (Eds.), *Family caregiving in an aging society: Policy perspectives* (pp. 64–91). Thousand Oaks, CA: Sage Publications.

Lombardo, N. (1991). Cognitive impairment: Policy implications for service design. *The American Journal of Alzheimer's Care and Related Disorders & Research, 6*(2), 4–18.

Lombardo, N.E., & Aronson, M.K. (1995). Caregiving research: An overview. In K. Iqbal, J.A. Mortimer, B. Winblad, & H.M. Wisniewski (Eds.), *Research Advances in Alzheimer's Disease and Related Disorders.* New York: John Wiley & Sons.

Mandelblatt, J.S., Fryback, D.G., Weinstein, M.C., Russell, L.B., Gold, M.R., & Hadorn, D.C. (1996). Assessing the effectiveness of health interventions. In Gold, M.R., Siegel, J.E., Russell, L.B., & Weinstein, M.C. (Eds.), *Cost-Effectiveness in Health and Medicine: Report of the Panel on Cost-Effectiveness in Health and Medicine.* New York: Oxford University Press.

Mandelblatt, J.S., Fryback, D.G., Weinstein, M.C., Russell, L.B., & Gold, M.R. (1997). Assessing the effectiveness of health interventions for cost-effectiveness analysis. *Journal of General Internal Medicine, 12*(9), 551–558.

Majchrzak, S. (1984). *Methods for Policy Research. Applied Social Research Methods Series, Vol.3.* Newbury Park, CA: Sage Publications, Inc.

Max, W., Webber, P., & Fox, P. (1995). Alzheimer's disease: The unpaid burden of caring. *Journal of Aging and Health, 7,* 179–199.

Mechanic, D. (1986). *From advocacy to allocation.* New York: The Free Press, Macmillan, Inc.

Mittelman, M.S., Ferris, S.H., Steinberg, G., Shulman, E., Mackell, J.A., Ambinder, A., & Cohen, J. (1993). An intervention that delays institutionalism of Alzheimer's disease patients: Treatment of spouse caregivers. *Gerontologist, 33*(6), 730–740.

Monheit, A. (1994). Underinsured Americans: A review. *Annual Review Public Health, 15,* 461–484.

National Committee to Preserve Social Security and Medicare. (1996, May). *Social Security Privatization.* Washington, D.C.

Neumann, P.J., & Johannesson, M. (1994). From Principle to Public Policy: Using Cost-Effectiveness Analysis. *Health Affairs Summer,* 206–214.

Nichol, K.L., Margolis, K.L., Wuorenmna, J., & von Sternberg, T. (1994). The efficacy and cost effectiveness of vaccination against influenza among elderly persons living in the community. *New England Journal of Medicine, 331,* 778–784.

Oktay, J.S., & Volland, P.J. (1990). Post-hospital support program for the frail elderly and their caregivers: A quasi-experimental evaluation. *American Journal of Public Health, 80*(1), 39–46.

Osterbusch, S.E., Keigher, S.M., Miller, B., & Linsk, N.L. (1987). Community care policies and gender justice. *International Journal of Health Services, 17*(2), 217–232.

Petitti, D.B. (1994). *Meta-analysis decision analysis and cost-effectiveness analysis: Methods for quantitative synthesis in medicine.* New York: Oxford University Press.

Quadagno, J. (1996). Social Security and the myth of the entitlement "crisis." *Gerontologist, 36*(3), 391–399.

Ricci, D.M. (1993). *The Transformation of American Politics, The New Washington and The Rise of Think Tanks.* New Haven: Yale University Press.

Rice, D.P., Fox, P.J., Max, W., Webber, P.A., Lindeman, D.A., Hauck, W.W., & Segura, E. (1993). The economic burden of Alzheimer's disease care. *Health Affairs, 12*(2), 164–176.

Ripich, D.N. (1994). Functional communication with AD patients: A caregiver training program. *Alzheimer Dis Assoc Disord, 8,* Suppl 3, 95–109.

Rivlin, A.M., Wiener, J.M., Hanley, R., & Spence, D.A. (1988) *Caring for the Disabled Elderly Who Will Pay?* Washington, DC: The Brookings Institute.

Robert Wood Johnson Foundation. (1997). *State Health Care Reform: Looking Back Toward the Future.* Princeton, N.J.

Robinson, K., & Yates, K. (1994). Effects of two caregiver-training programs on burden and attitude toward help. *Archives Psychiatric Nursing, (8)*5, 312–319.

Ross-Degan, D., Soumerai, S., Avorn, J., Bohn, R., Bright, R., & Aledort, L. (1995). Hemophilia home treatment. Economic analysis and implications for health policy. *International Journal of Technology Assessment in Health Care, 11*(2), 327–344.

Rossi, P.H., & Freeman, H.E. (1993). *Evaluation: A Systematic Approach, 5th edition.* California: Sage Publications, Inc.

Siegel, J.E., Weinstein, M.C., & Torrance, G.W. (1996). Reporting cost-effectiveness studies and results. In M.R. Gold, J.E. Siegel, L.B. Russell, & M.C. Weinstein (Eds.), *Cost-Effectiveness in Health and Medicine: Report of the Panel on Cost-Effectiveness in Health and Medicine.* New York: Oxford University Press.

Simion-Rusinowitz, L., Mahoney, K.J., & Benjamin, A.E. (1988). Payments to families who provide care: An option that should be available. *Generations, 22*(3), 69–75.

Stone, R.I., & Kemper, P. (1989). Spouses and children of disabled elders: How large a constituency for long-term care reform? *The Milbank Quarterly, 67*(3–4), 485–506.

Tennstedt, S.L., Crawford, S.L., & McKinlay, J.B. (1993). Is family care on the decline? A longitudinal investigation of the substitution of formal long-term care services for informal care. *The Milbank Quarterly, 71*(4), 601–624.

Thurber, C.F. (1997). Quality and managed care: Where is the fit? *American Journal of Medical Quality, 12*(4), 177–182.

Toseland, R.W., & Rossiter, C.M. (1989). Group interventions to support family caregivers: A review and analysis. *Gerontologist, 29*(4), 438–448.

Toseland, R.W., Rossiter, C.M., Peak, T., & Smith, G.C. (1990). Comparative effectiveness of individual and group interventions to support family caregivers. *Social Work, May,* 209–217.

Toseland, R.W., Labrecque, M.S., Goebel, S.T., & Whitney, M.H. (1992). An evaluation of a group program for spouses of frail elderly veterans. *Gerontologist, 32*(3), 382–390.

Toseland, R.W., Rossiter, C.M., & Labrecque, M.S. (1989). The effectiveness of three group intervention strategies to support family caregivers. *Am J Orthopsychiatry, 59*(3), 420–429.

Toseland, R.W., & Smith, G.C. (1990). Effectiveness of individual counseling by professional and peer helpers for family caregivers of the elderly. *Psychol Aging, 5*(2), 256–263.

U.S. Congress, Senate. (1986). *Statistical Policy for an Aging Society.* Joint Hearing of the Subcommittee on Aging, Committee on Governmental Affairs, and the Subcommittee on Energy, Nuclear Proliferation and Government Processes. 99th Congress, 2nd Session. Washington, D.C.

U.S. Office of Technology Assessment. (1987). *Losing a million minds: Confronting the tragedy of Alzheimer's Disease and other dementias.* OTA-BA-323. Washington, DC: U.S. Government Printing Office.

U.S. Preventive Services Task Force. (1996). *Guide to clinical preventive services,* 2nd ed. Baltimore: Williams & Wilkins.

Waller, M., & Batt, S. (1995). Advocacy groups for breast cancer patients. *Canadian Medical Association Journal, 152,* 829–833.

Weinberger, M., Gold, D., Divine, G.W., Cowper, P.A., Hodgson, L.G., Schreiner, P.J., & George, L.N. (1993). Expenditures in caring for patients with dementia who live at home. *Journal of Public Health, 83,* 338–341.

Weinstein, M.C., & Feinberg, H.V. (1980). *Clinical Decision Analysis.* Philadelphia: W.B. Saunders Company.

Weinstein, M.C., & Stason, W.B. (1977). Foundations for cost-effectiveness analysis for health and medical practices. *New England Journal of Medicine, 296,* 716–721.

Young, G., & Cohen, B. (1991). Inequities in Hospital Care, the Massachusetts experience. *Inquiry, 28,* 255–262.

Zarit, S.H., Anthony, C.R., & Boutselis, M. (1987). Interventions with caregivers of dementia patients: A comparison of two approaches. *Psychology and Aging, 2,* 225–232.

Zarit, S.H., Orr, N., & Zarit, J.M. (1985). *The Hidden Victims of Alzheimer's Disease: Families Under Stress.* New York: New York University Press.

Zarit, S.H., & Zarit, J.M. (1982). Families under stress: Interventions for caregivers of senile dementia patients. *Psychotherapy: Theory, Research, and Practice, 19,* 461–471.

Zarit, S.H. (1991). Intervention with frail elders and their families: Are they effective and why? In M.A.P. Stephens, J.H. Crowther, S.E. Hobfoll, et al. (Eds.), *Stress and coping in later life families.* Washington, DC: Hemisphere.

# 9

# Future Directions in Caregiving: Implications for Intervention Research

*Sara J. Czaja, Carl Eisdorfer, and Richard Schulz*

## INTRODUCTION

The aging of the population creates tremendous challenges for families, communities, and society at large. One of the most important issues confronting the 21st century is developing strategies to meet the needs of and enhance the quality of life of older adults and their families. Although increased life expectancy is associated with many positive benefits such as the increased potential for intergenerational relationships, increased longevity can also place burdens on family and societal resources.

Generally, the prevalence of chronic limiting conditions or illnesses such as dementia, diabetes, heart disease, or stroke increases with age and consequently older adults (especially the "oldest old") are more likely to need some form of care or assistance. Approximately, 7 million people aged 65+ years have mobility or self-care limitations. The risk for dementia and other types of chronic illness doubles every 5 years beyond age 65 (Eisdorfer, 1996). People over aged 85 have the highest rates of disability, nursing home use, and multiple chronic conditions. This is significant given that the number of adults in this age group is expected to increase to 19 million by 2050 (Klein, 1997).

Currently, about 4 million Americans suffer from AD and by the year 2040 this number is expected to increase to 9 million or about 1 in 30 Americans (Brody & Cohen, 1989). Currently, knowledge about the risk factors for AD indicate that the only factors consistently associated with risk for AD include advanced age and family history of dementia. Other factors associated with AD include gender; AD occurs in women more frequently than males; and genetic factors, ApoE-e4 is associated with increased risk of AD (Demirovic, 1998). The implications of the increased prevalence of AD are vast and of significant magnitude. Annual costs of caring for Alzheimer's patients range from $70 to $90 billion. These costs only reflect direct medical costs and do not include costs associated with family disruptions, loss productivity, or increased health care costs among family caregivers (Cohen, Andersen, & Cairl, 1998). The majority of people with AD (~ 80%) live at home and are cared for by family members such as spouses, daughters, or daughter-in-laws (chapter 1). Currently, approximately 3 million caregivers in the United States provide care for family members with Alzheimer's disease (AD). Although family members are typically willing to provide care for relatives with AD many do so at increased personal sacrifice especially since periods of care are longer than ever before (Zarit, Johansson, & Jarrott, 1998). Today, the average woman can expect to spend 17 years caring for a child and 18 years caring for an elderly patient (Family Caregiving Alliance, 1998).

Alzheimer's disease is a complex, neurodegenerative disorder of long duration with changing and unpredictable symptomatology. The consequences of the disease are devastating for the patient and for family members who provide care. Patient care places considerable physical, economic, and emotional demands on families. Caregivers have to provide assistance with basic activities such as toileting or dressing, manage finances and medications, answer repetitive questions, and control wandering and agitated behavior. Generally, the demands placed on the caregiver change and increase as the disease progresses. Primary caregivers of AD patients report that they spend between 60–75 hours per week on caregiving responsibilities (Haley, 1997).

Clearly, caring for a family member with dementia creates significant challenges and many caregivers experience considerable stress and burden which affects their physical and mental health and subsequent ability to provide care (see chapters 1 and 3). The negative consequences associated with caregiving are well-documented and include depression and anxiety, increased use of psychotropic medications, immunological dysfunction, and increased use of medical services. Family routines and dynamics are frequently disrupted and many caregivers become isolated from family members and friends. Furthermore, caregivers are continually confronted with the loss of a loved one and in some cases (e.g., children caregivers) adaptation to a new familial role. There are also considerable financial burdens due to medical costs (caregiver and patient), costs associated with respite care, and costs associated with placement in long-term care facilities. Recent estimates suggest that the cost of caring for a dementia patient at home is approximately $26,000 per year (Stommel, Collins, & Given, 1994).

Caregiving is not always associated with negative outcomes, and recent studies have focussed on identifying positive outcomes associated with caregiving. These outcomes include improved family cohesiveness, increased perception of self-worth and self-esteem, and enhanced opportunities for personal growth. The extent to which a caregiver experiences negative versus positive outcomes is influenced by caregiver variables (e.g., gender, ethnicity), care recipient variables (e.g., degree of behavioral agitation), and social and physical environment variables (e.g., family support). For example, among spousal caregivers wives are more likely to suffer from depression than are husbands, and White American caregivers generally report more burden and depression than African-American caregivers. Patient behavioral problems also appear to have a significant impact on caregiver burden and depression as opposed to cognitive or activities of daily living (ADL) limitations. The amount and adequacy of social support available to the caregiver is also a mediator of burden. To develop strategies to alleviate caregiver burden and effectively maintain the AD patient at home, the characteristics of patients, caregivers, and the environment that alleviate or exacerbate the "costs" associated with caregiving must be understood. There appear to be considerable individual differences in caregiver outcomes; some caregivers adapt to the demands of caregiving overtime whereas others experience continued stress and burden. In a recent review of the caregiving literature, Schulz, O'Brien, Bookwala, and Fleissner (1995) found overwhelming evidence that caregiving is burdensome and distressing to caregivers; however, the cause of the distress is not entirely clear. Psychiatric morbidity is associated with a multitude of factors including patient behavior problems, income, self-related health, perceived stress, and life satisfaction. Physical morbidity is associated with patient problem behaviors and cognitive impairment, caregiver depression, anxiety, and perceived social support. The authors concluded that more complex interactive and mediational models are needed to explain factors that are associated with caregiver distress as different causes of distress require different prevention or treatment approaches.

During the past decade there have been a substantial number of studies directed towards development of interventions for family caregivers. These interventions include community and family support groups, respite care programs, and psychoeducational programs such as skills training. However, despite the proliferation of these intervention programs they have only met with limited success for a variety of reasons. Services are not always available to caregivers, and many caregivers are unwilling to use available community services because of cost, logistic problems, or feelings of guilt regarding receiving help outside of the family structure. In addition, the impact of these programs on caregiver outcomes such as depression are equivocal (Bourgeois, Schulz, & Burgio, 1996). Given that most caregivers prefer to care for their demented relative at home and the care recipient generally prefers to be cared for at home (Segall & Wykle, 1989), there is a need to develop innovative interventions for AD patients and family care providers. This need is underscored by the fact that family caregiving is likely to become more prevalent as formal health care services become more constrained. Furthermore, despite our advances in knowledge regarding the pathophysiology and symptoms of the disease, a prevention or cure for AD still appears to be in the distant future.

Generally, the ability of caregivers to provide care for the patient at home is influenced by the interrelationship among four variables: caregiver/patient relationship, caregiver values, coping resources and strategies, and discontinuities in patient behavior (Miller & Eisdorfer, 1989). As shown in Figure 9.1, willingness to provide care at home is determined by the balance among these variables such that if discontinuities in patient behavior outweigh the positive variables, there is an increased likelihood of institutionalization. Clearly caregiving is a complex, multidimensional issue and the development of effective intervention strategies necessitates understanding the dynamic relationships among caregiver, care recipient, and social/physical environment variables, and the linkages between these relationships and caregiver outcomes. The need for this level of understanding is particularly pertinent for future generations of caregivers given the changes in demographic and social structures. For example, many children of AD patients live in other states and are not able to actively participate in the patient's treatment plan. Today, nearly 7 million Americans are long-distance caregivers for older relatives (Wagner, 1997). The number of minority elderly are also increasing and there appear to be ethnic differences in perception

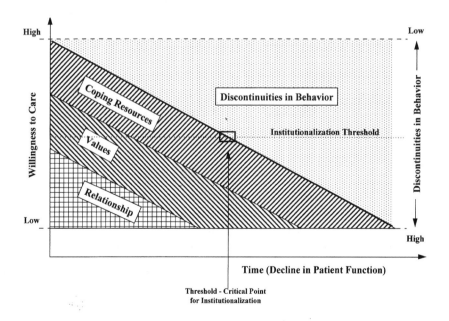

FIGURE 9.1  A model of the willingness to provide care.

of caregiving responsibilities and receptivity to available support services. Finally, newer medications such as the cholinesterase inhibitors may alter the course of the disease and prolong caregiving responsibilities. Intervention research needs to consider the "broad picture" of caregiving and take into account social and environmental contexts. Intervention approaches also need to be multifaceted and encompass the continuum of the caregiving experience from initial diagnosis through placement and death.

This chapter will discuss emerging demographic trends, which have implications for caregiving as well as potential interventions, such as information technologies, which hold promise for improving the lives of caregivers and care recipients. The chapter will also outline needed areas of future research. The overall goal of the chapter is to describe future directions in caregiving patterns and the implications of these directions for intervention approaches. An additional goal is to underscore the need for research in this area and stimulate interest in family caregiving among health care providers, policy makers, and social and behavioral scientists. Caregiving is affecting an increasingly large segment of the population and unless significant advances are made in the prevention and treatment of diseases, such as Alzheimer's disease, the number of caregivers will significantly increase as our population ages.

## CHANGES IN SOCIETAL CONTEXTS AND PATTERNS OF CAREGIVING

### Ethnic Considerations

Culture plays an important role in caregiving and the increased ethnic diversity of the population points to the need to devote attention to ethnic differences in attitudes towards caregiving and responses to caregiving responsibilities. By 2030 elders from minority populations will account for approximately 25% of older Americans. The number of Hispanic elderly is expected to increase from 4% to 16% and the number of Black elderly will account for 10% of those aged 65+. As discussed in chapter 5 there are vast differences among ethnic groups in health beliefs, health care utilization, health risks, and patterns of interactions among family members. For example, Black caregivers are less likely than White caregivers to seek information about AD and use formal support services. They are more likely to derive support from extended family members (nonfamilial kin) and to express more confidence in their abilities to handle the demands of caregiving (Eisdorfer, 1996). A number of studies have also shown that Black caregivers typically report less stress and burden than White caregivers (Fredman, Daly, & Lazur, 1995). It is suggested that this may be related to differences in cultural values and role expectations and the fact that Black elderly adults have stronger social networks than White caregivers.

Hispanic caregivers also have different perceptions of family and health than do White Americans. Among Hispanic families caregiving is perceived as a natural family responsibility and seeking help outside of the family is often perceived as a failure to meet family obligations. Similar to Black caregivers, Hispanic caregivers are less likely than their White counterparts to use formal support services. However, it is important to recognize that there is wide diversity among Hispanic cultures and thus caution is needed when making generalizations about this ethnic group. Furthermore, although Hispanic caregivers may accept caregiving as unquestioned family responsibility it does not mean that caregiving does not result in burden, stress, or emotional consequences. A recent study of Mexican-American caregivers (John & McMillian, 1998) found that although the study participants viewed caregiving as a responsibility and a privilege they also experienced emotional stress, frustration, and isolation from the outside world. Furthermore, institutionalization of family members was deemed as unacceptable. Mintzer and colleagues (1992) assessed differences in caregiver response among Cuban American and White non-Hispanic daughters caring for a parent suffering from AD and found that Cuban-American patients were more likely to reside in their daughter's home while the White non-Hispanic patients were more likely to be in institutional settings. The Cuban-American patients also had higher levels of depression than the White American patients and there was a similar trend among their daughters.

Finally as noted by Miranda (1991), endorsement of generic assumptions about cultural groups may be misleading. Cultural values and beliefs vary with generations and are changing. For example,

Cuban Americans born and raised in the United States may have different beliefs and values than their Cuban-born ancestors. Hispanic families similar to other cultural groups are experiencing changes in family structure, such as geographic dispersion, that are associated with higher educational attainment, career advancements, and geographic mobility.

It is critical that research directed towards family caregiving recognize the cultural distinctions among families. Failure to do so can produce misleading information and less effective policies and programs. There is a clear need for research on caregiver burden among minority groups in order to elucidate factors which influence burden and other outcomes such as depression. There is also a need to investigate if the efficacy of intervention strategies varies as a function of ethnicity of the caregiver. For most minority groups including Black Americans, Hispanics, Asians, and Native Americans information on caregiving is minimal or nonexistent.

## The Influence of Cohort

Cohort differences also have important ramifications for family caregiving. Individuals from different cohorts may have different values and assumptions regarding familial responsibilities. For example, earlier born cohorts have greater expectations that older family members should live with their children and are entitled to care. Census data indicates that the proportion of older adults living in the same households as their adult children has decreased significantly especially among White Americans and this trend is expected to continue into the future. Thus there will be increasing numbers of older people who live alone and are in need of care. Older people living alone may also be problematic for their adult children who may experience guilt because of perceived failure to meet family expectations and obligations and/or stress because of a lack of knowledge about or access to alternative forms of care for their aging parents. Both living at home with the AD patient and having the patient in a long-term care facility have been associated with depression and psychological distress in caregivers (Cohen & Eisdorfer, 1988). Generally reactions to caregiving are influenced by a complex array of factors including the relationship between the caregiver and the patient and the consensus in values and beliefs that they share over time.

Women are particularly influenced by generational changes in values and expectations. It is fairly well established that women are more likely than men to become caregivers of spouses, parents, or parent-in-laws. Among recent cohorts of women, this may create conflicts between issues such as employment and elder care and stress due to the need to "juggle" multiple roles—caregiver, wife, mother, and employee. Many middle-aged women are expected to have successful careers and to be nurturers of children and older parents. This conflict may exacerbate both physical (e.g., having to be "two places at once") and mental demands (e.g., feelings of failure in one or more roles) on female caregivers. In fact, the literature generally suggests that women caregivers experience more anxiety and depression than male caregivers and the potential for stress and depression is increased if they experience pressure in an alternate role (e.g., mother, employee). In some cases alternative roles may serve as a source of relief for the caregiver. The high rate of labor force participation among women is likely to continue and the issue of burden among female caregivers will continue to be an issue for future generations of caregivers. Caregiving cannot be understood in isolation from the social context of caregivers. Most caregivers have connections to other social institutions which generate demands and responsibilities. Current models of caregiving (e.g., Pearlin, Mullan, Semple, & Skaff, 1990) distinguish between primary stressors which relate to caregiving activities and secondary stressors—problems outside of caregiving. Understanding primary and secondary stressors is essential to the development of effective interventions as the total burden of care encompasses both sources of stress (Aneshensel, Pearlin, Mullen, Zarit, & Whitlatch, 1995). Interventions must target personal and external resources of caregivers. Interventions such as psychoeducational training for caregivers may need to be augmented by interventions directed towards employers—e.g., educating employers about the demands of caregiving and the need to institute flexible working situations to accommodate "elder care" as well as "child care."

An additional factor that is important with respect to generational differences in caregiving is the expected length of the caregiving role. Today adult children have triple the amount of contact with living parents than did children in the prior century which means that they have more opportunity for shared experiences but also greater potential for assuming responsibility for aging parents (VandenBos, 1998). The increased number of older adults reaching 80+ years means that families may have to provide assistance for older adults for extended periods of time. This issue may become especially pertinent with advances in medications which slow the progression of the disease. Currently, AD patients typically survive 10 to 20 years after diagnosis (Aneshensel et al., 1995). Extended care may increase the financial and emotional burden on families. In contrast, family members may learn effective coping strategies and burden and stress associated with caregiving may diminish as the caregiver acclimates to their role. To date, there have only been a few longitudinal studies of the impact of family caregiving. Shaw and associates (1997) evaluated health decline longitudinally among a sample of spousal caregivers of AD patients and married control participants. They found evidence that providing extended caregiving has health implications for caregivers and health decline is accelerated by greater ADL responsibility. Kielcolt-Glaser, Dura, Speicher, Trak, and Glaser (1991) examined longitudinal changes in immune function and health among a sample of spousal caregivers and found that caregivers experienced more decrements in immune functioning, and a greater incidence of depressive disorders and days of illness relative to controls. They also found that caregivers who reported lower levels of social support showed the most distress and negative health outcomes. Whitlatch, Feinberg, and Sebesta (1997) examined predictors of caregiver depression and adaptation over time among a sample of family caregivers. They found that the strongest predictors of caregiver depression one year after baseline were initial levels of depression, worsening of burden and caregiver health, and short-term sporadic use of in-home respite assistance. These findings have implications for the development of intervention programs. For example, diagnosing and treating caregiver depression "early on" or encouraging continued use of respite services may prevent the depression from worsening over the course of caregiving. The results of these studies also indicate the importance of examining the impact of caregiving over time. The demands of caregiving change and continue over time and to fully understand the impact of caregiving it is necessary to observe caregiving experiences longitudinally.

## The Impact of Family Structure

The family is the basic unit of society across most populations and as discussed throughout this book the family plays a critical role in maintaining disabled elderly in the community. Current estimates suggest that three-quarters of the help received by impaired elderly is provided by family members (Aneshensel et al., 1995). One challenge facing future generations of older adults is that family structures are changing; the American family can no longer be conceptualized as an extended family with three generations sharing the same household. For example, the numbers of married couples with no children is expected to increase to 7 million by the year 2010 and the average family size is expected to decline by approximately 10 percent (U.S. Bureau of the Census, 1997). By the year 2030, the average number of children per family will be approximately two as compared to three children per family in 1990 (Zedtewski & McBride, 1992). Furthermore, geographic mobility and career demands increase the likelihood that adult children will not be in the same geographic location as their older parents. Thus, there will be fewer younger family members available to provide care and support. As shown in Figure 9.2, there will be an approximately three-fold increase in the parent support ratio (number of persons 85+ per 100 persons age 50 to 64 years). By the year 2050, there will only be four potential caregivers for every elderly person. The number of "nontraditional" families is also expected to increase as alternative forms of partnerships become socially acceptable. These partnerships include couples who cohabitate without marriage and lesbian and gay partnerships. Also many marriages end in divorce and, although significant proportion of people remarry there are many who choose to remain single (Burgess, Schmeeckle, & Bengtson, 1997).

Changes in family structure have significant implications for caregiving and for older people. Issues of responsibility of care among family members take on added significance and the meaning of "family" may need to be redefined. Family conflict may also increase as there is more ambiguity regarding family roles and obligations. Also in the future many older adults are likely to enter old age either without a spouse or in new or recent remarriages or cohabitations. These arrangements may weaken spousal support systems and more

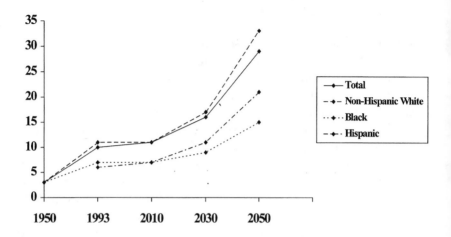

**FIGURE 9.2    Projected parent support ratio by ethnic group for the period of 1950–2050.**

Note: Parent support ratio = number of persons age 85 and over for every 100 persons age 50 to 64 years old.

of the care burden may fall on children or other family members (Burgess et al., 1997).

In summary, there are a number of demographic trends that will impact caregiving including changing family structures such as fewer children, divorce, geographic distance among family members, and nontraditional relationships that may decrease family resources available to older adults and increase the need for community-based interventions. Diversity in family structure also has policy implications. A central issue is the degree to which the family or the state should be responsible for providing care to older people.

## EMERGING INTERVENTIONS

A number of interventions designed to lessen the burden of caring for a family member have been described in the literature. These interventions include treatments aimed at the care recipient, the caregiver, and the social/physical environment. They include pharmacological interventions, psycho/educational approaches, community service interventions, and environmental modifications. Although many of these interventions hold promise for decreasing the burden and distress associated with caregiving, generally the data on the effectiveness of these strategies are equivocal. In this regard, several new intervention approaches are emerging and include pharmacological treatments, cognitive skills training, and the use of technology. This section will describe some recent developments in intervention research. The discussion of the intervention approaches will be organized according to the primary entity targeted by the intervention: care recipient (e.g., medications), caregiver (e.g., interactive technology), and the physical/social environment (e.g., environmental modifications).

When considering the effectiveness of an intervention strategy, it is important to take into account the changing nature of the disease. Different strategies may be helpful to caregivers at different stages of the disease course. As shown in Table 9.1, in the presymptomatic stage, information about the disease may be particularly important for caregivers whereas in the middle to late stages, they may benefit from respite care and family therapy. A combination of interventions may also be appropriate.

Also, interventions should continue through placement and death of the care recipient. Several studies have shown that caregiving roles are not abandoned when relatives are institutionalized and placement does not necessarily alleviate caregiver distress. Family members typically remain involved in decision making and ADL assistance. In a recent study, Boman, Mukhersee, and Forinsky (1998) compared emotional strain among family caregivers of nursing home and community older persons. They found no differences in global strain, competing demands, or emotional upset between community and nursing home family caregivers. The nursing home caregivers reported caregiving to be emotionally disturbing, and intrusive on their lives. Bereavement is also part of the caregiving experience. Although the death of a family member with dementia may represent relief from the chronic strain of providing care, many caregivers experience intense grief and would benefit from some type of support.

**TABLE 9.1 Summary of Potential Interventions Strategies According to Stage of Alzheimer's Disease**

| Primary target of intervention | Stages of disease/disability | | | | |
|---|---|---|---|---|---|
| | Presymptomatic (Primary Prevention) | Early stages (Secondary and Tertiary Prevention) | Middle to late stages (Secondary and Tertiary Prevention) | Institutionalization | Death |
| Patient | Patient education, life planning (e.g., long term care insurance), drug therapies (e.g., AD) | Education (e.g., coping strategies; using assistive devices), counseling, drug therapies, in-home services, support groups | Education, psychological therapies (e.g., counseling, music therapy), drug therapies, behavioral management, in-home respite services, cognitive training, respite care, music therapy, support groups | Drug therapies, cognitive training, behavior management, psychological therapies (e.g., counseling, music therapy) | |
| Caregiver | Education, life planning | Education, in-home respite services, assistive devices, support groups | In-home services, counseling, support groups, education, technology | Support services (e.g., transportation), education, support groups, counseling | Drug therapies (e.g., for depression), post-bereavement counseling |

**TABLE 9.1** *(continued)*

| Primary target of intervention | Stages of disease/disability | | | | |
|---|---|---|---|---|---|
| | Presymptomatic (Primary Prevention) | Early stages (Secondary and Tertiary Prevention) | Middle to late stages (Secondary and Tertiary Prevention) | Institutionalization | Death |
| Social environment | Family education, life planning, professional caregiver training | Family education, professional caregiving training | Family therapy, professional caregiver training | Family therapy, professional caregiver training | Family therapy |
| Physical environment | Environmental modifications | Environmental modifications | Environmental modifications | Environmental modifications | |

## Patient-Based Interventions

*Pharmacological Interventions.* Pharmacological approaches to the treatment of AD can be grouped into four categories: 1) treatments which target the cognitive symptoms of the illness (e.g., memory, attention); 2) treatments which attempt to slow the progress of the illness; 3) treatments which target the behavioral symptoms associated with the illness (e.g., agitation, depression); and 4) treatments which attempt to delay the time to onset of the illness (Schneider & Tariot, 1994).

*Cognitive Interventions.* Over the past decade, strides have been made in developing drugs to enhance memory functioning in AD patients. One class of drugs which has emerged as the most frequently used drugs for AD patients are acetylcholinesterase inhibitors. These drugs act to inhibit the action of acetylcholinesterase, an enzyme which limits the amount of acetylcholine, a neurotransmitter involved in nerve cell communication, available in the brain. Research has shown that there is an insufficient amount of acetylcholine in the brains of AD patients. It is hoped that by inhibiting the enzyme that breaks down acetylcholine higher concentrations will be available, thereby increasing nerve cell communication and enhancing cognitive function. One of the earliest medication of this type was COGNEX which was approved by the FDA in 1993. Although COGNEX was considered a breakthrough in AD treatments it is associated with a number of side effects (e.g., liver toxicity, digestive problems) that limit its use among older patients. ARICEPT, which was introduced in 1997, has fewer side effects than COGNEX and is a commonly prescribed treatment. Exelon is a similar medication, also associated with fewer side effects, which should be available by the near future. All of these drugs have been found to be moderately effective in enhancing the cognitive function of some patients in the early stages of the disease.

Drugs currently being tested in terms of their efficacy in slowing down or stopping the progression of the disease include lazabemide, deprenyl, and idebenone. Lazabemide inhibits the production of an enzyme, monoamine oxidase (MAO-B). It has been suggested that elevated levels of MAO-B may increase levels of neurotoxins and that the inhibition of MAO-B may preserve the surviving neurons of AD patients, thus retarding the progression of the disease. The reduction of MAO-B activity may also enhance monoamine levels (e.g., dopamine) which are important to cognitive functioning. Deprebyl is an MAO inhibitor which acts to increase levels of dopamine. It is currently marketed for Parkinsonian patients and has been effective in maintaining motor function. Vitamin E is an "alternative" antioxidant treatment which holds promise with respect to slowing down the progress of AD or delaying the onset of the disease.

Idebenone is a nerve growth–based approach (Nerve Growth Factor, NGF) to treatment which attempts to stimulate NGF activity. Animal studies suggest that NGR counteracts colinergic atrophy (Schneider & Tariot, 1994; Kennedy, Kwentus, Kumar, & Schmidt, 1998). The administration of a NGF-like medication to AD patients is an attempt to attenuate the rate of degeneration of surviving cholinergic neurons and enhance their functional performance. This is assumed to retard the progression of cognitive impairment.

The cholinergic system is one of the brain's most important regulatory neural systems. However, the role of the abnormally functioning cholinergic system in AD patients is not completely understood nor is the potential effectiveness of this type of treatment in delaying the progression of the illness.

Other treatments which are being investigated include anti-inflammatory agents (e.g., indomethacin), and hormone replacement therapy (estrogen). The catalyst for the anti-inflammatory medications is based on studies which have found that rheumatoid arthritis patients who take anti-inflammatory medications had a lower than expected frequency of Alzheimer's disease. There is limited evidence that indomethacin may enhance cognitive functioning in AD patients. However, there are also potential adverse side effects, such as gastrointestinal illnesses, associated with this medication (Dysken & Hoover, 1998).

Recently there has been interest in the potential of hormone replacement therapy, particularly estrogen, in delaying the onset of AD. Several studies have shown that estrogen replacement therapy (ERT) can be effective in improving cognitive functions such as memory, orientation, analytic skills, and verbal fluency (Sherwin, 1997; Robinson, Friedman, Marcus, Tinklenberg, & Yesavage, 1994; Jacobs, Tang, Stern, Sano, et al., 1998). Studies have also shown that the loss of estrogen after menopause is a risk factor for AD and ERT is associated with a reduction in risk for the disease (Birge, 1996; Schneider, Farlow, & Pogoda, 1997). The mechanisms underlying the effects of estrogen on cognitive functioning are not completely understood however, it is thought that estrogen has a potential effect on glucose metabolism which is a primary energy source of the brain. There is also some speculation that Ginko Biloba may increase gluscose metabolism and enhance cognitive functioning.

Currently there are no treatments which prevent the onset of AD. The development of these treatments is obviously dependent on a more complete understanding of the etiology and pathogenesis of the illness. In this regard, there have been tremendous advances towards understanding the role of genetic factors, protein molecules, and transport mechanisms in terms of risk for AD. Recent evidence (Laino, 1998) suggests that folic acid and B12 supplements may prevent the onset of AD. Research has shown that folic acid and B12 can lower levels of homocystein in the blood. Elevated levels of homocystein may predispose an individual to the development of brain plaques which are characteristic of AD (Laino, 1998).

The developments of treatments to enhance the cognitive functioning of AD patients and slow the progress of the disease have significant implications for family caregiving. For example, these medications may serve to extend the period of caregiving which may place greater burden on family resources and increase stress and depression among caregivers. These treatments may also create false hopes and expectations on the part of caregivers and patients which may in turn lead to adverse emotional reactions. Obviously, these medications also have many potential benefits such as extending periods of productivity and independence among AD patients which may in turn reduce caregiver burden. They may also prolong periods of meaningful and positive interactions between patients and caregivers thereby strengthening family relationships. There is a clear need for more research in the area of medical intervention and a need for more clinical trials to test the efficacy of these approaches. Research in this area must also consider the psychosocial impact of these treatment approaches and the implications for family caregiving. There is also a need to investigate the role of other potential factors such as nutrition or exercise in the onset or progression of AD. A number of studies have such that exercise improves both physical and cognitive functioning. As will be discussed later in this chapter, some investigators have shown that AD patients show an improvement in cognition as the result of an exercise intervention.

*Behavioral Management Interventions.* Pharmacological approaches are also directed towards the management of the behavioral symptoms of AD. Most of these treatments attempt to decrease depression, agitated behavior, and paranoia, which are common symptoms among AD patients. The prevalence rates for depression and AD vary widely due to a number of factors including differences in diagnostic methodology, residence of the patient (home vs. nursing home), and difficulty in diagnosis due to overlap of symptoms between dementia and depression. However, it is safe to assert that a large number of AD patients suffer from comorbid depression. This is an important consideration as AD patients who are depressed tend to function at lower levels and have a higher rate of mortality (Meyers & Tirumalasetti, 1998). Surprisingly, there have been only a few studies which have systematically evaluated treatment responses of AD patients to commonly used antidepressant medications, such as the serotonin re-uptake inhibitors (SSRIs, e.g., Prozac, Zoloft). These treatments have proven effective in alleviating depression among older adults without cognitive impairment. There are also case studies which indicate that antidepressant medications are effective in AD patients (e.g., Burke, Folks, Roccaforte, & Wengel, 1994). However, these reports are typically based on small samples. Large, controlled clinical studies are needed to assess the efficacy and safety of antidepressant medications in the treatment of depression in AD patients.

Medications have proven also effective in treating other common symptoms of AD, such as paranoia and agitated behavior. Medications used to treat behavioral problems of the AD patient include: antipsychotic (such as haloperidol, risperidone), antianxiety drugs (e.g., benzodiazepines (diazepam, lorazepam), buspirone) and beta-blocking agents. The choice of medication must be based on the nature and pathophysiology of the behavioral disturbance and risks to the patient. To date, as is the case with antidepressant medications, there have been relatively few large controlled clinical trials which have evaluated the efficacy and tolerability of these medications for AD populations.

Research is also needed to evaluate the effectiveness of nonpharmacological interventions such as behavioral and environmental interventions in treating behavioral disturbances. For example, behavioral approaches, based on the principles of operant conditioning, have proven effective in treating behavioral problems such as agitation, wandering, and socially inappropriate behavior (Gugel, 1994). Wandering and agitation may also be remediated by environmental modifications such as providing an enclosed area for the patient to walk and reducing the amount of clutter in the environment. Mayers and Griffen (1990) found that stimulus objects such as fabric books stimulated interest among AD patients and reduced boredom and agitation. Rentz (1995) found evidence that a reminiscense intervention was effective in improving the affect of AD patients. Several studies (e.g., Brotons & Pockett-Cooper, 1996; Glynn, 1992) have also shown that music therapy is effective in reducing behavior agitation of Alzheimer's disease patients. Investigation of interventions which reduce behavioral problems in AD patients should receive high priority given the link between behavioral symptoms and caregiver depression. Behavioral management strategies may both improve the quality of life of the patient and the caregiver.

*Cognitive Retraining.* Recent efforts for improving the cognitive functioning of AD patients also include cognitive retraining programs. These programs, which generally involve memory training approaches, have met with limited success. However, the results are encouraging. For example, in a series of studies, Backman and colleagues (1991) demonstrated that when a substantial amount of cognitive support is provided for both the encoding and retrieval of information, AD patients exhibit improvements in episodic memory. Camp and Schaller (1989) have shown that a technique known as "spaced retrieval" is effective in allowing patients with dementia to learn face-name, object-location information and recall this information across clinically meaningful periods of time (days, weeks). "Spaced retrieval" is based on work by Landauer and Bjork (1978) and involves retrieval of the same information at increasingly longer retention intervals. If a memory failure occurs individuals receive feedback and return to the previously successful retention interval. Sandman (1993) examined the effectiveness of four-week memory rehabilitation programs on a small sample of AD patients. The program was developed with an emphasis on recall of names, faces, places, and events. Procedures were designed to amplify sensory information and an emphasis was placed on rehearsal, stimulating interest, and increasing the interaction between the patient and the environment. Generally, the results were encouraging and indicated that the ability of the patients to recall name-face relationships and event information was significantly improved.

In contrast, studies have also found that cognitive rehabilitation strategies are not effective in improving the functioning of AD patients. Training procedures which have involved imagery (Backman, Josephsson, Herlitz, Stigsdotters, & Viitanen, 1991) or organization of information (Yesavage, 1982) have only reported minimal or nonexistent gains in memory improvement. Backman (1992) suggests that the design of the cognitive rehabilitation program has a significant impact on degree of effectiveness. He outlined four features of memory training approaches which have proven to be effective in AD patients: 1) the training is based on skills that are relatively well-preserved in AD (e.g., implicit memory, motor abilities), 2) the training programs are fairly extensive, 3) caregivers are involved in the training, and 4) the retrieval process is strongly supported.

Clearly, the data suggests that there is some plasticity in cognitive functioning in AD patients. Efforts directed at cognitive rehabilitation is a fertile area of research. It may be interesting to examine the degree to which information technologies can be used to augment or enhance the memory functioning of AD patients. For example, voice mail or computer messages can be sent to remind people of appointments, or personal databases can be constructed to remind patients/ caregivers of medication schedules. Computers may also be used for cognitive retraining. For example, Chute and Bliss (1994) have developed a software application, Prosthesesware, to augment the cognitive abilities of patients who have cognitive limitations due to brain injury. The software provides instruction on the procedural elements of basic ADL/IADL activities. This type of application may prove to be beneficial for patients with dementia. Recent developments in interactive videotechnology also hold promise with respect to improving both the cognitive and behavioral symptoms of AD patients. Lund, Hill, Caserta, and Wright (1995) evaluated Video Respite, a series of videotapes specifically designed for patients with dementia, as a mechanism to provide respite time for caregivers. Preliminary findings indicate that the videotapes were helpful in providing relief for caregivers and they also seemed to reduce behavioral agitation in patients.

Telemedicine is another emerging technology which may be effective in terms of improving the quality of life for both caregivers and AD patients. Telemedicine technology has shown to be effective in terms of providing care to patients who are unable to access health care due to chronic conditions or logistic factors, facilitating information exchange among health care providers, and as a teaching tool for health care professionals. With respect to the AD patient, telemedicine may serve as a mechanism for the clinician to monitor the patient's behavior, and provide information, advice, and support to caregivers. Freidman, Stollerman, Mahoney, and Rozenblyum (1997) have recently designed a telecommunications technology which links voice and database components, to be used as an alternative to and a supplement for office visits for ambulatory care. Preliminary evaluation of the system indicates that it is well-accepted by patients and health care providers and is efficacious with respect to clinical outcomes (e.g., medication adherence). In the current REACH project the use of computer/telephone technology as an intervention mechanism for caregivers is being investigated at two sites: Boston and Miami. These efforts will be described later in this chapter.

*Exercise-Based Interventions.* The efficacy of physical exercise in alleviating the symptoms of AD is also being evaluated. The available data suggests that exercise may play an important role in moderating the symptoms associated with dementia. For example, in a recent study (Palleschi, Vetta, DeGennaro, Idone, Sottosanti, Gianni, & Marigliano, 1996) found that a three-month aerobic training program enhanced the performance of a sample of 15 male AD patients on measures of cognitive performance. Friedman and Tappen (1991) found that a 10-week walking program improved the communication skills of AD patients. Namazi, Zarofozny, and Gwinnup (1995) found preliminary evidence that a light exercise program improved the sleep behavior of AD patients. Other studies (e.g., Mace, 1987; Beck, Modlin, Heithoff, & Shue, 1992) have shown that exercise can be effective in reducing behavioral problems associated with AD. Finally it has been suggested (Kanamori, Kondo, Isse, Shido, Niino, Sugita, & Kobayashi, 1994) that physical exercise may also help prevent the onset of the disease.

Theoretical explanation for the potential benefits of AD patients include that physical exercise: 1) stimulates cortical activity in the brain due to greater cerebral blood flow and/or activation and stimulation of the reticular activating system; 2) promotes functioning of the immune system; and 3) moderates the arteriosclerotic aspects of the disease process. The issue of exercise and Alzheimer's Disease poses many exciting research opportunities including the 1) examination of the extent to which exercise can improve the functioning of AD patients and/or prevent the onset or progression of the disease, 2) specification of the link between exercise and functional improvement, 3) determination of exercise programs which are safe and effective for AD populations, and 4) determination of strategies which facilitate the implementation of these types of interventions. As discussed by Bonner and Cousins (1996), one of the most important challenges facing researchers in this area is finding ways to successfully implement these programs with staff and caregivers.

## Caregivers-Based Interventions

Numerous efforts have been directed towards the development of interventions to alleviate burden and negative reactions among caregivers of AD patients. These efforts have included support programs, respite care programs, and psychoeducational programs. A review of these interventions and their effectiveness will not be done in this chapter as excellent and thorough reviews of existing programs and strategies have already been conducted (e.g., Bourgeois, Schulz, & Burgio, 1996), and this topic is covered in detail in chapter 2. Generally, the outcomes of these reviews have suggested that despite the proliferation of intervention programs and treatments they have only met with limited success. In this regard one of the goals of the REACH project is to comparatively evaluate the relative effectiveness of alternative intervention strategies (e.g., skills training, family therapy, technology-based interventions) on family caregiver outcomes. Clearly, innovative and creative caregiver intervention approaches are needed. The following section will discuss some potentially innovative caregiver intervention approaches. The emphasis of the discussion will be on family systems approaches and technologically based approaches.

*Family System Approaches.* Current thinking in intervention research is recognizing that dementia is an illness that impacts on the whole family and that the AD patient is a member of a family system, that in turn is part of broader systems within society. Family members provide most of the care for dementing relatives. It is widely recognized that family members who provide ongoing care for patients with dementia are at increased risk for medical and emotional difficulties (Zarit Todd, & Zarit, 1986; Poulshock & Deimling, 1984). Caregiver adaptation has been shown to vary with the course of illness (Eisdorfer, 1990; Fitting, Rabins, Lucas, & Eastham, 1986; Haley & Pardo, 1989), but it is also clear that caregivers are at high risk for psychiatric morbidity, particularly depression, impaired health status, and decreased immune functioning, distress and burden, and changing work and social roles (George & Gwyther, 1986; Morrissey, Becker, & Rubert, 1990; Pagel, Becker, & Coppel, 1985). Furthermore, caregiver distress and morbidity, including immune dysfunction, persist in a significant group of caregivers even after the patient has died or been institutionalized (George & Gwyther, 1986; Pagel, Becker, & Coppel, 1985; Stephens, Kinney, & Ogrocki, 1991).

In the course of providing care, caregivers are faced with many decisions and encounter many problems which are complex and multifaceted. These problems are often new to the family and typically the family does not have the knowledge or resources to deal with them effectively. While family members are recognized as being a vital source of development, influence, and assistance to individuals within the family system, family relationships are also a source of stress and dysfunction (Sherlock & Gardner, 1993). Although many family members adapt to their situation successfully, an overview of the literature suggests that the majority of family members have difficulty, including significant psychological distress and health problems (Drinka, Smith & Drinka, 1987; Dura, Stukenburg, & Kiecolt-Glaser, 1991; Kiecolt-Glaser et al., 1987; Morris, Morris, & Britton, 1988; Cohen & Eisdorfer, 1988).

For these reasons working with the families of caregivers has great potential to impact the functional effectiveness, health, and well-being of caregivers. The primary assumption of family-based intervention research is that, with rare exceptions, primary caregivers have resources within themselves as well as their families and communities that can be harnessed to reduce or solve problems associated with caring for a demented patient. The challenge of family-based intervention research is to identify the specific problems caregivers are experiencing, the efficacy of family problem-solving styles and solutions, the range of useable family resources available to the caregiver, the range of useable community resources available and accessible to the family, and the capacity of caregivers and their families to collaborate in the caregiving effort. In this regard the systematic program and structural methods for family systems therapy developed and tested by Szapocznik and colleagues (1989) with Cuban-American families has received considerable recognition in the treatment research field (e.g., Alexander, Holtzworth-Monroe, & Jameson, 1994; Kardin, 1993, 1994). Because these approaches have proven effective with a broad range of problems in families, and because of the early promising work using structural family systems concepts with Cuban elders, the Miami site of the REACH project is investigating the efficacy of this approach for caregivers of dementia patients and families.

*Technology-Based Interventions.* One challenge in intervention research is developing innovative techniques that facilitate the ability of caregivers to use available support services. Often logistical factors, such as difficulty arranging alternative help, inaccessible meeting places, or scheduling conflicts prevent family caregivers from attending support group meetings (Wright, Lund, Pett, & Caserta, 1987). In this regard, computer and communication technologies can be effectively used to provide support and deliver services to caregivers and other family members. Computer networks can be developed to link caregivers to each other, health care professionals, community service, and educational programs. This will not only help the caregiver by providing needed information, but it will also help alleviate the loneliness and isolation that often accompanies caregiving. Furthermore, it will enhance the ability of caregivers to participate in both formal support groups and informal supportive relationships with other caregivers, which will help to provide needed emotional support.

A recent study by Czaja, Guerrier, Nair, and Landauer (1993), which involved installing personal computers in the homes of a sample of elderly people, found that one of the primary reasons the participants used the computer was that it provided them with a means to meet and interact with new people. The results also showed that older adults are willing and able to use home computers and perceive them as useful. Leirer, Morrow, Tanke, and Pariante (1991) found that a computer network, "ComputerLink," enhanced the instrumental and emotional support provided by nurses to caregivers of persons with dementia. Smyth and Harris (1993) are currently evaluating the utility of a telecomputing information and support system for caregivers. Their system allows caregivers to access information about dementing disorders and to communicate with one another via a caregiver forum.

Currently two of the REACH sites (Miami and Boston) are evaluating technology-based interventions. The Miami site is evaluating the effectiveness of a computer-telephone system in enhancing the family therapy intervention. The intent of the intervention is to augment the family therapy intervention by facilitating the caregivers ability to access formal and informal support services. The system enables caregivers to communicate with therapists, family members, and friends using an individual or conference format; participate in on-line support groups; send and receive messages; and access information databases such as the Alzheimer's Association resource guide. The system is menu-based (voice and text) and is individualized for each caregiver.

The Boston site is also investigating the impact of an automated telecommunications system, Telephone-Linked Care for Alzheimer's Disease (TLC-AD). TLC-AD speaks over the telephone to caregivers using a computer-controlled human voice system. Caregivers press designated keys on the touch tone keypad of their home telephone to communicate with TLC-AD. TLC-AD will 1) monitor the primary caregiver's stress and health status weekly and make recommendations and referrals if necessary, 2) provide a voice-mail caregiver support network to reduce social isolation, 3) provide an "ask the expert" call option for recalcitrant caregiving problems, and 4) offer a distraction conversation for caregivers to use when they desire a mini-respite break from the person with AD.

The Internet and other innovations in telephony and cable television networks may also enhance the abilities of caregivers to provide care. The expansion of the Internet allows caregivers to access information on a wide variety of topics related to caregiving, communicate with other caregivers and health care providers, and perform tasks such as billing, paying, and shopping. Future innovations will expand voice and video exchange over network devices. While these technologies hold promise in terms of providing support for caregivers, a significant challenge exists for researchers in ensuring that these technologies are usable by caregivers especially those who are elderly. Currently the Internet frustrates many users and many people, especially those with limited experience with computer technology or those who have sensory cognitive or physical limitation. They find the internet difficult to use and thus access to resources and databases is limited for this group. Research that can promote a better understanding of what works in terms of making interfaces more useful, useable, and accessible for caregiver populations is needed. Issues surrounding privacy and quality control of information and the cost effectiveness of these types of systems also needs to be investigated.

*Community Programs.* Interventions aimed at caregivers also include community services and programs that provide aid to the patient and respite for the caregiver. Community programs typically include: adult day care, in-home help, short-term nursing care, and caregiver support groups. The intent of these services is to provide relief to the caregiver and ease the burden of caregiving. A secondary goal is to provide aid to the AD patient, e.g., many adult day-care facilities have programs and activities to stimulate interest and interaction among participants.

Although services of this type are available in most communities, caregivers who might benefit from these services do not use them or use them infrequently for a variety of reasons. More effort needs to be directed towards understanding the reasons that prevent use of these programs so that more effective programs and services can be developed. As discussed, information technologies may provide a vehicle to link caregivers to community resources. Strategies also need to be developed to more effectively integrate formal and informal care and to ensure that health care providers work with caregivers to maximize the benefits of these programs. As discussed by Zarit, Johansson, and Jarrott (1998) a challenge for the future is to strike a balance for pooling family and community resources to form effective partnerships for care provision.

## Physical and Social Environment

In contrast to interventions which attempt to change the patient (medication therapy, cognitive rehabilitation exercise), environmental interventions attempt to alter the situational context so that it is supportive of the patient and caregiving activities. In terms of Lawton's "environmental press model," these approaches attempt to reduce the demands of the environment so that they are commensurate with the capabilities/limitations of the AD patients. In other words, these approaches attempt to increase "environmental mastery or competency." On the basis of the environmental press model, Lawton (1980) was one of the pioneers of examining the effects of the environment on AD population.

Most of the efforts of environmental design have been directed at residential facilities and have involved efforts to increase spatial orientation of patients, facilitate recall of object-places locations, and provide outlets for behaviors such as wandering. Other environmental modifications have involved providing areas of stimulation for patients, to increase their interest and attention. Finally, many of these efforts have been directed towards enhancing the safety of AD patients, prevention of wandering off the premises and becoming "lost," and reducing risks for falls/injury. Many of these techniques have proven to be effective in reducing behavioral problems among and enhancing care of AD patients. Over the past decade many residential facilities have designed special care units (SCU) for AD patients. The underlying model for most of these efforts is consistent with Lawton's notion that the environment must be modified to maximize the functional capacity of AD patients and support caregiving tasks. The evidence generally suggests that SCUs are effective in terms of enhancing quality of care and functioning of AD patients. However, large-scale systematic studies to test the effectiveness of SCUs have been limited. Furthermore, the results of studies examining the effects of SCU on residents have been mixed. Currently, there are many different philosophies, staffing strategies, environmental modifications, and programming among nursing home SCUs (Maas, Swanson, Specht, & Buckwalter, 1994). Thus, it is difficult to evaluate "what works" and "what does not work" with respect to enhancing patient functioning or mitigating patient behavioral problems. Zairt, Zarit, and Rosemberg-Thompson (1990) describe a special care unit in a residential facility which combines medical, behavioral, and environmental features. They suggest that this combination of intervention strategies are especially effective in facilitating the management of and enhancing the functioning of AD patients. Systematic evaluation of the effects of SCU interventions on staff and family members has also been limited. In this regard, the National Institute on Aging recently founded an initiative to evaluate the impact of SCUs on patients, families, and staff members. The study is also investigating the cost-effectiveness of SCUs in nursing home. The National Institute for Nursing Research is funding a similar initiative. A particular focus of this initiative is the examination of the impact of SCUs on family involvement in caregiving. Policy issues have also emerged regarding regulations and reimbursement for SCU programs.

Recently the efficacy of environmental modifications for AD patients have also been evaluated in home settings. For example, in home environments simple strategies such as labeling household objects and locations and organization of clothing have proven to be effective in maintaining competence of older adults with dementia (Corcoran & Gitlin, 1991). Other strategies include reducing clutter and ambiguity in the environment and increasing support through personalization and reminiscence (e.g., photos of family members). The Philadelphia site of the REACH project is examining the effectiveness of home environment modifications on caregiver outcomes.

As discussed, one of the primary factors associated with caregiver distress is availability of social support. Research has consistently shown that caregivers who have higher levels of social support report less burden and less distress. Unfortunately, many caregivers also report dissatisfaction with social support as ties with other family members and friends often become severed during the course of the disease. In this regard interventions such as family therapy or community support groups may be an effective intervention for caregivers. As discussed, recent developments in technology may make it easier for caregivers to maintain contact with family and friends and to access community support groups. In the Miami REACH program, the "on-line" support groups are one of the most successful features of the technology intervention.

## CONCLUSIONS/RECOMMENDATIONS

Family caregiving is a burgeoning social and clinical issue. The aging of population will place an increased burden on family resources and innovative approaches are needed to aid family members in the provision of care for their elder family members. Currently, about 15% of U.S. adults are providing care for a seriously ill or disabled relative (Otten, 1991).

Using a public health model, three different levels of activities are required: 1) *primary prevention*—developing mechanisms that prevent the onset of dementia, 2) *secondary prevention*—developing more reliable and accurate diagnostic instruments and mechanisms which minimize or delay the progression of the disease, and 3) *tertiary prevention*—developing mechanisms that ameliorate the consequences of the disease for patients, family members, and caregivers. In this regard, research in the following areas is warranted:

- Epidemiological studies which identify risk factors for the development of Alzheimer's Disease, and differences in caregiving patterns and caregivers' responses to the demands of caregiving. It is important that studies in this area emphasize ethnic differences in these variables.
- Studies directed towards understanding the pathogenesis of AD so that more effective treatment mechanisms can be developed.
- Large-scale, controlled clinical studies which evaluate the efficacy and safety of medications in treating the behavioral symptoms of AD.
- Large-scale, controlled clinical studies which evaluate alternative treatment mechanisms (e.g., vitamin therapy) for AD patients.
- Studies which evaluate the effectiveness of combinations of treatment and which evaluate the efficacy of interventions across the continuum of care. Emphasis should be given to the potential usefulness of information technology as an intervention mechanism.
- Research directed towards the development of more cost-effective diagnostic strategies.
- Research directed towards identifying how much we can transfer from what we have learned from caregivers of other populations (e.g., stroke patients) to AD caregivers.
- Studies which examine innovative research and analytic methods. The conceptual model and analytic approach plan for the REACH project is a good initial step in this direction.

In addition to more research directed towards caregiving, there are also a number of policy issues which need to be addressed. Currently the bulk of support to older adults who are in need of assistance is provided by family members. Clearly, solutions to problems of caregiving will require a macro level response through government policy and private sector programs. An important question is the degree to which the government and state should provide care to older adults. Many community and long-term care services are not covered by health insurance programs such as Medicare. Public policy issues should also encompass needs of family members and staff training issues with respect to quality of long-term care for AD patients. Other issues concern resource allocation along the course of the illness. Inclusion of minority patients in service systems is also a central issue (Niederehe, 1993).

In summary, there are tremendous opportunities and challenges in family caregiving. However, for advances in this field to emerge, research in this area should be a priority among policy makers, funding agencies, and behavioral and social science researchers. Caregivers represent a critical component of health care and more attention needs to be directed towards their problems and concerns. The importance of caregiving will continue to increase given current demographic trends such as the increased number of women in the labor force, more older adults living alone, and fewer children available to provide care. Furthermore, caregiving is not just restricted to older adults; caregiving is provided to people of all ages.

## REFERENCES

Alexander, J.F., Holtzworth-Mohroe, A., & Jameson, P.B. (1994). Research on the process and outcome of marriage and family therapy. In A.E. Bergin & S.L. Garfield (Eds.), *Handbook of psychotherapy and behavioral change* (pp. 595–630). New York: Wiley and Sons.

Aneshensel, C.S., Pearlin, L.I., Mullan, J.T., Zarit, S.H., & Whitlatch, C.J. (1995). *Profiles in caregiving: The unexpected career.* San Diego: Academic Press.

Backman, L. (1992). Memory training and memory improvement in Alzheimer's disease: Rules and exceptions. *Acta Neurologica Scandinavica, Suppl. 139,* 84–89.

Backman, L., Josephsson, S., Herlitz, A., Stigsdotter, A., & Viitanen, M. (1991). The generalizability of training gains in dementia: Effects of an imagery-based mnemonic on face-name retention duration. *Psychology and Aging, 6,* 489–492.

Beck, C., Modlin, T., Heithoff, K., & Shue, V. (1992). Exercise as an intervention for behavior problems. *Geriatric Nursing, (September/October),* 273–275.

Birge, S.J. (1996). Is there a role for estrogen replacement therapy in the prevention and treatment of dementia? *Journal of American Geriatric Society, 44,* 860–870.

Bonner, A.P., & Cousins, S.O. (1996). Exercise and Alzheimer's disease: Benefits and barriers. *Activities, Adaptation & Aging, 20,* 21–34.

Bowman, K.F., Mukherjee, S., & Fortinsky, R.H. (1998). Exploring strain in community and nursing home family caregivers. *The Journal of Applied Gerontology, 17,* 371–392.

Brody, J., & Cohen, D. (1989). Epidemiologic aspects of Alzheimer's disease: Facts and gaps. *Journal of Aging and Health, 1,* 139–147.

Brotons, M., & Pickett-Cooper, R. K. (1996). The effects of music therapy intervention on agitation behaviors of Alzheimer's disease patients. *Journal of Music Therapy, 33,* 2–18.

Bourgeois, M.S., Schulz, R., & Burgio, L. (1996). Interventions for caregivers of patients with Alzheimer's disease: A review and analysis of content, process, and outcomes. *International Journal of Aging and Human Development, 43,* 35–92.

Burgess, E.O., Schmeeckle, M., & Bengtson, V.L. (1997). Aging individuals and societal contexts. In I.H. Nordhus, G.R. VandenBos, S. Berg, & P. Fromholt (Eds.), *Clinical Geropsychology* (pp. 15–31). Washington, DC: American Psychological Association.

Burke, W.J., Folks, D.J., Roccaforte, W.H., & Wengel, S.V. (1994). Serontonin-reuptake inhibitors for the treatment of coexisting depression and psychosis in dementia of the Alzheimer's type. *American Journal of Geriatric Psychiatry, 2,* 352–354.

Camp, C.J., & Schaller, J.R. (1989). Epilogue: Spaced-retrieval memory training in an adult day-care center. *Education Gerontology, 15,* 81–88.

Chute, D.L., & Bliss, M.E. (1994). Prosthesis ware: Concepts and caveats for microcomputer-based aids to everyday living. *Experimental Aging Research, 20,* 229–238.

Cohen, D., Andersen, B., & Cairl, R. (1998). Management of families caring for relatives with dementia: Issues and interventions. In V. Kumar & C. Eisdorfer (Eds.), *Advances in the diagnosis and treatment of Alzheimer's Disease* (pp. 351–375). New York: Springer Publishing Company.

Cohen, D., & Eisdorfer, C. (1988). Depression in family members caring for a relative with Alzheimer's Disease. *Journal of American Geriatric Society, 36,* 885–889.

Corcoran, M., & Gitlin, L.N. (1991). Environmental influences on behavior of the elderly with dementia: Principles for intervention in the home. *Physical & Occupational Therapy in Geriatrics, 9,* 5–22.

Czaja, S.J., Guerrier, J.H., Nair, S.N., & Landauer, T.K. (1993). Computer communication as an aid to independence for older adults. *Behaviour & Information Technology, 12,* 197–207.

Demirovic, J. (1998). Epidemiology of Alzheimer's disease. In V. Kumar & C. Eisdorfer (Eds.), *Advances in the diagnosis and treatment of Alzheimer's disease* (pp. 3–30). New York: Springer Publishing Company.

Drinka, T.J., Smith, J.C., & Drinka, P.J. (1987). Correlates of depression and burden for informal caregivers of patients in a geriatric referral clinic. *Journal of the American Geriatrics Society, 35,* 522–525.

Dura, J., Stukenberg, K., & Kiecolt-Glaser, J. (1991). Anxiety and depressive disorders in adult children caring for demented parents. *Psychology and Aging, 6,* 467–473.

Dysken, M.W., & Hoover, K.M. (1998). Noncholinergic drugs in the treatment of memory problems in Alzheimer's disease patients. In V. Kumar & C. Eisdorfer (Eds.), *Advances in the diagnosis and treatment of Alzheimer's Disease* (pp. 264–297). New York: Springer Publishing Company.

Eisdorfer, C. (1990). Caregiving: An emerging risk factor for emotional and physical pathology. *Bulletin of the Menninger Clinic, 55,* 238–247.

Eisdorfer, C. (1996). Families in distress: Caring is more than loving. *Psychiatric Annals, 26,* 285–288.

Family Caregiving Alliance. (1997). *Annual report: California's caregiver resource center system fiscal year 1996–1997.* San Francisco, CA: Family Caregiver Alliance, March, 1998.

Fitting, M., Rabins, P.M., Lucas, J., & Eastham, J. (1986). Caregivers for demential patients: A comparison of husbands and wives. *The Gerontologist, 26,* 248–252.

Fredman, L., Daly, M.P., & Lazur, A.M. (1995). Burden among white and black caregivers to elderly adults. *Journal of Gerontology: Social Sciences, 50B,* S110–S118.

Friedman, R., & Tappen, R.M. (1991). The effect of planned walking on communication in Alzheimer's Disease. *American Geriatrics Society, 39,* 650–654.

Friedman, R.H., Stollerman, J.E., Mahoney, D.M., & Rozenblyum, L. (1997). The virtual visit: Using telecommunications technology to take care of patients. *Journal of the American Medical Informatics Association, 4,* 413–425.

George, L.K., & Gwyther, L.P. (1986). Caregiver well-being: A multidimensional examination of family caregivers of demented adults. *The Gerontologist, 26,* 253–259.

Glynn, N.J. (1992). The music therapy: Assessment tool in Alzheimer's patients. *Journal of Gerontological Nursing, 18,* 3–9.

Gugel, R.N. (1994). Behavioral approaches for managing patients with Alzheimer's disease and related disorders. *Medical Clinics of North America, 78,* 861–867.

Haley, W.E. (1997). The family caregiver's role in Alzheimer's disease. *Neurology, 48,* S25–S29.

Haley, W.E., & Pardo, K.M. (1989). Relationship of severity of dementia to caregiving stressors. *Psychology Aging, 4,* 389–392.

Jacobs, D.M., Tang, M.X., Stern, Y., Sano, M., Marder, K., Bell, K.T., Schofield, P., Dooneief, G., Gurland, B., & Mayeux, R. (1998) Cognitive function in nondemented older women who took estrogen after menopause. *Neurology, 50,* 368–373.

John, R., & McMillian, B. (1998). Exploring caregiver burden among Mexican Americans: Cultural prescriptions, family dilemmas. *Journal of Aging and Ethnicity, 1,* 93–111.

Kanamori, M., Kondo, K., Isse, K., Shido, K., Niino, M., Sugita, M., & Kobayashi, M. (1994). Epidemiological results of risk factors for senile dementia of Alzheimer type in two districts of Japan, *Proceedings of the XVth Congress of the International Association of Gerontology, Budapest, Hungary,* 673–676.

Kardin, A.E. (1993). Psychotherapy for children and adolescents. *American Psychologist, 28,* 644–657.

Kardin, A.E. (1994). Psychotherapy for children and adolescents. In A.E. Bergin & S.L. Garfield (Eds.), *Handbook of psychotherapy and behavior change.* New York: John Wiley and Sons.

Kennedy, J.S., Kwentus, J.A., Kumar, V., & Schmidt, D. (1998). Cholinergic system therapy for Alzheimer's Disease. In V. Kimar & C. Eisdorfer (Eds.), *Advances in the diagnosis and treatment of Alzheimer's disease* (pp. 409–415). New York: Springer Publishing Company.

Kiecolt-Glaser, J., Dura, J.R., Speicher, C.E., Trak, O.J., & Glaser, R. (1991). Spousal caregivers of dementia victims: Longitudinal changes in immunity and health. *Psychosomatic Medicine, 53,* 345–362.

Kiecolt-Glaser, J., Glaser, R., Shuttleworth, E.C., Dyer, C.S., Ogrocki, P., & Speicher, C.E. (1987). Chronic stress and immunity in family caregivers of Alzheimer's disease victims. *Psychosomatic Medicine, 49,* 523–535.

Klein, S.M. (1997). *A national agenda for geriatric education.* New York: Springer Publishing Company.

Laino, C. (1998). Could vitamins fend off Alzheimer's? *MSNBC-Health.* [Online]. Available: http://www.msnbc.com/news/206428.asp.

Landauer, T.K., & Bjork, R.A. (1978). Optimal rehearsal patterns and name learning. In M.M. Gruneberg, P.E. Harris, & R.N. Sykes (Eds.), *Practical aspects of memory* (pp. 625–632). New York: Academic Press.

Lawton, M.P. (1980). Psychosocial and environmental approaches to the care of senile dementia patients. In J.O. Cole & J.E. Barrett (Eds.), *Psychopathology in the aged.* New York: QV Raven Press.

Leirer, V.O., Morrow, D.G., Tanke, E.D., & Pariante, G.M. (1991). Elders won adherence: Its assessment and medication reminding by voice mail. *The Gerontologist, 31,* 514–520.

Lund, D.A., Hill, R.D., Caserta, M.S., & Wright, S.D. (1995). Video respite: An innovative resource for family, professional caregivers, and persons with dementia. *Gerontologist, 35,* 683–687.

Maas, M.L., Swanson, E., Specht, J., & Buckwalter, K.C. (1994). Alzheimer's special care units. *Nursing Clinical North America, 29,* 173–194.

Mace, N. (1987). Principles of activities for persons with dementia. *Physical & Occupational Therapy in Geriatrics, 5,* 13–27.

Mayers, K., & Griffin, M. (1990). The play project: Use of stimulus objects with demented patients. *Journal of Gerontological Nursing, 16,* 32–37.

Meyers, B.S., & Tirumalasetti, F. (1998). Diagnosis and treatment of Alzheimer's disease and combined depression. In V. Kumar & C. Eisdorfer (Eds.), *Advances in the diagnosis and treatment of Alzheimer's disease* (pp. 233–246). New York: Springer Publishing Company.

Miller, M., & Eisdorfer, C. (1989). A model of caregiver's willingness to provide care. *Caring, December,* 10–13.

Mintzer, J.E., Rubert, M.P., Loewestein, D., Gomez, E., Millor, A., Quinteros, R., Flores, L., Miller, M., Rainerman, A., & Eisdorfer, C.E. (1992). Daughters caregiving for Hispanic and non-Hispanic Alzheimer patients: Does ethnicity make a difference? *Community Mental Health Journal, 28,* 293–301.

Miranda, M. (1991). Mental health services and the Hispanic elderly. In M. Sotomayor (Ed.), *Empowering Hispanic families: A critical issue for the 90's* (pp. 141–153). Milwaukee, WI: Family Service America.

Morris, R.G., Morris, L.W., & Britton, P.G. (1988). Factors affecting the emotional well-being of the caregivers of dementia sufferers. *British Journal of Psychiatry, 153,* 147–156.

Morrissey, E., Becker, J., & Rubert, M.P. (1990). Coping resources and depression in the caregiving spouses of Alzheimer patients. *British Journal of Medical Psychology, 63,* 161–171.

Namazi, K.H., Zarofozny, C.A., & Gwinnup, P.B. (1995). The influence of physical activity on patterns of sleep behavior of patients with Alzheimer's Disease. *International Journal of Aging and Human Development, 2,* 145–153.

Niederehe, G. (1993). Public policy issues related to SHMO demonstrations and Alzheimer's Disease. In S.H. Zarit, L.I. Pearlin, & K.W. Schaie (Eds.), *Caregiving systems: Formal and informal helpers* (pp. 201–216). New Jersey: Lawrence Erlbaum Associates.

Otten, A. (1991). About 15% of U.S. adults care for ill relatives. *Wall Street Journal,* April 22, B1.

Pagel, M.D., Becker, J., & Coppel, D.B. (1985). Loss of control, self-blame, and depression: An investigation of spouse caregivers of Alzheimer's disease patients. *Journal of Abnormal Psychology, 94,* 169–182.

Palleschi, L., Vetta, F., De Gennaro, E., Idone, G., Sottosanti, G., Gianni, W., & Marigliano, V. (1996). Effects of aerobic training on the cognitive performance of elderly patients with senile dementia of the Alzheimer type. *Archives of Gerontology and Geriatrics, S5,* 47–50.

Pearlin, L., Mullan, J., Semple, S., & Skaff, M. (1990). Caregiving and the stress process: An overview of concepts and their measures. *Gerontologist, 30,* 583–589.

Poulshock, S.W., & Deimling, G.T. (1984). Family caring for elders in residence: Issues in the measurement of burden. *Journal of Gerontology, 39,* 230–239.

Rentz, C.A. (1995). Reminiscence: A supportive intervention for the person with Alzheimer's disease. *Journal of Psychosocial Nursing, 33,* 15–20.

Robinson, D., Friedman, L., Marcus, R., Tinklenberg, J., & Yesavage, J. (1994). Estrogen replacement therapy and memory in older women. *Journal of American Geriatric Society, 42,* 912–922.

Sandman, C.A. (1993). Memory rehabilitation in Alzheimer's disease: Preliminary findings. *Clinical Gerontologist, 13,* 19–33.

Schneider, L.S., Farlow, M.R., & Pogoda, J.M. (1997). Potential role for estrogen replacement in the treatment of Alzheimer's dementia. *American Journal of Medicine, 103,* 46S–50S.

Schneider, L.S., & Tariot, P.N. (1994). Emerging drugs for Alzheimer's disease: Mechanisms of action and prospects for cognitive enhancing medications. In C. Eisdorfer & E.J. Olsen (Eds.), *The Medical Clinics of North America, 78,* 911–934.

Schulz, R., O'Brien, A., Bookwala, T., & Fleissner, K. (1995). Psychiatric and physical morbidity effects of dementia caregiving: Prevalence, correlates, and causes. *The Gerontologist, 35,* 771–791.

Segall, M., & Wykle, M. (1989). The black family's experience with dementia. *Journal of Applied Social Science, 13,* 170–188.

Shaw, W.S., Patterson, T.L., Semple, S.J., Ho, S., Irwin, M.R., Hauger, R.L., & Grant I. (1997). Longitudinal analysis of multiple indicators of health decline among spousal caregivers. *Annal of Behavioral Medicine, 19,* 101–109.

Sherlock, J., & Gardner, I. (1993). Systematic family intervention. In A. Chapman & M. Marshall (Eds.), *Dementia: New skills for social workers* (pp. 63–79).

Sherwin, B.B. (1997). Estrogen effects on cognition in menopausal women. *Neurology, 48,* S21–S26.

Smyth, K.A., & Harris, P.B. (1993). Using telecomputing to provide information and support to caregivers of persons with dementia. *Gerontologist, 33,* 123–127.

Stephens, M.A., Kinney, J.M., & Ogrocki, P.K. (1991). Stressors and well-being among caregivers to older adults with dementia: The in-home versus nursing home experience. *Gerontologist, 31,* 217–223.

Stommel, M., Collins, C.E., & Given, B.A. (1994). The costs of family contributions to the care of persons with dementia. *Gerontologist, 34,* 199–205.

Szapocznik, J., Rio, A., Murray, E., Cohen, R., Scopetta, M., Rivas-Vasquez, A., Hervis, O., Posada, V., & Kurtines, W. (1989). Structural family versus psychodynamic child therapy for problematic Hispanic boys. *Journal of Consulting and Clinical Psychology, 57,* 571–578.

U.S. Bureau of the Census. (1997). *Statistical abstract of the United States: 1997* (117th edition). Washington, D.C.

VandenBos, G.R. (1998). Life-span developmental perspectives on aging: An introductory overview. In I.H. Norrdhus, G.R. VandenBos, S. Berg, & P. Fromholt (Eds.), *Clinical geropsychology* (pp. 1–14).

Wagner, D.L. (1997). Long-distance caregiving for older adults. *Health Care and Aging,* National Council on Aging, Spring.

Whitlatch, C.J., Feinberg, L.F., & Sebesta, D.S. (1997). Depression and health in family caregivers. *Journal of Aging and Health, 9,* 222–243.

Wright, L.K., Clipp, E.C., & George, L.K. (1993). Health consequences of caregiving stress. *Medicine, Exercise, Nutrition, and Health, 2,* 181–195.

Wright, S.D., Lund, D.A., Pett, M.A., & Caserta, M.S. (1987). The assessment of support group experience by caregivers of dementia patients. *Clinical Gerontologist, 6,* 35–59.

Yesavage, J.A. (1982). Degree of dementia and improvement with memory training. *Clinical Gerontologist, 1,* 77–81.

Zarit, S.H., Johansson, L., & Jarrott, S.E. (1998). In I.H. Nordhus, G.R. VandenBos, S. Berg, & P. Fromholt (Eds.), *Clinical geropsychology* (pp. 345–360). Washington, DC: American Psychological Association.

Zarit, S.H., Todd, P.A., & Zarit, J.M. (1986). Subjective burden of husbands and wives of caregivers: A longitudinal study. *The Gerontologist, 26,* 260–266.

Zarit, S.H., Zarit, J.M., & Rosemberg-Thompson, S. (1990). A special treatment unit for Alzheimer's disease: Medical, behavioral, and environmental features. *Clinical Gerontologist, 9,* 47–63.

Zedtewski, S.R., & McBride, T.D. (1992). The changing profile of the elderly: Effects of future long-term care needs and financing. *The Milbank Quarterly, 70,* 247–275.

# Index

*320*